Paramedic Care
Principles & Practice
Trauma

Workbook

Fourth Edition

Paramedic Care
Principles & Practice
Trauma

Workbook

Fourth Edition

ROBERT S. PORTER

REVISED BY

LYNN WEBSTER, BS, MBA, EMT-P

President, Medical Education and Consulting Services of NC
EMS Instructor
Durham Technical Community College
Randolph Community College
Chapel Hill, NC

BRYAN E. BLEDSOE, DO, FACEP, FAAEM, EMT-P

Professor of Emergency Medicine
Director, Prehospital and Disaster Medicine Fellowship
University of Nevada School of Medicine
Attending Emergency Physician
University Medical Center of Southern Nevada
Medical Director, MedicWest Ambulance
Las Vegas, Nevada

ROBERT S. PORTER, MA, EMT-P

Senior Advanced Life Support Educator
Madison County Emergency Medical Services
Canastota, New York

RICHARD A. CHERRY, MS, EMT-P

Director of Training
Northern Onondaga Volunteer Ambulance
Liverpool, New York

PEARSON

Boston   Columbus   Indianapolis   New York   San Francisco   Upper Saddle River
Amsterdam   Cape Town   Dubai   London   Madrid   Milan   Munich   Paris   Montréal   Toronto
Delhi   Mexico City   São Paulo   Sydney   Hong Kong   Seoul   Singapore   Taipei   Tokyo

Publisher: *Julie Levin Alexander*
Publisher's Assistant: *Regina Bruno*
Editor-in-Chief: *Marlene McHugh Pratt*
Senior Managing Editor for Development: *Lois Berlowitz*
Editorial Project Manager: *Triple SSS Press Media Development, Inc.*
Assistant Editor: *Jonathan Cheung*
Director of Marketing: *David Gesell*
Marketing Manager: *Brian Hoehl*
Marketing Specialist: *Michael Sirinides*
Managing Editor for Production: *Patrick Walsh*
Production Liaison: *Faye Gemmellaro*
Production Editor: *Muralidharan Krishnamurthy/S4Carlisle Publishing Services*
Manufacturing Manager: *Ilene Sanford*
Cover Design: *Kathryn Foot*
Cover Image: *© corepics/Shutterstock*
Composition: *S4Carlisle Publishing Services*
Cover and Interior Printer/Binder: *Edward Brothers Malloy*

NOTICE ON CARE PROCEDURES

It is the intent of the authors and publisher that this Workbook be used as part of a formal Paramedic program taught by qualified instructors and supervised by a licensed physician. The procedures described in this Workbook are based upon consultation with EMS and medical authorities. The authors and publisher have taken care to make certain that these procedures reflect currently accepted clinical practice; however, they cannot be considered absolute recommendations.

The material in this Workbook contains the most current information available at the time of publication. However, federal, state, and local guidelines concerning clinical practices, including, without limitation, those governing infection control and universal precautions, change rapidly. The reader should note, therefore, that the new regulations may require changes in some procedures.

It is the responsibility of the reader to familiarize himself or herself with the policies and procedures set by federal, state, and local agencies as well as the institution or agency where the reader is employed. The authors and the publisher of this Workbook disclaim any liability, loss, or risk resulting directly or indirectly from the suggested procedures and theory, from any undetected errors, or from the reader's misunderstanding of the text. It is the reader's responsibility to stay informed of any new changes or recommendations made by any federal, state, and local agency as well as by his or her employing institution or agency.

NOTICE ON CPR AND ECC

The national standards for cardiopulmonary resuscitation (CPR) and emergency cardiovascular care (ECC) are reviewed and revised on a regular basis and may change slightly after this manual is printed. It is important that you know the most current procedures for CPR and ECC, both for the classroom and your patients. The most current information may be obtained from the appropriate credentialing agency.

Brady
is an imprint of

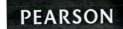

www.bradybooks.com

10 9 8 7 6 5 4 3
ISBN 10: 0-13-211158-6
ISBN 13: 978-0-13-211158-4

Dedication

This workbook is dedicated to the important people in your life: your wife/husband, mother, father, sister, brother . . . and friends who support you and the time and passion you devote to emergency medical services.
Without them, this endeavor would be lonely and much less rewarding.

–ROBERT S. PORTER

CONTENTS

INTRODUCTION

Welcome to the self-instructional Workbook for *Paramedic Care: Principles & Practice*. This Workbook is designed to help guide you through an educational program for initial or refresher training that follows the guidelines of the 2009 *National EMS Education Standards*. The Workbook is designed to be used either in conjunction with your instructor or as a self-study guide you use on your own.

This Workbook features many different ways to help you learn the material necessary to become a paramedic, as discussed next.

Features

Review of Chapter Objectives

Each chapter of *Paramedic Care: Principles & Practice* begins with objectives that identify the important information and principles addressed in the chapter reading. To help you identify and learn this material, each Workbook chapter reviews the important content elements addressed by these objectives as presented in the text.

Case Study Review

Each chapter of *Paramedic Care: Principles & Practice* includes a case study, introducing and highlighting important principles presented in the chapter. The Workbook reviews these case studies and points out much of the essential information and many of the applied principles they describe.

Content Self-Evaluation

Each chapter of *Paramedic Care: Principles & Practice* presents an extensive narrative explanation of the principles of paramedic practice. The Workbook chapter (or chapter section) contains between 10 and 50 multiple-choice questions to test your reading comprehension of the textbook material and to give you experience taking typical emergency medical service examinations.

Special Projects

The Workbook contains several projects that are special learning experiences designed to help you remember the information and principles necessary to perform as a paramedic. Special projects include contacting local agencies and services, Internet research, and a variety of other exercises.

Content Review

The Workbook provides a comprehensive review of the material presented in this volume of *Paramedic Care: Principles & Practice*. After the last text chapter has been covered, the Workbook presents an extensive content self-evaluation component that helps you recall and build upon the knowledge you have gained by reading the text, attending class, and completing the earlier Workbook chapters.

Patient Scenario Flash Cards

This Workbook contains scenario flash cards, each of which presents a patient scenario with signs and symptoms. On the reverse side you will find the appropriate field diagnosis and the care steps you should consider providing for the patient. These cards will help you recognize and remember common serious trauma emergencies, their presentation, and the appropriate care that would be given.

HOW TO USE THIS SELF-INSTRUCTIONAL WORKBOOK

The self-instructional Workbook accompanying *Paramedic Care: Principles & Practice* may be used as directed by your instructor or independently by you during your course of instruction. The following recommendations are intended to guide you in using the Workbook independently.

- Examine your course schedule and identify the appropriate text chapter or other assigned reading.

- Read the assigned chapter in *Paramedic Care: Principles & Practice* carefully. Do this in a relaxed environment, free of distractions, and give yourself adequate time to read and digest the material. The information presented in *Paramedic Care: Principles & Practice* is often technically complex and demanding, but it is very important that you comprehend it. Be sure that you read the chapter carefully enough to understand and remember what you have read.

- Carefully read the Review of Chapter Objectives at the beginning of each Workbook chapter (or section). This material includes both the objectives listed in *Paramedic Care: Principles & Practice* and narrative descriptions of their content. If you do not understand or remember what is discussed from your reading, refer to the referenced pages and reread them carefully. If you still do not feel comfortable with your understanding of any objective, consider asking your instructor about it.

- Reread the case study in *Paramedic Care: Principles & Practice*, and then read the Case Study Review in the Workbook. Note the important points regarding assessment and care that the Case Study Review highlights and be sure that you understand and agree with the analysis of the call. If you have any questions or concerns, ask your instructor to clarify the information.

- Take the Content Self-Evaluation at the end of each Workbook chapter (or section), answering each question carefully. Do this in a quiet environment, free from distractions, and allow yourself adequate time to complete the exercise. Correct your self-evaluation by consulting the answers at the back of the Workbook, and determine the percentage you have answered correctly (the number you got right divided by the total number of questions). If you have answered most of the questions correctly (85 to 90 percent), review those that you missed by rereading the material on the pages listed in the answer key and be sure you understand which answer is correct and why. If you have more than a few questions wrong (less than 85 percent correct), look for incorrect answers that are grouped together. This suggests that you did not understand a particular topic in the reading. Reread the text dealing with that topic carefully, and then retest yourself on the questions you got wrong. If incorrect answers are spread throughout the chapter content, reread the chapter and retake the Content Self-Evaluation to ensure that you understand the material. If you don't understand why your answer to a question is incorrect after reviewing the text, consult with your instructor.

- In a similar fashion, complete the exercises in the Special Projects section of the Workbook chapters (or sections). These exercises are specifically designed to help you learn and remember the essential principles and information presented in *Paramedic Care: Principles & Practice*.

- When you have completed this volume of *Paramedic Care: Principles & Practice* and its accompanying Workbook, prepare for a course test by reviewing both the text in its entirety and your class notes. Then take the Content Review examination in the Workbook. Again, review your score and any questions you have answered incorrectly by referring to the text and rereading the page or pages where the material is presented. If you note groupings of wrong answers, review the entire range of pages or the full chapter they represent.

If, during your completion of the Workbook exercises, you have any questions that either the textbook or Workbook doesn't answer, write them down and ask your instructor about them. Prehospital emergency medicine is a complex and complicated subject, and answers are not always black and white. It is also common for different EMS systems to use differing methods of care. The questions you bring up in class, and your instructor's answers to them, will help you expand and complete your knowledge of prehospital emergency medical care.

GUIDELINES TO BETTER TEST-TAKING

The knowledge you will gain from reading the textbook, completing the exercises in the Workbook, listening in your paramedic class, and participating in your clinical and field experience will prepare you to care for patients who are seriously ill or injured. However, before you can practice these skills, you will have to pass several classroom written exams and your state's certification exam. Your performance on these exams will depend not only on your knowledge but also on your ability to answer test questions correctly. The following guidelines are designed to help your performance on tests and to better demonstrate your knowledge of prehospital emergency care.

1. Relax and be calm during the test.

A test is designed to measure what you have learned and to tell you and your instructor how well you are doing. An exam is not designed to intimidate or punish you. Consider it a challenge, and just try to do your best. Get plenty of sleep before the examination. Avoid coffee or other stimulants for a few hours before the exam, and be prepared.

Reread the text chapters, review the objectives in the Workbook, and review your class notes. It might be helpful to work with one or two other students and ask each other questions. This type of practice helps everyone better understand the knowledge presented in your course of study.

2. Read the questions carefully.

Read each word of the question and all the answers slowly. Words such as "except" or "not" may change the entire meaning of the question. If you miss such words, you may answer the question incorrectly even though you know the right answer.

Example:
The art and science of emergency medical services involves all of the following, EXCEPT

    A. sincerity and compassion.
    B. respect for human dignity.
    C. placing patient care before personal safety.
    D. delivery of sophisticated emergency medical care.
    E. none of the above.

The correct answer is C, unless you miss the "EXCEPT."

3. Read each answer carefully.

Read each and every answer carefully. Although the first answer may be absolutely correct, so may the rest, and thus the best answer might be "all of the above."

Example:
Indirect medical direction is considered to be

    A. treatment protocols.
    B. training and education.
    C. quality assurance.
    D. chart review.
    E. all of the above.

Although answers A, B, C, and D are each correct, the best and only acceptable answer is "all of the above," E.

4. Delay answering questions you don't understand and look for clues.

When a question seems confusing or you don't know the answer, note it on your answer sheet and come back to it later. This will ensure that you have time to complete the test. You will also find that other questions in the test may give you hints to answer the one you've skipped over. It will also prevent you from being frustrated with an early question and letting it affect your performance.

Example:
Upon successful completion of a course of training as an EMT-P, most states will

- A. certify you. (correct)
- B. license you.
- C. register you.
- D. recognize you as a paramedic.
- E. issue you a permit.

Another question, later in the exam, may suggest the right answer:

The action of one state in recognizing the certification of another is called:

- A. reciprocity. (correct)
- B. national registration.
- C. licensure.
- D. registration.
- E. extended practice.

5. Answer all questions.

Even if you do not know the right answer, do not leave a question blank. A blank question is always wrong, whereas a guess might be correct. If you can eliminate some of the answers as wrong, do so. It will increase the chances of a correct guess.

A multiple-choice question with five answers gives a 20 percent chance of a correct guess. If you can eliminate one or more incorrect answers, you increase your odds of a correct guess to 25 percent, 33 percent, and so on. An unanswered question has a 0 percent chance of being correct.

Just before turning in your answer sheet, check to be sure that you have not left any items blank.

Examples:
When a paramedic is called by the patient (through the dispatcher) to the scene of a medical emergency, the medical direction physician has established a physician/patient relationship.

- A. True
- B. False

A true/false question gives you a 50 percent chance of a correct guess.

The hospital health professional(s) responsible for sorting patients as they arrive at the emergency department is (are) usually the

- A. emergency physician.
- B. ward clerk.
- C. emergency nurse.
- D. trauma surgeon.
- E. both A and C (correct).

Paramedic Care

Principles & Practice

Trauma

Workbook

Fourth Edition

Trauma and Trauma Systems

Review of Chapter Objectives

After reading this chapter, you should be able to:

1. Define key terms introduced in this chapter.

Knowing and being able to apply the key terms in each chapter is critical to understanding chapter concepts. Write the list of key terms. Then write the definition of each one in your own words. Check your understanding by confirming the definitions in the text glossary. Correct any misunderstandings. Create a study aid by writing each key term on the front of an index card and the definition on the back. Use the cards to quiz yourself, or to have someone quiz you.

2. Describe the epidemiology of trauma in general, and with respect to trauma that results in requests for emergency medical care. **p. 3**

Trauma is the third leading cause of death in the United States, and the number-one killer for persons under the age of 44. It accounts for 177,000 deaths per year and may be the most expensive medical problem of society today because of lost productivity for victims. Motor vehicle crashes (MVCs) account for 34,500 deaths, and gunshot wounds (GSWs) account for another 31,500 deaths.

Overall, 30 percent of EMS responses are to trauma calls. Of these, 47 percent are for falls, 28 percent for on-the-road vehicle collisions, 13 percent for other blunt trauma, 3 percent for off-the-road vehicle collisions, and 2 percent for intentional lacerations/stabbings.

3. Compare the role of a paramedic caring for a patient with life-threatening injuries to the role of a paramedic caring for a patient with non-life-threatening injuries. **pp. 3–4**

The nature and severity of trauma can range from a slight abrasion to multiple-system injuries. Although trauma may pose a serious threat to life, its presentation may mask the patient's true condition. When assessing a trauma patient, you must look beyond obvious injuries for evidence that suggests a life-threatening condition.

Serious life-threatening conditions occur in fewer than 10 percent of trauma patients. Prehospital care cannot definitively stabilize these patients. Prehospital care entails immobilizing the cervical spine, securing the airway, ensuring adequate ventilation, controlling any significant external hemorrhage, and rapidly transporting the patient to a definitive trauma care center. Some 90 percent of trauma patients do not have serious life-threatening injuries. You can best care for these patients by providing thorough on-scene assessment and care followed by conservative transport to the nearest general hospital or other appropriate health care facility.

4. **Apply the five-step public health model to injury prevention.** pp. 4–6

Modern-day EMS began with the publication of the white paper "Accidental Death and Disability: The Neglected Disease of Modern Society." It is only since the development of this paper that trauma has been viewed and managed as a disease. Modern medicine uses a five-step approach to prevent or reduce the impact of disease which is known as the public health model. The public health model uses surveillance, risk analysis, intervention development, implementation, and evaluation to identify, examine, and address disease and prevention of disease. Surveillance is the collection of data to identify the existence, significance, and characteristics of disease. Risk analysis looks at disease and determines the various factors that impact the development, course, and consequences. A helpful tool to identify risk elements associated with trauma is the Haddon Matrix. This tool identifies elements occurring before the event (pre-event), during the incident (event), and after the incident (post-event). Intervention development creates or modifies programs to reduce both the incidence and the seriousness of trauma. Implementation is putting an intervention into practice. Finally, evaluation is repeating the surveillance process that took place before an intervention to determine the degree of success of the intervention and to modify future offerings. Injury prevention is an evolving role of the modern EMS system.

5. **Describe the capabilities of the various levels of designated trauma centers.** pp. 7–8

A well-designed EMS system allocates trauma resources in a way that provides patients with the most efficient and effective care. Such a system utilizes hospitals with special resources and a commitment to trauma patient care. These hospitals are designated as trauma centers.

Level I or Regional Trauma Center. This is a hospital, usually a university teaching hospital, that is prepared and committed to handle all types of serious trauma 24 hours a day and 7 days a week. It also provides leadership and resource support to other trauma center levels within the regional trauma system.

Level II or Area Trauma Center. This is a facility with a high commitment to trauma patient care with 24-hour surgical care capability. A Level II center can handle all but the most seriously injured specialty and multisystem trauma patients.

Level III or Community Trauma Center. This is a general hospital with a commitment to special staff training and specific resource allocation for the care of trauma patients. Such centers are generally located in rural areas and will stabilize more serious trauma patients for transport to higher-level trauma centers.

Level IV Trauma Center. In some remote areas there is a Level IV trauma facility, which receives trauma patients and stabilizes them for transport to a more distant higher-level facility, often by helicopter.

6. **Given a variety of scenarios, conduct trauma assessments that result in categorization of patients as critical, unstable, potentially unstable, or stable.** pp. 8–10

Trauma assessment follows the general format for all patients, including the scene survey, primary assessment, secondary assessment, and periodic reassessment. Key areas where it differs from medical patient assessment include an increased likelihood of scene hazards, need to analyze mechanism of injury (MOI), consideration of environmental impacts, application of trauma triage guidelines, and determination of an appropriate patient destination. You will assign the patient a preliminary priority for further assessment, care, and transport at the end of the primary assessment using the CUPS categorizations of patient severity. Patients who do not make it out of the primary assessment because you are unable to stabilize airway, breathing, or circulation are considered critical (C). Those who present with limited injuries but are breathing well and have strong pulses are stable (S). Those in between are either unstable (U) or potentially unstable (P).

©2013 Pearson Education, Inc.
Paramedic Care: Principles & Practice, Vol. 5, 4th Ed.

7. **Discuss the role of time to definitive care in the outcomes of trauma patients.** p. 10

Time is a critical consideration for the survival of a seriously injured trauma patient. For some patients, research shows that survival rates increase dramatically as time from a trauma incident to surgical intervention is reduced. The current goal for incident-to-surgery time is about 1 hour, often referred to as the Golden Period. Many time-consuming factors, which are beyond your control, consume a portion of the Golden Period. Therefore, it is vital to minimize time spent on factors within your control. Ideally you should provide the primary and secondary assessments, emergency stabilization, patient packaging, and initiation of transport in less than 10 minutes.

8. **Apply trauma triage criteria to identify patients who should be transported to a trauma center.** pp. 11–12

Trauma triage criteria include a listing of mechanisms of injury and physical findings suggestive of serious injury. Patients likely to benefit from the care offered by the Level I or II trauma center are identified using the "guidelines for field triage of injured patients." The guidelines use a step-by-step approach to identification.

Step One: Physiologic Criteria

- Glasgow Coma Scale (GCS) score ≤ 13, or
- systolic blood pressure (SBP) of < 90 mmHg, or
- respiratory rate of < 10 or > 29 breaths per minute (< 20 in infant aged < 1 year), or need for ventilatory support.

Step Two: Anatomic Criteria

- all penetrating injuries to head, neck, torso, and extremities proximal to elbow or knee;
- chest wall instability or deformity (e.g., flail chest);
- two or more proximal long-bone fractures;
- crushed, degloved, mangled, or pulseless extremity;
- amputation proximal to wrist or ankle;
- pelvic fractures;
- open or depressed skull fractures; or
- paralysis.

Step Three: Mechanism of Injury

- falls
  - adults: > 20 feet (one story = 10 feet)
  - children: > 10 feet or two to three times the height of the child
- high-risk auto crash
  - intrusion, including roof: > 12 inches occupant site; > 18 inches any site
  - ejection (partial or complete) from automobile
  - death in same passenger compartment
  - vehicle telemetry data consistent with a high risk for injury;
- automobile versus pedestrian/bicyclist thrown, run over, or with significant (> 20 mph) impact; or motorcycle crash > 20 mph

Step Four: Special Considerations

- older adults
  - risk for injury/death increases after age 55 years
  - SBP < 110 might represent shock after age 65 years
  - low-impact mechanisms (e.g., ground-level falls) might result in severe injury
- children
  - should be triaged preferentially to pediatric capable trauma centers

- anticoagulants and bleeding disorders
  - patients with head injury are at high risk for rapid deterioration
- burns
  - without other trauma mechanism: triage to burn facility
  - with trauma mechanism: triage to trauma center
- pregnancy > 20 weeks
- EMS provider judgment

9. **Describe the purposes of data collection in injury prevention, the trauma registry, and quality improvement.** pp. 11, 13

Injury prevention is one of the most cost-effective means to reduce trauma morbidity and mortality. Data collection provides an important role in identifying injury patterns and developing safety programs. In trauma systems, regional trauma centers collect a uniform set of data that becomes part of a national trauma registry. Data are analyzed to describe the types of patients and injuries we respond to, determine how well the system is performing and identify factors that may improve patient survival. Accurate prehospital care reports support these research efforts. Trauma system quality improvement (QI) is another data-driven means for examining system performance with the goal of providing improved patient care. In the QI process, committees look at selected care indicators to determine if designated care standards are being met. If shortfalls are identified, the committees may recommend continuing education, EMS equipment modifications, or protocol revisions. True QI is not punitive, but rather a method to assess system quality and provide for improvement.

Case Study Review

Reread the case study on pages 2 and 3 in Paramedic Care: Trauma; *then, read the following discussion.*

This case study presents a good opportunity to examine the components of the trauma system and the role they fulfill in the provision of prehospital care. John's very life is dependent upon the trauma system functioning efficiently.

Paramedic Earl Antak responds to the incident alone in a vehicle with advanced life support (ALS) equipment but not designed to transport patients (sometimes called a "fly car"). This system configuration permits ALS to be more flexible and available to a larger geographic area. Less seriously injured patients may be transported by ambulance without the paramedic, making Earl more quickly available for another call, or in this case available immediately after the helicopter leaves with the patient.

As Earl arrives at the scene, he performs the elements of the scene size-up. He ensures the scene is safe and that the police are controlling traffic. Earl, in consideration of scene safety, will wear gloves because there are open wounds, and he avoids the glass around the vehicle door. As he approaches the patient, Earl evaluates the mechanism of injury (MOI) and notes that the bicyclist probably ran into the open car door. The MOI suggests significant impact and the probable need to enter the patient into the trauma system. Earl also notes that the rider was wearing a helmet, possibly the result of injury prevention programs in his local community, and suggesting a reduced incidence of head injuries, though not reducing the chances of spinal injury.

Earl's primary assessment reveals a well-developed young male who was unconscious but now is fully conscious and alert. Earl rules out any immediate airway, breathing, or circulation problem, applies oxygen, and ensures that the sheriff's department officer and then the ambulance crew continue to maintain immobilization of John's head and spine. As Earl moves on to the rapid trauma assessment, he notes neurologic signs that suggest a cervical spine injury. Earl also notes a likely clavicle fracture and carefully assesses for any associated respiratory injury. He also carefully watches for the early signs of shock, because clavicular injury can lacerate the subclavian artery. Vital signs are within normal limits for someone recently involved in heavy exercise and the emotional stress of trauma. Earl will, however, carefully record the vital signs and the results of his rapid trauma assessment during the reassessments (every 5 minutes for this patient) and compare them to detect any trends in the patient's condition.

©2013 Pearson Education, Inc.
Paramedic Care: Principles & Practice, Vol. 5, 4th Ed.

Earl contacts medical direction and is assigned a transport destination. This communication ensures that John is transported to an appropriate center and one that has the resources to care for his injuries. Should a particular center be overcrowded with patients or have essential services unavailable (for example, no surgeon immediately on hand), Earl would be directed to transport John to another facility. Time is a critical factor in caring for John, so Earl quickly performs the skills necessary to protect John's spine, then moves to transport him quickly. Earl also requests air medical services because the ground transport time is in excess of 30 minutes. He does not, however, await the helicopter but intercepts it at a predesignated landing zone. His intercept with the helicopter will likely reduce the transport time by minutes, an important factor with a seriously injured trauma patient. In this case, it is clearly to John's benefit to get to the trauma center as quickly as possible. The interactions between Earl and the police officer, the responding EMTs in the ambulance, the medical direction physician, the trauma triage nurse, and the flight crew ensure that the system works in a coordinated way and to the benefit of its patient, John.

Content Self-Evaluation

MULTIPLE CHOICE

_____ 1. Auto accidents account for how many deaths each year?
- A. 12,000
- B. 24,000
- C. 34,500
- D. 68,000
- E. 150,000

_____ 2. Although trauma poses a serious threat to life, its presentation often masks the patient's true condition.
- A. True
- B. False

_____ 3. Some 90 percent of all trauma patients do not have serious, life-endangering injuries.
- A. True
- B. False

_____ 4. Trauma triage criteria are mechanisms of injury or physical signs exhibited by the patient that suggest serious injury.
- A. True
- B. False

_____ 5. The legislation that helped establish guidelines, funding, and state-level leadership and support for trauma systems was the
- A. Highway Safety Act of 1966.
- B. Consolidated Emergency Services Act of 1971.
- C. Trauma Care Systems Planning and Development Act of 1990.
- D. Trauma Systems Act of 1963.
- E. National Readiness Act of 1960.

_____ 6. The trauma system is predicated on the principle that serious trauma is
- A. a frequent occurrence.
- B. usually a medical emergency.
- C. inevitable.
- D. a surgical disease.
- E. fatal if the patient is not seen by a qualified physician in less than 30 minutes.

7. A Level I trauma center is usually a(n)
   A. community hospital.
   B. teaching hospital with resources available full-time for emergency cases.
   C. emergency department with 24-hour service.
   D. nonemergency health care facility.
   E. stabilizing and transport facility.

8. The small community hospital or health care facility in a remote area, designated as a receiving facility for trauma, is Level
   A. I.
   B. II.
   C. III.
   D. IV.
   E. V.

9. Trauma centers may also be designated for provision of which of the following special services?
   A. Pediatric trauma center
   B. Burn center
   C. Neurocenter
   D. Hyperbaric center
   E. All of the above

10. You arrive on scene to find a 4-year-old child who has fallen out of a second-story window. The child responds to verbal stimulus. Respirations and pulse are within normal limits. You note a broken left arm but no other apparent injuries. Your index of suspicion for possible injuries includes
    A. internal bleeding.
    B. head injury.
    C. cervical spine injury.
    D. all of the above.

11. Your primary concern on the scene described in question 10 is
    A. obtaining patient medical history and medications.
    B. splinting the broken arm.
    C. rapid packaging and transport.
    D. completing a detailed physical exam.

12. The period of time between the occurrence of serious injury and surgery suggested as a goal for prehospital care providers is the
    A. platinum 10 minutes.
    B. Golden Period.
    C. trauma time differential.
    D. bleed-out equation.
    E. critical differential.

13. In applying trauma triage criteria, it is best to err on the side of precaution.
    A. True
    B. False

14. Trauma triage criteria are designed to overtriage trauma patients to ensure those with more subtle injuries are not missed.
    A. True
    B. False

15. You arrive on scene to find a 26-year-old male patient ejected from a motor vehicle. The patient is unconscious but breathing at a rate of 28. He is bleeding profusely from the head. You note an open femur fracture on the left leg. The trauma triage criteria that is most indicative of a serious injury is
    A. respiratory rate.
    B. head bleed.
    C. ejection from vehicle.
    D. open femur fracture.

©2013 Pearson Education, Inc.
Paramedic Care: Principles & Practice, Vol. 5, 4th Ed.

_____ 16. The reduction in the incidence and seriousness of trauma in recent years can be credited to
    A. better highway design.
    B. better auto design.
    C. use of auto restraint systems.
    D. development of injury prevention programs.
    E. all of the above.

_____ 17. The standardized data retrieval system used to evaluate and improve the trauma system is the
    A. prehospital care report system.
    B. trauma triage system.
    C. trauma registry.
    D. trauma quality improvement program.
    E. CISD.

_____ 18. Quality improvement is a significant method of assessing system quality and providing for its improvement.
    A. True
    B. False

2

Blunt Trauma

Review of Chapter Objectives

After reading this chapter, you should be able:

1. Define the key terms introduced in this chapter.

Knowing and being able to apply the key terms in each chapter is critical to understanding chapter concepts. Write the list of key terms. Then write the definition of each one in your own words. Check your understanding by confirming the definitions in the text glossary. Correct any misunderstandings. Create a study aid by writing each key term on the front of an index card and the definition on the back. Use the cards to quiz yourself, or to have someone quiz you.

2. Apply the laws of inertia and energy conservation to the kinetics of blunt impact.
pp. 18–19

Newton's two basic principles of kinetics are the laws of inertia and of energy conservation. Inertia is the tendency for objects at rest or in motion to remain so unless acted upon by an outside force. In some cases, that force is the energy exchange that causes trauma. For example, a moving vehicle colliding with a tree or a stopped vehicle being struck from behind both encounter outside forces. Energy conservation is the physical law stating that energy can neither be created or destroyed but can only be changed from one form to another. In a motor vehicle collision (MVC) the transformation of one form of energy to another causes the deformity to the auto and may cause blunt-force injury to the occupants.

3. Apply the concepts of force and kinetic energy exchange to the potential for injury.
pp. 19–20

Newton's second law of motion states that force strength is related to an object's weight (mass) and the rate of its change in velocity. Kinetic energy is the energy of an object in motion. It is a function of the object's mass and velocity. Changes in velocity have the greatest impact on the object's kinetic energy. The force formula, (Force = [Mass (Weight) × Acceleration (or Deceleration)] / 2), explains how energy is delivered to the structure of a vehicle, the occupants, and their organs and tissues. Once an object has significant energy, the rate of deceleration or acceleration then determines the force of impact and the severity of resulting injuries.

4. Associate the application of energy to various body tissues with biomechanical forces produced to predict injury patterns.
pp. 20–22

The biomechanics of trauma examine the injury process by looking at the kinetic energy forces as they progress from the body's exterior surface to the internal organs. Trauma is divided into two general categories when looking at the injury process: blunt and penetrating. Penetrating trauma is when an object physically enters the body and injures tissue, either directly or indirectly. Blunt trauma is when kinetic energy forces enter the body and damage tissue. Because not all organs are uniformly attached to the body and do not have a consistent density, elasticity, and strength, they vary in their ability to withstand biomechanical forces.

Blunt trauma results in three types of body tissue injuries: compression, stretching, and shearing. Compression is an injury resulting from a blunt impact that quickly halts a portion of the body while inertia causes the remaining structures to continue its motion. A stretch injury is when one part of the body is pulled away from another. A shear injury is seen along the edges of the impacting force or at organ attachments. The impacting force slows down a part of the body, but the tissue along the impact border continues its motion.

5. **Describe the events that occur in motor vehicle impacts.** pp. 22–24

There are basically five types of vehicle impacts: frontal, lateral, oblique, rear-end, and rollover impacts. Each type generally progresses through a series of five events. Vehicle collision: First, the vehicle impacts an object and comes to a rest. Body collision: Then, the vehicle occupants strike the vehicle interior, causing the occupants' kinetic energy to transform into initial tissue deformity. Organ collision: Meanwhile, various organs and structures within the occupants' bodies collide with one another, causing compression, stretching, and shear injury as the body comes to a halt. Secondary collisions: Objects within the vehicle may continue their forward motion until they impact the slowed or stopped occupant. Additional impacts: In some instances, secondary vehicle impacts occur. This secondary impact may induce additional injuries or increase the seriousness of those already received.

6. **Describe the effects of use of restraints and safety mechanisms on the potential for injuries in vehicle collisions.** pp. 24–26

Restraints such as seat belts, shoulder straps, air bags, and child safety seats have a profound effect on the injuries associated with motor vehicle collisions. Lap belts and shoulder straps control the deceleration of the vehicle occupant during a crash, slowing them with the auto. This lessens the likelihood of serious injury. They also reduce the chances that an occupant will be ejected from the vehicle. However, when they are improperly worn, serious injuries may result. Shoulder straps alone may account for serious neck injury, while the lap belt worn too high may injure the spine and abdomen.

Supplemental restraint systems (air bags) inflate explosively during an impact and provide a cushion of gas as the occupant impacts the steering wheel, dash, or vehicle side. This slows the impact, reduces the deceleration rate, and reduces injuries. Rapid inflation of the air bag, however, may impact the driver's fingers, hands, and forearms, possibly resulting in dislocations or fractures. Inflation may also cause nasal fractures, facial injury, and contusions in persons of small stature who are seated very close to the steering wheel or dash. Although air bags mounted on the steering wheel and dash only offer protection in frontal-impact collisions, manufacturers are installing supplemental restraint systems in the headliners and seat sides for protection in lateral-impact collisions. These may mitigate serious injury in lateral impacts.

Child safety seats provide much-needed protection for infants and small children for whom normal restraints do not work adequately by themselves because of the children's rapidly changing anatomical dimensions. The seat faces rearward for infants and very small children (up to two years of age), then should be turned to face forward as the child grows. This positioning permits the seat belt to provide restraint, similar to that provided for the adult. Child safety seats should not be positioned in front of air-bag restraint systems because inflation of those devices may push the rear-facing child forcibly into the seat.

Headrests are designed to prevent unopposed rearward motion of the head during a rear-end collision. A properly positioned headrest will prevent violent backward head rotation and neck extension, significantly reducing the incidence of whiplash injury to the spinal column, neck ligaments, and neck muscles in rear-end collisions.

7. **Describe the association between vehicle damage and injury potential** pp. 26–30

The degree and location of vehicle damage should heighten your index of suspicion for the seriousness of injury. Impacts may result in occupant compartment intrusion. This occurs when collision forces push through the vehicle's structure and deform the occupant compartment. Intrusion suggests that increased kinetic energy forces may have reached the occupant, causing substantial injury. Lateral impacts often are accompanied by vehicle intrusion because the associated crumple zone within the vehicle door is very limited. When a lateral impact occurs, the index of suspicion for serious and life-threatening internal injuries must be higher than vehicle damage alone might suggest. Frontal collisions interpose more space between the point of impact and the occupant compartment. Modern design uses this region (called the crumple zone) to absorb impact forces, making collapse of vehicle structures more gradual, reducing forces expressed upon occupants, and limiting occupant injury. In oblique or rotational impacts, because autos are often deflected from their path rather than being stopped abruptly, injuries are frequently less than vehicle damage might suggest. In rear-end collisions the degree of damage is dependent upon several factors, including whether the vehicle is stopped or moving and the speed at which it is struck. Rear structures are designed to crumple and absorb kinetic forces. While moderate-speed impacts may cause significant damage, as a rule, rear-impact collisions usually result in limited injuries. Rollovers can be especially violent because of limited crumple zones (as in the vehicle roof) and can result in serious injury. Severity is more directly related to vehicle damage.

8. **Describe injury patterns associated with various types of vehicle impacts.**   pp. 26–30

Frontal impacts are the most common type of auto collision and produce four pathways of patient travel and potential injury. **Restrained Pathway:** The use of lap belts and shoulder straps restrict movement of the occupant, limiting interior impacts. Injuries are typically associated with lap-belt placement, such as intra-abdominal, lumbar spine, and hip dislocation injuries. Shoulder belts may cause contusions and possible rib fractures. **Up-and-Over:** The unrestrained body's upper half pivots forward and upward. The steering wheel impinges the femurs, possibly causing bilateral fractures. Abdominal contents are also compressed, possibly causing hollow-organ rupture and liver laceration. If abdominal contents are forced against the diaphragm, it may rupture, allowing organs to enter the thoracic cavity. Chest injury may occur when the lower chest impacts the upper steering wheel. If the same forward motion propels the head into the steering wheel, skull or facial fractures, soft-tissue, neck, and internal head injuries may occur. **Down-and-Under:** The unrestrained occupant slides downward as the vehicle stops. Knee, femur, and hip dislocations or fractures occur as the knees strike the firewall. The upper body rotates forward, contacting the steering wheel. Chest injuries such as flail chest, blunt cardiac injury, and aortic tears result. The driver may demonstrate "paper-bag" syndrome with concordant pneumothorax or pulmonary contusion. If the neck strikes the steering wheel, tracheal and vascular injury may occur. **Ejection:** The up-and-over pathway may lead to ejection from the vehicle if the occupant is unrestrained. Victims experience two impacts: contact with the vehicle windshield and impact with an external surface or object such as the ground or a tree. Multiple, significant trauma and death can occur.

During **lateral impacts,** the occupant is turned 90 degrees to the impact, resulting in fractures of the hip, femur, shoulder girdle, clavicle, and lateral ribs. Internal injury may result to the aorta and spleen on the driver's side or liver on the passenger's side. Vertebral fractures may occur from the rapid lateral and twisting motion and skull fractures may result from the head striking the window. Lateral compression affecting the body cavity may cause diaphragm rupture and pulmonary contusion. An unbelted occupant may impact the other occupant, causing further injury.

Oblique impacts result from a vehicle being struck at an angle. This creates rotational movement that mediates the deceleration and reduces potential injury. Injury patterns resemble a mix of those associated with frontal, lateral and rear-end patterns. While injuries may be serious, the severity is generally less than the vehicle damage might suggest.

Rear-end impacts push the auto, auto seat, and finally the occupant forward. The head, however, may remain stationary while the shoulders move rapidly forward. This results in rapid extreme hyperextension of the head followed by hyperflexion, injuring the neck and cervical spine. Once the vehicle ends its acceleration, an unrestrained occupant may sustain other injuries as the body contacts the dash, steering wheel, or windshield. In general, rear-end impacts result in limited injuries, especially if the headrest is positioned properly.

Rollovers occur as the roadway elevation changes or a vehicle with a high center of gravity becomes unstable around a turn. As the vehicle rolls, it impacts the ground at multiple points, with the occupant sustaining an impact with each vehicle impact. These impacts can be especially violent because of limited crumple zones. Anticipated injuries relate to the specific vehicle impacts involved. Additionally, the initial collision is usually compounded by secondary impacts. The result may be serious injuries anywhere on the body or ejection of the occupants. Ejections may be partial with a limb, torso, or head trapped between the rolling vehicle and the ground. Mortality increases significantly with motor vehicle ejection.

9. **Given a variety of scenarios, conduct a vehicle collision analysis.** pp. 30–32

Vehicle collisions often produce hazards not only to the vehicle occupants but also to bystanders and care providers. A vehicle collision analysis takes into account a multitude of factors that will influence your actions on the scene as well as your care for the patients. Be alert for hazards during the scene size-up, such as hot engines, exhaust, transmission parts, hot fluids, caustic substances, sharp, jagged edges of torn metal, and broken glass. Pay attention to dangers from moving traffic and downed power lines. Evaluate the terrain for obstacles to patient access and movement. During the scene size-up examine the vehicle to determine the direction of impact and the amount of vehicle damage. Consider the relative size of the colliding vehicles or objects. Apply your knowledge of types of impacts to develop your index of suspicion for injuries. Examine the vehicles' interior compartments next. Look for spider-webbing of the windshield, deformed steering wheels, dented dashes, and deformed gas, brake, or clutch pedals. Note whether restraints were used and whether there was air-bag deployment. All these observations will direct your index of suspicion for injury. Check positioning of headrests and examine the interior for intrusion. Whenever you evaluate motor vehicle trauma you should consider the possibility of alcohol or drug intoxication. If you suspect either of these, your assessment must be even more diligent. Finally, view any evidence surrounding the collision and re-create it in your mind. Attempt to determine whether the driver tried to stop before the collision or took avoidance measures. If not, consider a medical cause that may have contributed to or caused the accident.

10. **Modify collision analysis to account for the characteristics of motorcycle and off-road vehicle collisions.** pp. 32–34

Motor and off-road vehicle collisions are becoming more frequent. These types of collisions often result in more serious injury to the victims because the vehicles do not have the structural protection offered by autos for absorbing much of the crash energy. Thus, you must take several additional factors into consideration when conducting a collision analysis. Upon arrival, after determining that the scene is safe, you should attempt to ascertain the type of impact and associated injury potential. Motorcycle impacts are of four types. Frontal or head-on impacts propel the rider upward and forward as the bike front dips downward. An angular impact occurs as the bike strikes an object at an oblique angle. Sliding impacts occur when an experienced rider "lays the bike down" to avoid an imminent collision. Ejections are common and usually result in serious injury. The type of impact should direct your index of suspicion for injury and subsequent care. Additionally, pay attention to the use of protective equipment, as it has a major effect on injury patterns. Determine whether the rider was wearing a helmet and/or face shield. Note whether the rider was wearing leather clothing or boots. Remember that even with protection, motorcycle impacts often result in serious trauma even at lower speeds. As with motorcycles, off-road riders do not have the benefit of structural protections or restraint systems found in autos. Your collision analysis for these types of emergencies must take into account accessibility to the victim. Delays in detecting the incident and difficulty in reaching and retrieving the victims may increase the seriousness of injuries and require special equipment. Pay attention to any protective equipment the rider was using, such as helmets, face shields, and clothing. When responding to snowmobile incidents, consider the possibility of cold exposure and hypothermia. With watercraft accidents, drowning and hypothermia must also be considered. Hybrid vehicles pose additional hazards.

11. **Describe the considerations in assessing a patient who has fallen.** pp. 34–35

Falls are the most common form of blunt trauma. Most at risk for fall injury are the very young and the elderly. Falls are a release of stored gravitational energy, resulting in an impact between the body and the ground or other surface. In evaluating a fall, determine the fall height, anatomical point of impact, force of the impact, nature of the impact surface, and possible transmission pathway of forces along the skeleton. Then anticipate fracture sites and possible internal injuries. Trauma resulting from a fall is dependent on the contact area and the energy transmission pathway. Injuries occur at the point of impact and along the pathway of transmitted energy, resulting in soft tissue, skeletal, and internal trauma. During the physical assessment, pay particular attention to areas where you expect trauma, looking for further signs of injury. Assess circumstances surrounding a fall and the magnitude of forces involved, remembering that some fractures in the elderly can occur without application of significant trauma force. In some cases, a fracture may cause a fall instead of the fall causing the injury.

12. **Describe the mechanisms of blast injury, blast-injury patterns, and special blast-injury care considerations.** pp. 35–40

The blast-injury process results in six distinct mechanisms of injury—pressure waves, blast wind, projectiles, displacement of persons near the blast, structural collapse, and burns.

Pressure injury occurs as the pressure wave moves outward, rapidly compressing and then decompressing anything in its path. A victim is impacted by the wave, and air-filled body spaces such as the lungs, auditory canals, sinuses, and bowels may be damaged. Hearing loss is the most frequent result of pressure injury, though lung injury is most serious and life threatening. The pressure change may damage or rupture alveoli, resulting in dyspnea, pulmonary edema, pneumothorax, or air embolism. Care includes provision of high-concentration oxygen, gentle positive-pressure ventilation (PPV), and rapid transport. The patient with hearing loss needs careful reassurance and simple instruction.

Blast wind follows behind a pressure wave. This is an outward movement of heated and expanding combustion gases from the explosion epicenter. It is less strength but greater duration than a pressure wave and causes less direct injury. However, it may propel debris or displace victims, which, in turn, will produce injuries.

Projectiles may be fragments from the exploded casing or debris put in motion by the pressure of the explosion. They may impale or enter the body, resulting in hemorrhage, amputations, and internal injury. Projectiles may also be coated with agents to increase hemorrhage or toxins to interfere with wound healing.

Personnel displacement occurs as the pressure wave and blast wind propel the victim through the air away from the blast's epicenter. The victim then impacts the ground or other surface. Blunt and penetrating trauma may result.

In confined-space explosions the pressure wave maintains energy longer than in other conventional explosions. Confining structures can increase the blast's projectile content and result in increased, deadly, blast overpressure.

Collapse of a structure after a blast may entrap victims under debris and result in crush and pressure injuries. The collapse may make victims hard to locate and then extricate.

Burns secondary to heat may result directly from the explosion or as a result of secondary combustion of debris or clothing. Generally, the initial explosion will cause only superficial damage because of the short duration of the heat release and the fluid nature of the body. However, incendiary agents and burning debris or clothing may result in severe full-thickness burns.

There are four types of blast injury patterns: primary, secondary, tertiary, and quarternary. In a primary blast the injuries are caused by the heat of the explosion and the overpressure wave. They most often damage air-filled body spaces such as the ears, sinuses, bowel, and lungs. Secondary blast injuries are caused by projectiles and can be more severe than primary blast injuries. Tertiary blast injuries result from personnel displacement and structural collapse. Injuries can be extensive and result in soft, skeletal, nervous, and vascular tissue and organ destruction. Quarternary blast injuries include any other injuries caused by the explosion.

When caring for a patient experiencing blast injuries, first try to determine if the blast was a result of terrorist action, as the explosive devices may be set to injure rescuers and may contain radioactive contamination. Also be aware of secondary hazards such as gas leaks, disrupted electrical wiring, and possible structural collapse, which can endanger the scene. The most common life-threatening trauma associated with explosions is lung injury, so anticipate this for any patient with significant signs or symptoms of blast injury. Also evaluate your patient's breath sounds and look for any developing breathing problems, or drop in oxygen saturation. If you need to ventilate a patient with a blast injury, understand that there may be complications from the mechanism of injury. Even with the ventilation risks, always provide positive-pressure ventilations to any patient with serious dyspnea.

A blast-injury patient may also experience injuries to the abdomen, though these do not require special attention in the early stages of care. The only exception is when the blast is extremely powerful or the patient was close to detonation. In these situations be aware of developing shock and provide rapid transport and fluid resuscitation as necessary. Ear injuries are also common for blasts. Hearing loss is frequently temporary but may be permanent. Because these injuries will likely improve over time, direct your care to supporting your patient and make sure the ear canal remains uncontaminated. If a blast patient presents with any penetrating wounds or burns, the care is the same as you would perform in any other situation.

13. **Describe the considerations in assessing a patient injured during a sporting event.** pp. 40–41

Sports injuries are most commonly produced by extreme exertion, fatigue, or direct trauma. Injuries may be secondary to acceleration, deceleration, compression, rotation, hyperextension, or hyperflexion. These forces can result in soft tissue damage to the skin and muscles, tendon and ligament injuries, skeletal trauma, spinal injury, and internal damage to hollow or solid organs. Any athlete experiencing a head injury with associated loss of consciousness, neurologic deficit, or lowered level of orientation should be seen in an emergency department. Protective gear often mitigates injury; however, in some cases it can be the cause of an injury, as when cleats force a body to turn on an immobile foot. In other cases, protective gear can hinder assessment and care. Helmets may make spinal immobilization difficult, but removing a helmet may cause greater cervical spine injury.

14. **Describe the considerations for assessing crush injuries.** p. 41

Crush injuries may result from a variety of mechanisms that direct significant force to soft tissue and bones, compressing surfaces together while stretching semifluid soft tissues laterally. Both internal and external hemorrhage may result. If the compressing force remains in place for an extended period of time the pressure can disrupt blood flow through the limb, allowing the accumulation of toxins. This toxic buildup may then be carried back to the central circulation when the pressure is released, inducing cardiac arrhythmias or serious damage to the kidneys. Hemorrhage from many disrupted blood vessels at the wound site may be hard to control. In some instances, sodium bicarbonate may be administered to counteract the toxic effects.

15. **Identify mechanisms with a potential for producing compartment syndrome.** p. 41

A type of blunt trauma associated with crush injury is compartment syndrome. Blunt trauma to a large muscle mass, like the calf, thigh, forearm, or arm, may cause the muscle to swell more quickly than the surrounding connective tissue. As pressure increases, blood flow to the muscle is reduced, causing the muscle to stiffen and become painful. Unless recognized and promptly treated, it may cause permanent and debilitating injury.

Case Study Review

Reread the case study on pages 17 and 18 in Paramedic Care: Trauma; *then, read the following discussion.*
 This scenario represents a typical serious auto collision in which knowledge of the kinetics of trauma assists in analyzing the mechanism of injury and helps guide assessment and care. Using this approach results in a better understanding of the potential injuries. It also provides for an orderly scene approach in which the patients are quickly assessed, prioritized, and immediately stabilized and then quickly transported. The incident is evaluated carefully, using an analysis of the mechanism of injury to anticipate both the nature and severity of patient injuries. This information is then used in combination with the data gathered through the patient assessments to develop a clear picture of what happened to the auto passengers and to determine which resources will be distributed to each patient.

The information given by the dispatcher allows Kris and Bob to begin planning for arrival at the scene. The dispatch information describes a severe accident with the potential for several seriously injured patients. While still en route, Kris and Bob locate equipment in the ambulance and set it out on the stretcher for quick transport to their patients' side. Lactated Ringer's solution in 1,000-mL bags might be readied in the ambulance with trauma tubing, pressure infusers, and large-bore catheters, just in case the decision is made to rapidly transport any of the patients. Kris and Bob may also use this time to review their responsibilities, which begin with arrival at the scene.

©2013 Pearson Education, Inc.
Paramedic Care: Principles & Practice, Vol. 5, 4th Ed.

Given the police update, the team begins thinking about the kinetic energy associated with the collision and the injuries that it is likely to cause. One auto was stopped and was hit from behind by a vehicle at "highway speed." In the auto hit, the suspected injuries should include cervical spine injury, with the rest of the body well protected except for secondary impacts. Kris and Bob should anticipate the need for spinal precautions and ready a collar, vest-type immobilization device, and long spine board.

The auto traveling at highway speed most likely impacted the other frontally. If the occupants were unrestrained, they may have traveled either through the down-and-under or up-and-over pathway. If they were restrained, the lap, lap and shoulder, or air-bag restraint systems may have protected them. (Remember that the air-bag restraint system is beneficial only for the initial frontal impact.) Internal head injuries, chest trauma, and shock are the leading trauma killers. The team will anticipate these types of injuries and treat the patients accordingly.

Kris and Bob gain a great deal of information quickly during the scene size-up. Potential hazards, the number of patients, the resources needed, and the mechanism of injury all are identified. From analysis of the mechanism of injury, they anticipate the nature and extent of injuries for each of the three expected patients. By examining what happened, how badly the autos are damaged, and from what direction the impacts came, the team can garner enough information to anticipate which patient is likely to be the most seriously injured.

In this collision, the green car struck the red one from behind. The red car sustained severe rear-end damage, reflecting a strong impact. The passenger would have been pushed forward with great acceleration by the auto seat, while the unsupported head rotated backward, extending the cervical spine. An important observation was that the headrest was in the "up" position. This positioning probably limited the forceful hyperextension of the head and neck and reduced the potential for injury. The seat belt also limited the danger of secondary impact, ensuring the driver came to rest with the vehicle, not afterward.

The second car (the green one) sustained front-end damage and two spider-web cracks in the windshield. This suggests an unrestrained driver and passenger, the up-and-over pathway, and a potential for severe head, neck, thoracic, and abdominal injuries. The deformed steering wheel also provides evidence that the driver may have sustained a chest injury. Using the analysis of the mechanism of injury, Kris and Bob have a good preliminary picture of the collision process and the likely injuries it produced. As they leave their vehicle and approach the scene, they don gloves and ensure the scene is safe for them, their patients, fellow rescuers, and bystanders. They also request anticipated resources (another ambulance) to handle the multiple patients they expect. Because the mechanism of injury analysis suggests the most serious patients will be found in the green car, Kris and Bob head there first.

Assessment confirms the injuries anticipated by review of the impact and the degree of auto damage. As reported by the police officer, the driver of the red car appears only shaken up, with a possible spine injury. His vitals are within normal limits, given the circumstances. The choice is made to leave him with an Emergency Medical Responder while Kris and Bob remain with the patients in the green car. While it would be more preferable to have a paramedic by the side of each patient, this decision is justified based upon the findings at the scene. Bob and Kris will have another Emergency Medical Responder hold spinal immobilization for the driver of the green car as they attend to the unconscious passenger.

The primary assessment reveals that the occupants of the green auto are in serious condition. The driver has sustained chest trauma and is experiencing dyspnea, though her breath sounds are clear at this time. She is stable for now. However, she has the potential to deteriorate rapidly at any time. Her passenger is moving rapidly into hypovolemic shock, presumably due to pelvic and femur fractures and internal hemorrhage. She is also unconscious, either due to the hypovolemia or the head impact. The passenger is critical and a candidate for immediate transport. The driver, though more stable, is a candidate for immediate transport also.

This case study demonstrates the value a good scene analysis can have in triaging, anticipating the findings of assessment, and determining the care needed by the patient or patients. Although the mechanism of injury analysis does not give definitive information regarding the nature and extent of patient injuries, it can complement the overall assessment of both the scene and each individual patient.

Content Self-Evaluation

MULTIPLE CHOICE

_____ 1. The study of impact is related to a branch of physics called
- **A.** kinetics.
- **B.** velocity.
- **C.** ballistics.
- **D.** inertia.
- **E.** heuristics.

_____ 2. The anticipation of injuries based upon the analysis of the collision mechanism is referred to as the
- **A.** mechanism of injury.
- **B.** index of suspicion.
- **C.** trauma triage criteria.
- **D.** mortality potential.
- **E.** RTS.

_____ 3. Penetrating trauma is the most common type of trauma associated with patient mortality.
- **A.** True
- **B.** False

_____ 4. The tendency of an object to remain at rest or remain in motion unless acted upon by an external force is
- **A.** kinetics.
- **B.** velocity.
- **C.** ballistics.
- **D.** inertia.
- **E.** deceleration.

_____ 5. Two autos accelerate from a stop sign to a speed of 30 miles per hour, the first one by normal acceleration and the second when it was struck from behind by another vehicle. Assuming that both vehicles have the same weight, which vehicle gained the most kinetic energy?
- **A.** The vehicle in normal acceleration gained the most kinetic energy.
- **B.** The vehicle struck from behind gained the most kinetic energy.
- **C.** Both vehicles gained the same kinetic energy.
- **D.** Cannot be determined because the kinetic energy is not known.
- **E.** Cannot be determined because the force is not known.

_____ 6. Which of the following is an example of energy dissipation from an auto accident?
- **A.** Sound of the impact
- **B.** Bending of the structural steel
- **C.** Heating of the compressed steel
- **D.** Internal injury to the occupant
- **E.** All of the above

_____ 7. Which of the following increases the kinetic energy of an object most quickly?
- **A.** The temperature of the object
- **B.** Increasing object speed
- **C.** Decreasing object speed
- **D.** Increasing object mass
- **E.** Decreasing object mass

_____ 8. Blunt trauma may cause
- **A.** rupture of the bowel.
- **B.** bursting of the alveoli.
- **C.** crushing of blood vessels.
- **D.** contusion of the liver or kidneys.
- **E.** all of the above.

_____ 9. Which of the following is a common cause of blunt trauma?
- **A.** Auto collisions
- **B.** Falls
- **C.** Sports injuries
- **D.** Pedestrian impacts
- **E.** All of the above

©2013 Pearson Education, Inc.
Paramedic Care: Principles & Practice, Vol. 5, 4th Ed.

10. In which order do the events of an auto collision usually occur?
   A. Body collision, vehicle collision, organ collision, secondary collisions
   B. Organ collision, vehicle collision, body collision, secondary collisions
   C. Vehicle collision, secondary collisions, body collision, organ collision
   D. Vehicle collision, body collision, organ collision, secondary collisions
   E. Body collision, vehicle collision, secondary collisions, organ collision

11. The major effect of the seat belt during the auto collision is to slow the passenger with the auto.
   A. True
   B. False

12. A supplemental restraint system (SRS) refers to which of the following?
   A. Shoulder belts   *prim*
   B. Air bags   *second*
   C. Lap belts   *prim*
   D. Child seats   *prim*
   E. All of the above

13. Which of the following restraint systems is likely to induce hand fractures?
   A. Shoulder belts
   B. Passenger air bags
   C. Driver-side air bags
   D. Child seats
   E. Lap belts

14. While less convenient than a child carrier, holding a child in the arms is relatively safe except in the most severe of crashes.
   A. True
   B. False

15. The type of auto impact that occurs most frequently is
   A. lateral.
   B. oblique.
   C. frontal.
   D. rear-end.
   E. rollover.

16. Which type of auto impact occurs least frequently?
   A. Lateral
   B. Rear-end
   C. Frontal
   D. Oblique
   E. Rollover

17. The down-and-under pathway is most commonly associated with which type of auto collision?
   A. Lateral
   B. Rear-end
   C. Frontal
   D. Oblique
   E. Rollover

18. When analyzing the lateral-impact injury mechanism, you must assign a higher index of suspicion for serious life-threatening injury than with other types of impact.
   A. True
   B. False

19. Which of the following injuries are associated with significant lateral impact?
   A. Aortic aneurysms
   B. Clavicular fractures
   C. Pelvic fractures
   D. Vertebral fractures
   E. All of the above

20. With oblique impacts, the seriousness of injury is often less than vehicle damage would suggest.
   A. True
   B. False

_____ 21. The most common injury associated with the rear-end impact is to the
    A. abdomen.
    B. pelvis.
    C. aorta.
    D. femur.
    E. head and neck.

_____ 22. Which of the following is a hazard commonly associated with auto collisions?
    A. Hot liquids
    B. Caustic substances
    C. Downed power lines
    D. Sharp glass or metal edges
    E. All of the above

_____ 23. With modern vehicle construction that incorporates crumple zones, you can dependably use the amount of vehicular damage to approximate the patient injuries inside.
    A. True
    B. False

_____ 24. In fatal collisions, about what percentage of the drivers are legally intoxicated?
    A. 10 percent
    B. 20 percent
    C. 35 percent
    D. 50 percent
    E. 83 percent

_____ 25. The most common body area associated with vehicular mortality is the
    A. head.
    B. chest.
    C. abdomen.
    D. extremities.
    E. spine.

_____ 26. In motorcycle accidents, the highest index of suspicion for injury should be directed at the
    A. neck.
    B. head.
    C. extremities.
    D. pelvis.
    E. femurs.

_____ 27. Use of a helmet in a motorcycle crash reduces the incidence of head injury by about
    A. 25 percent.
    B. 35 percent.
    C. 50 percent.
    D. 75 percent.
    E. 85 percent.

_____ 28. In an auto-versus-child pedestrian accident, you would expect the victim to turn toward the impact.
    A. True
    B. False

_____ 29. In addition to the danger of trauma, the boating collision patient is also likely to suffer possible hypothermia and drowning.
    A. True
    B. False

_____ 30. Severe injury is generally associated with a fall from
    A. three times the patient's own height.
    B. twice the patient's own height.
    C. greater than 12 feet.
    D. more than 6 feet.
    E. none of the above.

_____ 31. Which of the following mechanisms can cause patient injury in a blast?
    A. The pressure wave
    B. Flying debris
    C. The patient being thrown into objects
    D. Heat
    E. All of the above

_____ 32. Underwater detonation of an explosive generally increases its lethal range by
    A. 10 percent.
    B. 25 percent.
    C. 100 percent.
    D. 300 percent.
    E. 500 percent.

©2013 Pearson Education, Inc.
Paramedic Care: Principles & Practice, Vol. 5, 4th Ed.

_____ 33. A victim's orientation to the blast does not affect the nature and severity of the injuries he sustains from an explosion.
   A. True
   B. False

_____ 34. The arrow-shaped projectiles in military-type explosives that are designed to extend the injury power of a bomb are called
   A. ordinance.
   B. casing material.
   C. flechettes.
   D. oatmeal.
   E. granulation.

_____ 35. When victims are within a structure that contains an explosion, such as a building, the effects of the blast are concentrated and the severity of the expected injuries increases.
   A. True
   B. False

_____ 36. Which of the following are secondary blast injuries?
   A. Heat injuries
   B. Pressure injuries
   C. Projectile injuries
   D. Injuries caused by structural collapse
   E. Both A and B

_____ 37. If you suspect that a blast was a terrorist act, you should be cautious of secondary explosive devices intended to injure rescue personnel.
   A. True
   B. False

_____ 38. The most serious and common traumas associated with explosions affect the
   A. heart.
   B. bowel.
   C. auditory canal.
   D. lungs.
   E. brain.

_____ 39. When ventilating the victim of a severe blast, you should use forceful deep ventilations with the bag-valve mask because doing this will ensure good chest expansion.
   A. True
   B. False

_____ 40. Sports injuries are frequently associated with
   A. fatigue.
   B. extreme exertion.
   C. compression.
   D. rotation.
   E. all of the above.

Special Project

Mechanism of Injury Analysis

Study the accompanying photographs of each accident scene. For each photo, identify the type of impact that has occurred and list at least three injuries that you would expect to have occurred.

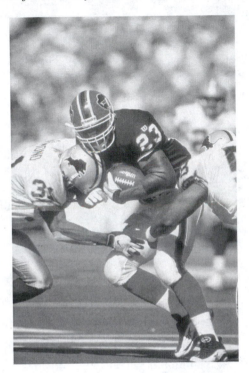

A.   Mechanism of injury _____

   Anticipated injuries
   _____
   _____
   _____
   _____
   _____
   _____
   _____
   _____

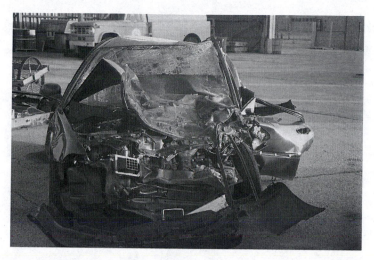

B. Mechanism of injury _____

Anticipated injuries

_____
_____
_____
_____

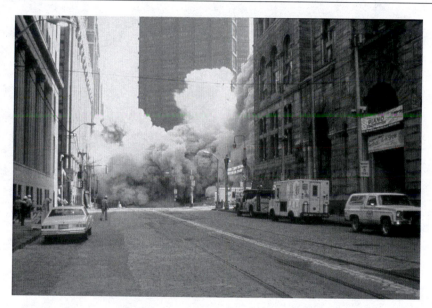

C. Mechanism of injury _____

Anticipated injuries

_____
_____
_____
_____

Personal Benchmarking—Analyzing Mechanisms of Injury

Next time you are in a vehicle for some time, take a look at your position with regard to the interior of the auto in relation to your anatomy. Visualize the forces of impact and what your body will strike during that impact. Identify protections offered by crumple zones and the likely injuries resulting from serious impact, and then determine what effect restraints will have on injury patterns (nature and seriousness).

> Frontal impact
> Lateral impact
> Rear-end impact
> Rotational impact
> Rollover impact

The next time you go to an auto collision, use this information to help you "relive" the auto impact and anticipate patient injuries.

©2013 Pearson Education, Inc.
Paramedic Care: Principles & Practice, Vol. 5, 4th Ed.

3

Penetrating Trauma

Review of Chapter Objectives

After reading this chapter, you should be able to:

1. **Define the key terms introduced in this chapter.**

   Knowing and being able to apply the key terms in each chapter is critical to understanding chapter concepts. Write the list of key terms. Then write the definition of each one in your own words. Check your understanding by confirming the definitions in the text glossary. Correct any misunderstandings. Create a study aid by writing each key term on the front of an index card and the definition on the back. Use the cards to quiz yourself, or to have someone quiz you.

2. **Apply the laws of inertia and energy conservation to the kinetics of penetrating trauma.** pp. 46–47

   Recall that the law of inertia states that an object at rest or in motion will remain so unless acted upon by an outside force. Energy conservation is the physical law stating that energy can neither be created or destroyed but can only be changed from one form to another. The kinetic energy of a penetrating object is dependent on its mass and even more so on its velocity according to the kinetic energy formula, $\left(KE = \dfrac{M \times V^2}{2} \right)$. Therefore, the greater the mass or speed of an object, the greater its kinetic energy. This relationship between mass and velocity explains why very small and relatively light bullets traveling at high speed have potential to do great harm. It also clarifies why different weights of bullets traveling at different speeds can cause differing degrees of damage. The Law of Conservation of Energy explains that a projectile's kinetic energy is transformed into damage as it slows. The kinetic energy lost by the projectile as it passes through an object and slows is transferred into tissue displacement, converted to physical tissue damage, and a small amount of heat.

3. **Apply the concepts of force and kinetic energy exchange to the potential for injury.** pp. 46–47

   Recall that Newton's second law of motion states that force strength is related to an object's weight (mass) and the rate of its change in velocity (acceleration or deceleration). The forces causing trauma are related to this force formula. A projectile's kinetic energy is dependent upon its mass and velocity. The more quickly an object slows, the more rapidly it gives up its kinetic energy. Therefore, the damage a projectile causes within human tissue is directly related to the rate of energy exchange. A large projectile traveling at high speed has the kinetic potential to cause significant injury. How the projectile behaves within the body will determine the extent of damage.

4. Apply principles of ballistics to the prediction of injury patterns.   pp. 47–49

The study of projectiles in motion and their effects on objects they impact is described by the science of ballistics. Trajectory refers to the curved path that a bullet follows after it is fired from a gun. Gravity serves to pull a bullet downward. The longer the distance between a gun and an object hit and the slower a bullet, the greater the trajectory curves. The flatter the trajectory, either because of high speed or close range, the more damage the bullet will cause. A more significant aspect of projectile travel is the energy exchange between the bullet and the object. Factors that affect this energy exchange include drag, profile, stability, expansion, shape, and cavitation. Drag occurs from wind resistance and slows the movement of the projectile. The greater the drag, the greater the slowing effect. A bullet fired at close range has minimal drag and consequently causes more damage. Projectiles with high kinetic energy create a shock wave and a temporary cavity on entry. This is known as cavitation, which is related to a bullet's velocity and energy exchange rate. The energy exchange rate, in turn, is related to the projectile's contacting surface size, which is determined by its shape and profile. Profile is the cross section of the bullet along its direction of travel. A larger surface profile causes more extensive damage. Blunt-shaped bullets will release kinetic energy faster than pointed bullets.

The location of a bullet's center of mass affects its stability during flight and when it meets resistance. An unstable bullet will tumble or yaw (wobble). When it strikes human tissue the yaw or tumble may become more pronounced. This increases the presenting profile and thus its energy exchange rate, enhancing its potential for causing damage. Some projectiles may increase their profile and energy exchange rate by deforming when they strike an object. Bullets that mushroom out or fragment release their energy rapidly due to their increased surface area. This results in more serious injury. Energy exchange between a projectile and body tissue can also be affected by any object it strikes during travel. Degree of injury will depend on how much the projectile slows and whether the surface area becomes deformed. Bullet deformity caused by body armor may increase the energy exchange rate but the reduction in velocity and lost kinetic energy will more likely cause blunt trauma, with an overall reduction in injury potential.

5. Apply the characteristics of specific weapon types to the prediction of injury patterns.   pp. 49–50

Weapons such as handguns, domestic rifles, assault rifles, shotguns, bladed instruments, and arrows each have certain characteristics associated with the injuries it produces. **Handguns** are medium-velocity weapons that are most effective at close range. The lower energy limits its potential to cause damage. Injury severity is usually related to organs directly damaged by a bullet's passage. Civilian hunting **rifles** fire heavier projectiles with greater velocity. Bullets travel further with greater accuracy and retain more kinetic energy than in handguns. This results in extensive wounds, often extending beyond the bullet's immediate track. Because **assault rifles** are often automatic, multiple wounds and casualties can be expected. **Shotguns** can fire single projectiles or numerous pellets contained in a shell. A slug will cause a single entrance wound similar to a rifle bullet wound. In contrast to bullets, **knives, swords, arrows,** or other slow-moving penetrating objects generally cause damage to tissues coming in direct contact with the source. The penetration, however, can result in serious internal hemorrhage or injury to individual or multiple organs.

6. Associate the application of low-, medium-, and high-velocity penetrating mechanisms to various body tissues with the biomechanical forces produced to predict injury patterns.   pp. 50–54

High-velocity/high-energy projectiles (rifle bullets) are likely to cause the most extensive injury because they have the potential to impart the most kinetic energy to the patient. Rapid energy exchange causes the greatest cavitational wave and is most likely to produce bullet deformity and fragmentation. These characteristics cause more severe tissue damage to a greater area. The effects of these projectiles can be further enhanced if the bullet hits bone and causes it to shatter, creating additional projectiles that are driven into adjoining tissue.

©2013 Pearson Education, Inc.
Paramedic Care: Principles & Practice, Vol. 5, 4th Ed.

Medium-velocity/medium-energy projectiles (from handguns) are likely to cause only moderate injury beyond the direct pathway of the bullet because their reduced energy does not usually cause the bullet deformity, fragmentation, and extensive cavitation waves seen with rifle projectiles. The shotgun is a particularly lethal weapon at close range because its medium-energy projectiles are numerous and their numbers cause many direct injury pathways.

Low-velocity/low-energy penetrating objects are commonly knives, arrows, ice picks, and other objects traveling at low speeds. They generally cause only direct injury along the path of their travel. They may, however, be twisted, moved about, or inserted at an oblique angle. Therefore, the entrance wound may not reflect the actual organs and tissues damaged.

The passage of a projectile and its associated injury are related to its speed, path of travel, and, specifically, to the body region it passes through. Damage occurs through direct injury, the pressure wave, and cavitation. Direct injury is damage done by direct contact of the object with tissue. Damage with most medium- and low-velocity projectiles is limited to direct injury. High-velocity projectiles create a pressure wave on entry. Energy is transmitted forward and outward, pushing tissue in its path in those directions. As tissue moves away from the projectile's path, a temporary cavity is created. This is called cavitation. The natural elasticity of injured tissue and the adjoining tissue closes the cavity, but an area of disrupted tissue remains. This permanent cavity becomes filled with air, blood, fluids, and debris. The size depends on the amount of energy transferred during the passage of the object.

Damage caused by a bullet varies depending on the elasticity (resiliency) and density of the tissue the bullet strikes. Connective tissue is very resilient, stretches easily, and will somewhat resist cavitational injury. Solid organs such as the liver, spleen, and pancreas are dense and much less resilient than connective tissue. Injury is closely associated with the temporary cavity size. Although surrounding tissue may cause the organs to return to their original orientation, hemorrhage and damage are often severe. Hollow organs are resilient when not distended with fluid; if an organ is full, however, the cavitational wave may cause the organ to rupture, resulting in severe hemorrhage. Pericardial tamponade may result from slower and smaller projectiles penetrating the pericardial sac. With greater force, the heart and great vessels may perforate or rupture, with rapid exsanguination ensuing. Direct injury can also perforate an organ and permit spillage of its contents into surrounding tissue. Lung tissue is air-filled, which limits the cavitational wave and thus injury. Large penetrations of the thoracic wall, however, may permit air to escape into the thorax, causing a pneumothorax or tension pneumothorax.

Penetrating chest trauma may also affect the esophagus, trachea, and diaphragm. Tracheal tears may result in airway compromise, whereas esophageal tears may release gastric contents into the mediastinum, with potentially deadly results. Bone is extremely dense and inelastic. Direct contact with a bullet or, in some cases, just the cavitational wave, may shatter the ribs or other bones, driving bony fragments into surrounding tissue. Neck injuries may permit severe hemorrhage, disrupt the trachea, or allow air to enter the jugular veins and embolize the lungs. Head injuries may disrupt the airway or may penetrate the cranium and cause extensive, rarely survivable, injury to the brain.

7. **Describe the forces and characteristics associated with entrance and exit wounds from penetrating trauma.**
pp. 54–55

Entrance wounds may be smaller or larger than bullet caliber suggests. Entry wounds sustained at close range display special characteristics. Such wounds may be marked by elements of the barrel exhaust and bullet passage. These signs might include tattooing from propellant residue or a discoloration ridge from skin stretching. If barrel exhaust is pushed into the wound it may produce subcutaneous emphysema and crepitus. Burns may also be evident from the hot gases of barrel exhaust. Exit wounds may more accurately reflect the damage potential caused by a bullet than entrance wounds. Exit wounds are caused by the bullet's passage and cavitational wave. The wound may have a stellate appearance with tears radiating outward in a star-like fashion. If no exit wound is apparent the bullet may have expended all its kinetic energy and remain lodged within the body tissue. When documenting bullet wounds, refrain from identifying them as entrance or exit but provide a detailed description of the injuries.

8. **Describe special concerns for EMS provider safety that are associated with penetrating trauma.** p. 55

Penetrating trauma, especially when associated with shootings or stabbings, presents the danger of violence directed toward others (other rescuers, bystanders, your patient, and you). It is essential that you approach the scene with great caution and ensure that the police have secured it before you approach or enter. Stage your vehicle at least one block away and out of sight if law enforcement personnel are not yet on scene. Ensure there are no weapons within reach of the patient and that the patient does not have any concealed weapons before beginning an assessment.

9. **Given a penetrating trauma scenario, reconstruct events to gain additional information that can help predict injury patterns.** p. 55

During the scene size-up, you should evaluate the mechanism of injury, including the type of weapon, caliber, distance, the number of shots fired, and the angle between the shooter and the victim. For bladed weapon injuries, determine the gender and approximate the attacker's weight and height. Males and females display characteristic strike patterns. Make note of the weapon's length if it has been removed from the victim.

10. **Describe the medical-legal concerns specific to penetrating trauma situations.** p. 55

Although providing patient care is always of primary importance, try to preserve the crime scene. Do not unnecessarily disturb objects around the patient. Cut around bullet or knife holes in patient clothing. Give any clothing to the police for evidence. Be sure to use appropriate local protocols for handling deceased patients.

11. **Describe the special considerations in management of penetrating trauma to the face and chest, and of impaled objects.** pp. 56–57

Certain penetrating wounds need special attention. Facial gunshot wounds may endanger the airway and destroy landmarks, making endotracheal intubation difficult. Bubbling seen while the chest is compressed may help guide placement of the tube. Be prepared to perform a percutaneous cricothyrotomy if endotracheal intubation is unsuccessful. High-velocity bullets may create chest wounds large enough to permit air movement through the chest wall, causing an open pneumothorax. If frothy blood is present a tension pneumothorax may have developed. Cover any open chest wound with an occlusive dressing taped on three sides to allow air to escape. Needle decompression may be indicated to relieve pressure. If penetrating trauma causes heart and great vessel damage, the patient may develop pericardial tamponade. This condition requires immediate treatment in the emergency department, so rapid transport is essential. If a low-velocity object becomes impaled, attempting to remove it may cause more serious injury. Only remove objects that interfere with airway or cardiopulmonary resuscitation (CPR). Immobilize impaled objects in place using bulky dressings and splinting materials to stabilize the object. If the object is too large to transport, cut the object while minimizing patient movement.

Case Study Review

Reread the case study on page 45 in Paramedic Care: Trauma; *then, read the following discussion.*

This scenario involves a patient who has sustained a serious penetrating injury to the chest and provides the opportunity to apply an understanding of the kinetics of trauma to the wounding process. The case also allows us to review scene considerations that should be followed when violence is involved.

Weapon use in modern society represents violence and a danger to rescuers, bystanders, the patient, and the responding EMS team. Sandy is somewhat reassured by the dispatch information, which states that the patient is in custody, so as she arrives at the scene she notes the police officers surrounding the patient. However, she remains cautious and ensures that the patient is free of weapons before she begins her care.

©2013 Pearson Education, Inc.
Paramedic Care: Principles & Practice, Vol. 5, 4th Ed.

In assessing the patient, Sandy anticipates a serious injury, because police are generally equipped with relatively powerful handguns. She recognizes that the bullet delivered significant wounding energy to the thorax and may have fragmented as it hit the ribs and drove rib fragments into tissue as it passed. She anticipates lung damage along the bullet's path, probably more related to the damage seen at the exit wound, rather than at the entrance wound. Sandy is also concerned about the penetration of the chest wall and the pleura caused by the bullet's passage. Such a wound may permit air to enter the pleural space and cause the lung to collapse (an open pneumothorax). She seals both the entrance and exit wounds on three sides to allow any building air pressure (tension pneumothorax) to escape. She also carefully monitors breath sounds and respiratory effort to ensure that an unrecognized closed tension pneumothorax does not develop. Sandy anticipates that this patient's respirations will worsen as the edema associated with the injured lung tissue gets worse and with the continued loss of blood from the internal wound.

Because of the proximity of the wound to the heart, Sandy applies the electrocardiogram (ECG) electrodes and constantly monitors the patient's heart rate and rhythm. She also trends both the patient's level of consciousness and vital signs to ensure that the earliest signs of hypovolemia, shock, and decreased tissue perfusion are noted. This patient is clearly a candidate for rapid transport to the closest trauma center.

Content Self-Evaluation

MULTIPLE CHOICE

_____ 1. Approximately what number of deaths is attributable to shootings each year?
   A. 31,500
   B. 40,500
   C. 44,000
   D. 50,500
   E. 100,000

_____ 2. An object traveling at twice the speed of another object of the same weight has
   A. twice the kinetic energy.
   B. three times the kinetic energy.
   C. four times the kinetic energy.
   D. eight times the kinetic energy.
   E. ten times the kinetic energy.

$2^2 \quad 2 \times 2 = 4$
$4^2 \quad 4 \times 4 = 16$

_____ 3. Wounds from rifle bullets are considered two to four times more lethal than those from handgun bullets.
   A. True
   B. False

_____ 4. The curved tract a bullet follows during flight is called its
   A. ballistics.
   B. cavitation.
   C. trajectory.
   D. yaw.
   E. parabola.

_____ 5. The surface of a projectile that exchanges energy with the object struck is its
   A. caliber.
   B. profile.
   C. drag.
   D. yaw.
   E. expansion factor.

_____ 6. When a rifle bullet hits tissue, normally it will
   A. continue without tumbling.
   B. tumble once then travel nose-first.
   C. tumble quickly, then slowly rotate.
   D. wobble but not tumble.
   E. tumble 180 degrees then continue.

_____ 7. Although handgun bullets are made of relatively soft lead, their kinetic energy is generally not sufficient to cause significant deformity.
   A. True
   B. False

8. Civilian hunting ammunition is designed to expand dramatically on impact.
   A. True
   B. False

9. Which of the following statements accurately describes a rifle bullet in contrast to a handgun bullet?
   A. It is a heavier projectile.
   B. It travels at a greater velocity.
   C. It is more likely to expand.
   D. It travels further.
   E. All of the above.

10. The shotgun is limited in range and accuracy; however, injuries it inflicts at close range can be very severe or lethal.
    A. True
    B. False

11. Which element of the projectile injury process is related to the actual damage caused as the bullet contacts tissue?
    A. Direct injury
    B. Pressure wave
    C. Temporary cavity
    D. Permanent cavity
    E. Zone of injury

12. The formation of subatmospheric pressure behind the bullet as it passes through the body is a result of
    A. direct injury.
    B. the pressure wave.
    C. a temporary cavity.
    D. fragmentation.
    E. referred injury.

13. The passage of a projectile through the body results in a region where tissues are disrupted and not functioning normally known as the
    A. direct injury.
    B. pressure wave.
    C. temporary cavity.
    D. permanent cavity.
    E. zone of injury.

14. The temporary cavity formed as a high-velocity/high-energy bullet passes may be how large?
    A. Twice the bullet caliber
    B. Four times the bullet caliber
    C. Six times the bullet caliber
    D. 12 times the bullet caliber
    E. Rarely more than the bullet caliber

15. The tissue structure that is very resilient, yet dense, and usually sustains limited damage with the passage of a projectile is
    A. a solid organ.
    B. a hollow organ.
    C. connective tissue.
    D. bone.
    E. a lung.

16. The tissue structure that is likely to rupture and spill its contents when struck by a projectile is
    A. a solid organ.
    B. a hollow organ.
    C. connective tissue.
    D. bone.
    E. a lung.

17. Penetrating wounds to the extremities account for about 70 percent of all penetrating wounds yet account for less than 10 percent of fatalities related to this injury mechanism.
    A. True
    B. False

©2013 Pearson Education, Inc.
Paramedic Care: Principles & Practice, Vol. 5, 4th Ed.

18. The abdominal organ most tolerant to the passage of a projectile is the
    A. bowel.
    B. liver.
    C. spleen.
    D. kidney.
    E. pancreas.

19. Because of the pressure-driven dynamics of respiration, any large bullet wound to the chest is likely to seriously compromise breathing.
    A. True
    B. False

20. The body region in which a penetrating wound has the greatest likelihood of drawing air into the venous system is the
    A. abdomen.
    B. thorax.
    C. head.
    D. neck.
    E. none of the above.

21. Which of the following is NOT associated with an entrance wound?
    A. Tattooing
    B. A small ridge of discoloration around the wound
    C. A blown-outward appearance
    D. Subcutaneous emphysema
    E. Propellant residue on the surrounding tissue

22. The entrance wound is more likely to reflect the actual damaging potential of the projectile than the exit wound.
    A. True
    B. False

23. Which of the following information should you gain through the scene size-up, if possible?
    A. The gun caliber
    B. The angle of the gun to the victim
    C. The type of gun used
    D. Assurance that no other weapons are involved
    E. All of the above

24. As you care for a patient at a potential crime scene, actions you take to help preserve evidence should include
    A. cutting through, not around, bullet or knife holes in clothing.
    B. moving what you can away from the patient.
    C. removing obviously dead patients from the scene as quickly as possible.
    D. disturbing only the items necessary to provide patient care.
    E. all of the above.

25. Frothy blood at a bullet exit or entrance wound suggests a(n)
    A. simple pneumothorax.
    B. open pneumothorax.
    C. tension pneumothorax.
    D. pericardial tamponade.
    E. mediastinum injury.

Special Project

Label the Diagram

Demonstrate your knowledge of the process by which projectiles injure body tissue by identifying the labels A through E on the accompanying diagram showing a bullet's penetration of the body.

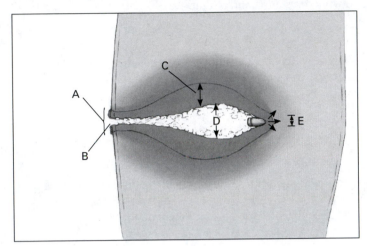

A. _____

B. _____

C. _____

D. _____

E. _____

©2013 Pearson Education, Inc.
Paramedic Care: Principles & Practice, Vol. 5, 4th Ed.

4

Hemorrhage and Shock

Review of Chapter Objectives

After reading this chapter, you should be able to:

1. **Define the key terms introduced in this chapter.**

   Knowing and being able to apply the key terms in each chapter is critical to understanding chapter concepts. Write the list of key terms. Then write the definition of each one in your own words. Check your understanding by confirming the definitions in the text glossary. Correct any misunderstandings. Create a study aid by writing each key term on the front of an index card and the definition on the back. Use the cards to quiz yourself, or to have someone quiz you.

2. **Apply concepts of anatomy, physiology of the circulatory system to explain the disruption of homeostasis that occurs in the face of hemorrhage, and the body's compensatory mechanisms for attempting to maintain homeostasis.**   pp. 62–63, 71–74

   The cardiovascular system is a closed system of interconnected tubes (blood vessels) that direct blood to the essential organs and tissues of the body. Arteries distribute blood to the various organs and tissues of the body. Arterioles determine the amount of blood perfusing the tissue of an organ and together constrict and increase peripheral vascular resistance or dilate and reduce peripheral vascular resistance. Progressive vasoconstriction can help maintain blood pressure and circulation to the most critical organs as the body loses blood during hemorrhage or fluid during other forms of shock. The venous system collects blood and returns it to the heart. It contains 64 percent of the total blood volume and, when constricted, can return a relatively great volume (up to 1 liter) to the active circulation.

   The cardiovascular system is powered by the central pump, the heart. It circulates the blood and, against the peripheral vascular resistance, drives the blood pressure. Its output is a factor of preload (the blood delivered to it by the venous system), stroke volume (the amount of blood ejected into the aorta with each contraction), rate, and afterload (the peripheral vascular resistance). The heart can help compensate for blood loss by attempting to maintain cardiac output by increasing its stroke volume (which is hard to do in hypovolemic states) or by increasing its rate. Finally, the cardiovascular system contains a precious fluid: blood. Blood provides oxygen and nutrients to the body cells and removes carbon dioxide and waste products of metabolism. Blood also contains clotting factors that will occlude blood vessels if they are torn or disrupted.

   The central nervous system provides control of the cardiovascular system using baroreceptors in the carotid arteries and aortic arch to sense fluctuations in blood pressure. It will maintain blood pressure by increasing heart rate, cardiac preload, and peripheral vascular resistance. Hormones from the kidneys and elsewhere help control blood volume and electrolytes as well as the production of erythrocytes.

3. **Describe the characteristics and concerns associated with venous, arterial, and capillary bleeding.** pp. 63–64

Hemorrhage is usually classified by the type of vessel injured. Capillary hemorrhage involves the smallest blood vessels. Blood oozes from the wound, clots quickly, and is generally bright red because it is well oxygenated. Venous hemorrhage flows more quickly. It can be extensive if a large vessel is involved but usually stops in a few minutes. The deoxygenated blood is generally dark red. Arterial hemorrhage is the most serious. Blood flows rapidly and may spurt. Blood is well oxygenated and appears bright red. The size of the arteries and the high pressure within them can result in significant blood loss.

4. **Describe the process of hemostasis and factors that can affect it.** pp. 64–66

Hemostasis is a complex three-step process. **Vascular phase:** Smooth muscle within the walls of a vessel begin to contract when the vessel is torn and bleeds. This causes the vessel to withdraw into the wound, thicken its wall, and reduce its lumen. **Platelet phase:** Injury disrupts the vessel's smooth interior lining, causing turbulent blood flow. Platelets adhere to each other and to collagen fibers exposed by the injury to the cell wall. This phase halts hemorrhage from capillaries and small veins and arteries. The clot formed is unstable. **Coagulation phase:** Clotting factors are activated and released into the bloodstream. These clotting factors trigger a series of chemical reactions that cause formation of strong protein fibers called fibrin. Fibrin strands stick together, forming a strong mesh that entraps red blood cells. This forms a stronger, more stable clot and takes about 7–10 minutes.

Numerous factors can affect the hemostatic process. Movement around the injury may cause clots to break loose and disrupt developing fibrin strands. Aggressive fluid therapy may adversely impact the effectiveness of hemostatic mechanisms. High fluid volume increases the pressure pushing against developing clots, worsening bleeding. Additionally, excess fluid dilutes clotting factors and platelets without replacing red blood cells. This reduces the blood's oxygen-carrying capacity. Body temperature also affects the hemostatic process. If body temperature falls below normal in shock states, clot formation is not as rapid or effective. Medications may also interfere with the clotting process and prolong or worsen hemorrhage. These include medications that inhibit platelet aggregation and protein fiber generation.

5. **Given a variety of scenarios involving external hemorrhage, demonstrate appropriate measures to control it.** pp. 66, 81–83

Most external hemorrhage is easy to recognize and control. Capillary and venous bleeding can generally be controlled by bandages and dressings. Hemorrhage from large veins or arteries requires direct pressure. Tourniquets may be employed for uncontrollable life-threatening bleeding.

Direct pressure: For most wounds, cover the wound with a wad of dressing material, apply a firm bandage, and focus finger pressure directly on the site. If bleeding saturates the dressing, apply another dressing and bandage and continue pressure. If bleeding still persists, remove dressings and reapply then direct pressure to the precise site of bleeding. Consider pneumatic splints to further control limb bleeding, as these immobilize and apply circumferential pressure. In cases of open skull fracture, do not apply pressure to the fracture site. Apply digital pressure to the scalp edges. If cerebral spinal fluid is draining from the ears or nose do not attempt to stop the flow. Cover the area with a soft, porous dressing and bandage loosely in place. For orbital injuries, never apply direct pressure to the eye globe. Apply pressure only to the intact and stable bony orbital rim. Neck lacerations will require firm digital pressure. Cover an open neck wound with an occlusive dressing, covered by a soft dressing and held firmly in place with bandaging. Avoid pressure on the larynx or other airway structures. Large gaping wounds will require using a mass of dressing material approximating the size of the wound. Place the material with the sterile, nonadherent side down into the wound and bandage firmly in place. Crush injuries are challenging to control. Place a dressing around and over the crushed tissue. Place a pneumatic splint over the dressing, and inflate to a pressure that holds the dressing firmly in place to control bleeding.

©2013 Pearson Education, Inc.
Paramedic Care: Principles & Practice, Vol. 5, 4th Ed.

Elevation and Pressure Points: Elevation may help staunch persistent bleeding where there is an isolated limb wound. If bleeding still persists, apply firm pressure to an arterial pulse point proximal to the wound. Maintain this pressure once applied.

Topical Hemostatic Agents: Hemostatic agents and dressings are applied directly or indirectly to active hemorrhage. These agents work by enhancing blood coagulation in different ways.

6. **Describe the indications, application, benefits, and consequences of tourniquet use.**   pp. 66–67, 83

Tourniquets are a last resort and should only be used to halt persistent, life-threatening bleeding that cannot be controlled by direct pressure. Military experience has demonstrated benefits in treating severe limb injuries from high-velocity gunshot wounds and blast-related amputations. In civilian situations tourniquets may be valuable in mass-casualty circumstances when resources are limited. Ideally, commercially available devices should be used. Alternatively, a wide cravat or blood pressure cuff may be employed. Devices that are too narrow will constrict and damage tissue. Tourniquets that are applied too loosely can increase hemorrhage. A tourniquet, although appropriately applied to halt all blood flow into a limb, allows toxins and metabolic waste to accumulate from anaerobic respiration. When the tourniquet is subsequently released, these toxins can move into central circulation, with severe consequences. Therefore, once applied, a tourniquet should be left in place until the patient is in the emergency department.

7. **Given a variety of scenarios, identify internal hemorrhage.**   pp. 67–68

Internal hemorrhage can involve capillary, venous, or arterial blood loss. It is associated with blunt and penetrating trauma but may also be caused by nontraumatic illness or disease. Generally blood loss is self-limiting; however, large contusions, massive soft tissue injuries, and large hematomas, especially affecting the thighs or buttocks, can result in moderate blood loss. Humerus and tibia/fibula fractures may account for 500–750 mL of loss. Femur and pelvic fractures can cause up to 1,500–2,000 mL of loss. Blood loss in the chest, abdomen, and is often uncontrollable and requires surgical intervention to stop the bleeding.

Carefully evaluate body orifices for evidence of internal bleeding. Nasal and oral cavity trauma can result in significant hemorrhage, obstruct the airway, and cause nausea/vomiting.

Chest trauma, tuberculosis, or cancer can cause hemorrhaging in the lower airways or alveoli. Patients may cough bright red blood or pink, frothy sputum.

Hemorrhage in the upper digestive system may cause accumulation of blood in the stomach. Causes may include trauma, caustic ingestion, cancer, ulcers, or ruptured esophageal varices. Stomach irritation may result in hematemesis. Blood that resembles wet coffee grounds has been in the gastrointestinal tract for a long time.

Lower gastrointestinal bleeding may result from trauma, cancer, hemorrhoids, or diverticulosis. Patients may bleed from the rectum or pass dark, tarry stools if the blood has remained in the bowel for some time.

Vaginal bleeding may be mild, moderate, or severe. Hemorrhage may result from trauma, sexual assault, degenerative disease, or complications of pregnancy.

Urethral bleeding may reflect injury to the genitourinary tract, infection, or other causes. Usually this bleeding is minor and blood may be present in urine.

8. **Given a variety of scenarios involving internal hemorrhage, develop appropriate patient management plans.**   pp. 67–68

Internal hemorrhage may be difficult or impossible to control. Local injury signs and early signs and symptoms of blood loss and shock are the best indicators of internal hemorrhage. Mechanism of injury alone may not be a reliable indicator of injury severity. Vital signs and level of responsiveness should guide treatment and transport priorities. Minimize movement and immobilize long bone fractures to assist natural control mechanisms. However, in multiple-system trauma, do not spend time splinting but immobilize the patient to a long spine board and begin transport. Patients with nasal or oral bleeding may require suction or nasal pressure with the patient in an upright or recovery position if spinal injury is not suspected. Assign priority to patients with internal bleeding based on their clinical presentation. Consider fluid resuscitation and keep the patient warm if he shows signs and symptoms of shock.

9. **Describe the pathophysiology and findings associated with the four stages of hemorrhage.**   pp. 68–69

Hemorrhage can be divided into four classes as a patient moves through compensated, decompensated, and irreversible shock.

Class I blood loss is a loss of up to 15 percent of the patient's blood volume. Blood pressure, pulse pressure, respiratory rate, and urine output remain constant. It generally presents with a slight increase in pulse rate, some nervousness, cool skin, and slight pallor. It is difficult to detect because the body compensates well for blood loss in this range.

Class II blood loss is a loss of up to 30 percent of the patient's blood volume. Signs and symptoms become more apparent as first-line compensation fails. Tachycardia, diminished pulses, and a narrowing pulse pressure become evident. Patients may display thirst, anxiety, restlessness, and cool and clammy skin.

Class III blood loss is a loss of up to 40 percent of the patient's blood volume. Classic signs of shock appear. Blood pressure begins to fall and tachycardia is more pronounced. A pulse is barely palpable. Patients display air hunger, tachypnea, and more severe thirst. Skin is pale, cool, and diaphoretic. Survival is unlikely without immediate intervention.

Class IV blood loss is a blood loss in excess of 40 percent of the patient's blood volume. The patient begins to display a deathlike appearance, with pulses disappearing and respirations becoming very shallow and ineffective. The patient becomes very lethargic and then unconscious. Survival is unlikely.

10. **Describe the effects of hemorrhage on categories of special patients, such as pregnant women, athletes, obese patients, children, and the elderly.**   pp. 69–70

Certain categories of patients react differently to blood loss. In pregnancy, blood volume increases by as much as 50 percent. The woman may compensate for blood loss longer but the fetus will be deprived of oxygen. Well-conditioned athletes have greater fluid and cardiac reserves. As a result, they may lose more blood than typical before moving through each stage of hemorrhage. Obese patients have lower blood volume as a percent of body weight. Apparently smaller blood losses may have a more serious effect. Infants and young children have a proportionately higher volume of blood than adults, but less developed compensatory mechanisms. They may show limited signs or symptoms of blood loss and then suddenly move into later stages of shock. The elderly are more seriously affected by blood loss than average adults. They have lower fluid reserves and compensatory mechanisms are less effective. Medications may limit their ability to maintain blood pressure or interfere with coagulation. Chronic cardiovascular inefficiency limits their tolerance for inadequate tissue perfusion. Reduced pain perception, lower levels of mental acuity, and less resistance to hypothermia all contribute to more serious consequences from hemorrhage.

11. **Describe the events of shock at the cellular level.**   pp. 70–71

Cells are the elemental building blocks of the body and ultimately carry out all body functions. They derive their energy from a three-step process. The first step, called glycolysis, requires no oxygen (anaerobic) and generates a small amount of energy. The second step, called the citric acid or Krebs cycle, occurs in the walls of the mitochondria. This step requires oxygen (aerobic). The third step, called the electron transport chain, occurs in the mitochondria, where residual compounds are converted into energy. The three-step aerobic process generates 36 ATP (energy) molecules. If oxygen and glucose are in ample supply, cells have enough energy to perform their functions. When oxygen is lacking, cells generate energy only through glycolysis, which results in excess lactic acid. In shock, which is inadequate tissue perfusion that does not adequately supply the cells with oxygen, anaerobic metabolism predominates, resulting in the dangerous condition called metabolic acidosis.

©2013 Pearson Education, Inc.
Paramedic Care: Principles & Practice, Vol. 5, 4th Ed.

12. **Describe the effects of shock on oxygen transport.** p. 71

Circulation carries oxygen-rich blood from the pulmonary system through the heart and then into the major arteries. There it is directed into the microcirculation by arterioles and precapillary sphincters bringing oxygen to the organs and tissues where internal respiration takes place. The cardiovascular system is often the system most affected by shock, thus causing disruption of oxygen delivery to cells. Oxygen delivery system disruption is the most critical and the most immediate life threat from trauma and shock.

13. **Describe the cardiovascular events that take place in shock.** pp. 73–75

As hemorrhage or vasodilation causes a reduction in preload (return of blood to the heart), the ventricles do not engorge, contractility decreases, and stroke volume drops, with a consequent reduction in blood pressure. Baroreceptors in the aorta and carotid arteries sense this reduction and signal the brain to increase heart rate, peripheral vascular resistance, and venous tone. Additionally, blood is diverted to critical organs. If volume deficits are corrected the cardiovascular system can compensate for the temporary loss. If deficits continue, the venous system becomes overwhelmed and loses its ability to maintain muscular tone. This triggers a further increase in peripheral vascular resistance in the arteries to maintain systolic pressure. Diastolic pressure now rises, narrowing the pulse pressure and weakening the pulse. Sympathetic stimulation causes hormone release, which further increases peripheral vascular resistance, consequently reducing blood flow to more tissues. Decreased circulation results in anaerobic respiration at the cellular level with a subsequent buildup of lactic acid and carbon dioxide, which relax precapillary sphincters. Postcapillary sphincters remain closed, however, forcing fluid into the interstitial spaces by hydrostatic pressure.

Edema further reduces cellular perfusion. Capillary walls and cell membranes break down while red blood cells become sticky and clump together. Rising acidosis causes postcapillary sphincter relaxation with a subsequent release of accumulated toxins into venous circulation, producing profound metabolic acidosis and micro-emboli. Cardiac output, blood pressure, and perfusion drop to zero and the body moves irreversibly toward death.

14. **Describe the transition from compensated to decompensated to irreversible shock.** pp. 75–76

Compensated shock is the first stage of shock where the body is still capable of meeting the critical metabolic needs through a series of progressive compensating actions. With prehospital interventions and rapid transports a patient is most likely to survive. Compensated shock ends with a sudden drop in blood pressure. You may also notice the patient's skin becoming pale, cyanotic, or ashen. Near the end of this stage, the patient may experience air hunger and tachypnea.

Decompensated shock begins when compensatory mechanisms are unable to respond to a continuing blood loss. This will present in the patient's inability to maintain a constant blood pressure, causing a precipitous drop in blood pressure. At this stage the heart begins to fail because of poor perfusion and the increased oxygen demands that are created by tachycardia and increased contractility. The brain also becomes hypoxic, resulting in the patient's responsiveness dropping, and other bodily functions such as respiration diminish, and the body takes on a death-like appearance.

Irreversible shock occurs when the body's cells are so badly injured and die in such quantities that organs can no longer carry out their normal functions. This organ failure ultimately results in organism failure. The transition between decompensated and irreversible shock is a clinical one and is impossible to differentiate by looking for signs or symptoms.

15. **Describe each of the following types of shock:** pp. 76–77

Shock can have many causes and is often classified based on its origin. Regardless of origin, shock will progress through the same three stages in a similar fashion.

Hypovolemic shock is caused by a significant reduction in the cardiovascular volume. Fluid loss may result from numerous causes such as plasma loss from extensive burns; fluid depletion from protracted vomiting, diarrhea, sweating, and urination; "third space" losses when fluid shifts into various body compartments; and severe blood loss.

Cardiogenic shock results from cardiac insufficiency. If the heart is deprived of oxygen or experiences reduced pumping action, cardiac output is profoundly affected. The underlying cause is often coronary artery blockage or myocardial infarct. This problem cannot be compensated for by other body systems and has an 80 percent mortality rate.

Neurogenic shock is a form of shock resulting from spinal or head injury. Nervous system control over vasculature distal to the injury is compromised, causing the vascular container to expand. Additionally, the body's compensatory mechanisms are affected and tachycardia and rising diastolic blood pressure may not occur.

Anaphylactic shock results from a massive histamine release that causes general vasodilation.

Septic shock results from massive infection where toxins interfere with the control of blood vessels.

16. **Demonstrate assessments that can identify patients with hemorrhage and shock.**   pp. 78–79

Altered mental status is often an early sign of shock. Agitation, restlessness, and reduced level of consciousness occur as the brain receives a reduced flow of oxygenated blood. The hypoxia causes the defense mechanisms of agitation and restlessness, followed by a noticeable reduction in the level of consciousness. Tachycardia is a compensatory cardiac action to maintain cardiac output when a reduced preload is present. A weak pulse reflects a narrowing pulse pressure and increasing peripheral vascular resistance to maintain systolic blood pressure. Cool, clammy skin is due to the redirection of blood to more critical organs than the skin. In spine-injured patients, skin below the injury may be warm and dry. Ashen, pale, or mottled skin may present as a result of hypoxia and peripheral vasoconstriction. Dull, lackluster eyes occur secondary to low perfusion and hypoxic states. Rapid, shallow respiration may occur as shock progresses, the respiratory muscles tire in the hypoxic state, and respiratory effort becomes less efficient. Dropping oxygen saturation may also provide evidence to support developing shock. As the peripheral circulation slows, the readings may drop or become erratic. Note a narrowing pulse pressure, as this precedes a drop in systolic pressure. Falling blood pressure heralds the progression from compensated to decompensated shock. As a late sign, it should not be used to determine the presence of shock.

17. **Demonstrate management plans for patients with hemorrhage and shock.**   pp. 84–86

Shock patient management begins with corrective actions taken during the primary assessment. The major goal of care is to maximize tissue oxygenation and carbon dioxide offload. Begin with airway and breathing management. Provide a secure, patent airway and good ventilations either with supplemental high-concentration oxygen (15 L via nonrebreather mask) or positive-pressure ventilations if breathing is inadequate. Maintain a hemoglobin oxygen saturation of at least 96 percent. Consider positive end-expiratory pressure (PEEP) and continuous positive airway pressure (CPAP) if indicated. Provide pleural needle decompression if there is any sign of tension pneumothorax. Also provide rapid control of any significant external hemorrhage. The objective of fluid resuscitation in the field is not the return of normal vital signs but the stabilization of vital signs until the patient reaches the trauma center. Isotonic fluid administration is indicated for any patient with the classic signs and symptoms of shock and controlled hemorrhage. Establish two large-bore IV lines and run normal saline or lactated Ringer's solution wide open until systolic blood pressure returns to 100 mmHg. Use aggressive fluid resuscitation if the blood pressure drops below 50 mmHg. For circumstances in which hemorrhage is not controlled, administer fluid boluses to maintain a blood pressure of 80 mmHg. Remember that for head injury patients even brief periods of hypotension are detrimental to good outcomes.

Overly aggressive fluid resuscitation in uncontrolled internal bleeding may lead to increased hemorrhage and hemodilution, making perfusion and clotting less effective. When hemorrhage is controlled, administer fluid to maintain vital signs with a stable blood pressure just around 100 mmHg. Conserving body temperature is another critical objective. Trauma patients commonly lose heat more rapidly and heat production is low. Hypothermia reduces the effectiveness of clotting mechanisms and can prolong hemorrhage. Cover the patient with a blanket and use room-temperature or warmed IV solutions. Pharmacological interventions are generally limited in shock patients. For hypovolemic, spinal, and obstructive shock, intravenous fluid is sufficient. In cases of cardiogenic or distributive shock, consider dopamine in conjunction with fluids.

Case Study Review

Reread the case study on pages 60 and 61 in Paramedic Care: Trauma; *then, read the following discussion.*

This case study presents an example of aggressive and appropriate care for a patient who, by mechanism of injury alone, is suspected of advancing into shock. It highlights the elements of shock assessment and care.

Arriving on the scene, Dave is presented with a situation that presents with no noticeable hazards and one patient with a mechanism of injury that indicates the potential for serious internal bleeding. The overturned bulldozer trapped the patient's legs and pelvis and may have fractured the pelvis and femurs. These injuries are frequently associated with severe internal blood loss and shock.

Dave suspects that as the vehicle is lifted off Ken, internal bleeding will occur more rapidly. In preparation, he ensures good oxygenation and assesses the visible portion of the patient. He gathers a baseline set of vital signs (all of which indicate that the patient is not yet in decompensated shock), including a pulse oximeter reading. He starts two IV lines using normal saline, both infusing slowly. Dave and his fellow rescuers converse with Ken not only to calm and reassure him, but also to maintain a continuous assessment of Ken's level of consciousness and determine a patient history.

As the bulldozer is removed, Ken is quickly assessed and then moved to the awaiting spine board. The pelvic, femoral, and tibial fractures suggest shock will develop quickly, so Dave applies the pelvic sling to stabilize the pelvis and help control the blood loss. Ken is carefully secured to the long spine board with straps and padding and both IV lines are run wide open to administer a 500-mL bolus of fluid. Ken is then transported rapidly to the ambulance.

The hospital is updated on the patient's condition so it can be ready with O-negative blood. Whole blood or packed red cells are required because the replacement of blood lost through hemorrhage with crystalloid dilutes the number of red blood cells and clotting factors available.

The hospital personnel are ready and waiting for the patient as the ambulance backs into the emergency department bay. The blood is hung and connected, and infusion is begun. The trauma surgeon makes his quick assessment, and the patient is en route to surgery in minutes.

If any one of a number of critical steps in the care of this patient had not been completed, this patient probably would not have survived the trip to the hospital. Dave moved quickly and decisively, performing the skills that stabilized his patient, yet omitting care that would have been provided had the patient not been critical. The paramedic must, through experience, be quickly able to distinguish the patient who needs rapid transport and aggressive care from the patient who will best benefit from meticulous care at the scene and during transport.

Content Self-Evaluation

MULTIPLE CHOICE

_____ 1. Which of the following most specifically slows the heart rate?
A. Autonomic nervous system
B. Sympathetic nervous system
C. Parasympathetic nervous system
D. Somatic nervous system
E. None of the above

_____ 2. Which of the following affects the stroke volume of the heart?
A. Preload
B. Afterload
C. Cardiac contractility
D. Ventricular wall stretching
E. All of the above

_____ 3. The heart maintains an efficient pumping function through a rate range of
A. 40–160 beats per minute
B. 50–180 beats per minute
C. 60–170 beats per minute
D. 60–100 beats per minute
E. 80–150 beats per minute

4. The normal cardiac output is about
   A. 4 liters.
   B. 5 liters. /min
   C. 8 liters.
   D. 10 liters.
   E. 12 liters.

5. The blood vessel layer that determines the artery's maximum diameter is the
   A. tunica intima.
   B. tunica media.
   C. tunica adventitia.
   D. escarpment.
   E. lumen.

6. Approximately what volume of blood is contained within the venous system?
   A. 13 percent
   B. 7 percent
   C. 64 percent
   D. 23 percent
   E. 45 percent

7. Venous constriction is able to return about what volume of blood to the active circulation?
   A. 500 mL
   B. 1,000 mL
   C. 2,000 mL
   D. 2,500 mL
   E. 3,000 mL

8. The percentage of the blood that consists of red blood cells is referred to as
   A. hemoglobin.
   B. viscosity.
   C. the erythrocytic count.
   D. the hematocrit.
   E. plasma.

9. The blood cells responsible for clotting and blood vessel repair are the
   A. erythrocytes.
   B. leukocytes.
   C. platelets.
   D. red blood cells.
   E. hematocrits.

10. Which of the following types of hemorrhage is characterized by bright red blood?
    A. Capillary bleeding
    B. Venous bleeding
    C. Arterial bleeding
    D. Both A and C
    E. Both A and B

11. Which of the following types of hemorrhage is characterized by dark red blood?
    A. Capillary bleeding
    B. Venous bleeding
    C. Arterial bleeding
    D. Both A and C
    E. None of the above

12. Which of the following is NOT a stage in the clotting process?
    A. Intrinsic phase
    B. Vascular phase
    C. Platelet phase
    D. Coagulation phase
    E. All of the above

13. Which of the following represents the phase of clotting where blood cells are trapped in fibrin strands?
    A. Intrinsic phase
    B. Vascular phase
    C. Platelet phase
    D. Coagulation phase
    E. Marrow phase

14. The clotting process normally takes about what length of time?
    A. 1 to 2 minutes
    B. 3 to 4 minutes
    C. 4 to 6 minutes
    D. 7 to 10 minutes
    E. 10 to 12 minutes

15. Cleanly and transversely cut blood vessels tend to bleed very heavily.
    A. True
    B. False   Easier to slow flow

_____ 16. Which of the following is likely to adversely affect the clotting process?
   A. Aggressive fluid resuscitation
   B. Hypothermia
   C. Movement at the site of injury
   D. Drugs such as aspirin
   E. All of the above

_____ 17. Bleeding from capillary or venous wounds is easy to halt because the pressure driving the hemorrhage is limited.
   A. True
   B. False

_____ 18. Fractures of the femur can account for a blood loss
   A. from 500 to 750 mL.
   B. up to 1,500 mL.
   C. in excess of 2,000 mL.
   D. less than 500 mL.
   E. in excess of 2,500 mL.

_____ 19. Intravascular fluid accounts for what percentage of the total body water?
   A. 7 percent
   B. 15 percent
   C. 35 percent
   D. 45 percent
   E. 75 percent

_____ 20. In which class of hemorrhage does the patient first display thirst?
   A. Class I
   B. Class II
   C. Class III
   D. Class IV
   E. Class V

_____ 21. In which class of hemorrhage does the patient first display air hunger?
   A. Class I
   B. Class II
   C. Class III
   D. Class IV
   E. Class V

_____ 22. Which of the following react differently to blood loss than the normal, healthy adult?
   A. Pregnant women
   B. Athletes
   C. The elderly
   D. Children
   E. All of the above

_____ 23. The late-pregnancy female is likely to have a blood volume
   A. much less than normal.
   B. slightly less than normal.
   C. slightly greater than normal.
   D. much greater than normal.
   E. that is normal and does not change with pregnancy.

_____ 24. Obese patients are likely to have a blood volume
   A. much less than normal.
   B. slightly less than normal.
   C. slightly greater than normal.
   D. much greater than normal.
   E. none of the above.

_____ 25. Elderly patients are more adversely affected by blood loss due to
   A. reduced pain perception.
   B. chronic cardiovascular inefficiency.
   C. lower fluid reserves.
   D. medications.
   E. all of the above.

_____ 26. The aerobic component of the cell's utilization of glucose to obtain energy is called
   A. the Kreb's cycle.
   B. glycolysis.
   C. glycogenolysis.
   D. the pyruvic acid cycle.
   E. the glyco cycle.

27. Which of the following is not a characteristic of interstitial fluid?
   A. It is rich in carbon dioxide.
   B. It has a lowered pH.
   C. It is separated from the blood by capillary walls.
   D. It contains hemoglobin.
   E. It has the lowest oxygen concentration in the body.

28. Blood fills the vascular space EXCEPT in shock states.
   A. True
   B. False

29. Which of the following is a result of parasympathetic nervous system stimulation?
   A. Decreased heart rate
   B. Decreased peripheral vascular resistance
   C. Decreased blood pressure
   D. Decreased respiratory rate
   E. All of the above

30. Which of the following is a catecholamine?
   A. Antidiuretic hormone
   B. Angiotensin II
   C. Aldosterone
   D. Epinephrine
   E. Erythropoietin

31. Which of the following is a hormone that induces an increase in peripheral vascular resistance and causes the kidneys to retain water?
   A. Angiotensin
   B. Aldosterone
   C. Norepinephrine
   D. Antidiuretic hormone
   E. Adrenocorticotropic hormone

32. Erythropoietin accelerates the production of
   A. platelets.
   B. leukocytes.
   C. red blood cells.
   D. hemoglobin.
   E. plasma.

33. The column of coagulated erythrocytes caused by capillary stagnation is called
   A. ischemia.
   B. rouleaux.
   C. capillary washout.
   D. hydrostatic reflux.
   E. compensated reflux.

34. Which list places the stages of shock in the correct order of their occurrence?
   A. Irreversible, decompensated, compensated
   B. Compensated, decompensated, irreversible
   C. Compensated, irreversible, decompensated
   D. Decompensated, irreversible, compensated
   E. Decompensated, compensated, irreversible

35. Which stage of shock ends with a precipitous drop in blood pressure?
   A. Compensated
   B. Decompensated
   C. Irreversible
   D. Hypovolemic
   E. None of the above

36. Which of the following does NOT occur during the compensated stage of shock?
   A. Increasing pulse rate
   B. Decreasing pulse strength
   C. Decreasing systolic blood pressure
   D. Skin becomes cool and clammy
   E. The patient experiences thirst and weakness

37. Once the patient becomes profoundly unconscious and loses his vital signs, he moves into irreversible shock.
   A. True
   B. False

38. All of the following can cause hypovolemic shock, EXCEPT
   A. burns.
   B. pancreatitis.
   C. cardiac dysrhythmias. *cardiogenic shock*
   D. ascites.
   E. gastritis.

39. Under which of the following shock types would anaphylactic shock fall?
   A. Hypovolemic
   B. Distributive
   C. Obstructive –
   D. Cardiogenic
   E. Respiratory

40. Under which of the following shock types would spinal injury fall?
   A. Hypovolemic
   B. Distributive
   C. Neurogenic
   D. Cardiogenic
   E. Respiratory

41. The sooner the signs and symptoms of shock appear in your patient, the greater the hemorrhage rate and the likelihood that the patient will move into the later stages of shock.
   A. True
   B. False

42. Which of the following suggests shock?
   A. A pulse rate above 100 in the adult
   B. A pulse rate above 140 in the school-age child
   C. A pulse rate above 160 in the preschooler
   D. A pulse rate above 180 in the infant
   E. All of the above

43. When using a pulse oximeter, you should use oxygen and ventilation to keep the reading above which oxygen saturation value?
   A. 45 percent
   B. 80 percent
   C. 85 percent
   D. 95 percent
   E. 99 percent

44. In the normotensive patient, the jugular veins should be full when the patient is in the supine position.
   A. True
   B. False

45. During assessment you note that the patient's lower extremities and lower abdomen are warm and pink while the upper extremities, thorax, and upper abdomen are cool and clammy. This presentation is consistent with which type of shock?
   A. Hypovolemic
   B. Neurogenic
   C. Obstructive
   D. Cardiogenic
   E. Respiratory

46. Fractures of the pelvis can account for a blood loss
   A. from 500 to 750 mL.
   B. up to 1,500 mL.
   C. in excess of 2,000 mL.
   D. up to 500 mL.
   E. of none, because the pelvis does not bleed.

47. A black, tarry stool is called
   A. hemoptysis.
   B. melena.
   C. hematuria.
   D. hematochezia.
   E. ebony stool.

48. A positive tilt test demonstrating orthostatic hypotension is positive when
    A. the blood pressure rises by at least 20 mmHg.
    B. the blood pressure falls by at least 20 mmHg.
    C. the pulse rate rises by at least 20 beats per minute.
    D. the pulse rate falls by at least 20 beats per minute.
    E. both B and C.

49. For the patient in compensated shock, you should perform a reassessment
    A. every 5 minutes.
    B. every 15 minutes.
    C. after every major intervention.
    D. after noting any change in signs or symptoms.
    E. all except B.

50. Which of the following is a technique used to help control hemorrhage?
    A. Direct pressure
    B. Elevation
    C. Pressure points
    D. Limb splinting
    E. All of the above

51. When applying a tourniquet, you should inflate the blood pressure cuff
    A. until the bleeding slows.
    B. to the diastolic blood pressure.
    C. to the systolic blood pressure.
    D. 20 to 30 mmHg above the systolic blood pressure.
    E. none of the above.

52. Which of the following may be an indication to employ overdrive respiration?
    A. Severe rib fractures
    B. Flail chest
    C. Diaphragmatic respirations
    D. Head injury
    E. All of the above

53. Which of these fluid replacement choices would be most desirable for the patient who is losing blood through internal bleeding?
    A. Packed red blood cells
    B. Fresh frozen plasma
    C. Whole blood
    D. Colloids
    E. Crystalloids

54. Most of the solutions used in prehospital care for infusion are
    A. hypotonic colloids.
    B. isotonic colloids.
    C. hypertonic colloids.
    D. hypotonic crystalloids.
    E. isotonic crystalloids.

55. Which of the following characteristics of a catheter will ensure that fluids run rapidly through it?
    A. Short length, small lumen
    B. Short length, large lumen
    C. Long length, small lumen
    D. Long length, large lumen
    E. Large lumen and either long or short length

56. In the patient who has internal bleeding and hypovolemia, the objective of fluid resuscitation is to maintain a systolic blood pressure
    A. of 120 mmHg.
    B. of 100 mmHg.
    C. of 80 mmHg.
    D. of below 50 mmHg.
    E. at a steady level.

©2013 Pearson Education, Inc.
Paramedic Care: Principles & Practice, Vol. 5, 4th Ed.

Special Projects

Scenario-Based Problem Solving

You are caring for a victim of a single stab wound to the left upper quadrant. He is a 36-year-old male who is conscious, alert, and oriented, though somewhat agitated. His initial vitals are blood pressure: 120/90, pulse: 110 and weak, respirations 20 with clear breath sounds, and his skin is somewhat cool and moist.

1. What organs might be injured by this mechanism?

   bowel diaphragm, spleen,

   _____

2. Why is the patient somewhat agitated?

   _____

   _____

   _____

3. If this patient's normal blood pressure is 120/80, what would explain the increased diastolic blood pressure?

   _____

   _____

4. What is the relationship between the increased diastolic blood pressure and the weak pulse?

   _____

   _____

   _____

5. Why is the skin somewhat cool and clammy?

   _____

   _____

   _____

5

Soft-Tissue Trauma

Review of Chapter Objectives

After reading this chapter, you should be able to:

1. **Define key terms introduced in this chapter.**

   Knowing and being able to apply the key terms in each chapter is critical to understanding chapter concepts. Write the list of key terms. Then write the definition of each one in your own words. Check your understanding by confirming the definitions in the text glossary. Correct any misunderstandings. Create a study aid by writing each key term on the front of an index card and the definition on the back. Use the cards to quiz yourself, or to have someone quiz you.

2. **Describe the epidemiology of soft tissue injuries.**   pp. 92–93

   Soft tissue injuries are by far the most prevalent type of traumatic injury, accounting for over 10 million visits to the emergency department annually. Most injuries require simple care; however, artery, nerve, or tendon damage can cause permanent disability. Open injuries to the skin may permit pathogens to enter resulting in infection. Significant wounds may cause cosmetic and, to some degree, functional disruption of the skin. School-age children and the elderly are most prone to soft tissue injury. Other risk factors include alcohol, drug abuse, and some occupations.

3. **Describe the anatomy and physiology of the skin and associated soft tissues.**   pp. 93–95

   The integumentary system, or skin, is the largest body organ, accounting for about 16 percent of weight. It provides the outer barrier for the body and protects it against environmental extremes, fluid loss, and pathogen invasion. The three-layer structure consists of:

   a. **Epidermis**
   The epidermis is the outermost superficial layer of the skin and consists of numerous layers of dead or dying cells. The epidermis contains sebum, a waxy substance, which keeps the outer layer flexible, strong, and resistant to penetration by water.
   b. **Dermis**
   The dermis holds the skin firmly around the body and permits articulation. Comprised of connective tissue, it contains blood vessels, sensory nerve endings, hair follicles, and glands, which are specialized skin cells that produce sweat and oil. Other cells attack invading organisms and foreign materials. The upper-level capillary beds allow for conduction of heat to the body's surface.

c. **Subcutaneous tissue**

The subcutaneous layer, although not a true part of the skin, works in concert with the skin to insulate the body from heat loss and the effects of trauma. It consists of connective and adipose (fatty) tissues.

d. **Blood vessels**

Blood vessels include arteries, arterioles, capillaries, venules, and veins. The larger vessels are comprised of three layers. The tunica intima is the smooth inner lining. The tunica media is the muscular component. The tunica adventitia is the tougher outer layer. Capillaries are one cell thick and provide oxygen to all cells of the body.

e. **Muscles**

Muscles lie below the skin surface and form points of attachment to bone via tendons. Comprised of strong contractile tissue, muscles allow for movement and protect vital organs and nerves.

f. **Fasciae**

Fasciae are strong, fibrous sheets of collagen that form compartments of muscle mass. These compartments have limited room for expansion.

4. **Describe the pathophysiology of open and closed soft tissue injuries.**   pp. 96–99

Soft tissue injuries either damage blood vessels and the structure of the soft tissue or open the envelope of the skin and may permit pathogens to enter and blood to escape. Blood loss may be external or internal and range in severity from minor to life threatening. Closed wounds include contusions, hematomas, and crush injuries. Open wounds include abrasions, lacerations, incisions, punctures, impaled objects, avulsions, and amputations.

Contusions are caused by blunt injury that crushes and damages small blood vessels. Leaking blood vessels cause the characteristic black-and-blue discoloration of bruising, called ecchymosis.

Hematomas are blunt soft tissue injuries in which blood vessels (larger than capillaries) are damaged and leak into the fascia, causing a pocket of blood. Large hematomas may accumulate up to 500 mL of blood, contributing significantly to hypovolemia.

Crush injuries involve compression to a body part that damages muscles, blood vessels, bones, and other internal structures. Damage can be massive and life threatening as the soft tissues are trapped between a compressing force and an unyielding object. Open crush injuries are frequently associated with severe infection.

Abrasions result from removal of the layers of the epidermis and upper dermis. Only superficial blood vessels are damaged, so bleeding is limited.

Lacerations involve penetration into the dermal layer. Underlying vessels, nerves, muscles, tendons, ligaments, and organs can sustain significant damage. Because it is an open wound, it carries with it the danger of infection and external hemorrhage.

Incisions are surgically smooth lacerations that may bleed freely.

Punctures are penetrating lacerations that may be deceiving because the wound generally seals itself, masking the underlying damage. Punctures carry an increased risk of infection because the penetrating object introduces bacteria deep into the body tissue.

Impaled objects enter and become lodged within the soft or other tissue. Removing the object may produce further damage to underlying structures or cause uncontrollable hemorrhage if the object is tamponading a large vessel.

Avulsions involve a partial tearing away of the skin and soft tissues. They are commonly associated with blunt skull trauma, animal bites, or machinery accidents. Degloving injuries expose underlying muscle, connective tissue, blood vessels, and bone. Contamination with subsequent infection may be serious.

Amputations involve partial or complete severance of a body part. The injury usually results in the complete loss of the limb distal to the site of severance; however, the severed limb can sometimes be successfully reattached or its tissue may be used for grafting to extend the length and usefulness of the remaining limb. Degree of hemorrhage depends on the contour of the wound.

5. **Describe the process of wound healing.**   pp. 100–101

Wound healing is an essential component of homeostasis. Wound healing can be divided into stages, as discussed later, but it is important to remember that these stages overlap considerably and are intertwined.

a. Hemostasis

Hemostasis is the process by which the body tries to restrict or halt blood loss. It begins with the constriction of the injured blood vessel wall to reduce the rate of hemorrhage. The injured tissue of the vessel wall and the platelets become sticky. The platelets then aggregate to further occlude the lumen. Finally, the clotting cascade produces fibrin strands that trap erythrocytes and form a more durable clot to halt all but the most severe hemorrhage.

b. Inflammation

Cells damaged by trauma or invading pathogens signal the body to recruit white blood cells (phagocytes) to the injury site. These cells engulf or attack the membranes of the foreign agents. The by-products of this action cause the mast cells to release histamine, which dilates precapillary vessels and increases capillary permeability. Fluid and oxygen flows into the region, resulting in an increase in temperature and edema.

c. Epithelialization

The stratum germinativum cells of the epidermis create an expanding layer of cells over the wound edges. This layer eventually joins almost unnoticeably, or, if the wound is too large, a region of collagen may show through (scar tissue).

d. Neovascularization

Neovascularization occurs as the capillaries surrounding the wound extend into the new tissue and begin to provide the new tissue with circulation. These new vessels are very delicate and prone to injury and tend to bleed easily.

e. Collagen synthesis

Collagen synthesis is the building of new connective tissue (collagen) in the wound through the actions of the fibroblasts. Collagen binds the wound margins together and strengthens the healing wound. The early repair is not as good as new, but by the fourth month the wound tissue is about 60 percent of the original tissue's strength.

6. **Describe the pathophysiology and risk factors for soft tissue injury complications, including:**

a. Infection   pp. 101–102

Infection is the most common, potentially serious complication of open wounds. They delay healing and may cause systemic infection, called sepsis. A variety of bacteria cause infection, with the most common being *Staphylococcus* and *Streptococcus*. Infection generally appears two to three days after the initial wound. Risk factors include the health and age of the host, the wound type and location, associated contamination, and treatment. Individuals with preexisting medical conditions or taking certain medications are at increased risk. Gangrene and tetanus pose serious complications from infection and may result in loss of limb, sepsis, and death.

b. Hemorrhage, impaired hemostasis, and rebleeding   p. 103

Certain diseases and several medications can interfere with clotting. Anticoagulants, aspirin, and clopidogrel all cause prolonged clotting time by various mechanisms. Hemophiliacs have protein abnormalities that interfere with hemostasis. All wounds are at risk for rebleeding and movement of the injured area, and dressings may dislodge clots. Partially healed wounds may reopen, and postoperative wounds may cause life-threatening hemorrhage.

c. Delayed healing   p. 103

Diabetics, the elderly, the chronically ill, and the malnourished are at greatest risk for prolonged healing. Wounds that become chronically infected or wounds in locations with limited blood flow take longer to heal and are easily reinjured.

d. **Compartment syndrome** p. 103

Compartment syndrome is a complication of fractures or crush injuries. Swelling increases the pressure within a fascial compartment of the body, restricting venous flow from the extremity, capillary flow through the affected portion of the limb, and arterial return to the central circulation. Untreated compartment syndrome may result in loss or shortening of the muscle mass and compromise limb function.

e. **Abnormal scarring** pp. 103–104

Abnormal scar tissue may develop during the healing process. Keloids are excessive scar tissue extending beyond the wound boundaries. Hypertrophic scar formation is an excessive accumulation of scar tissue within the injury border.

f. **Complications associated with pressure injuries** p. 104

Prolonged compression of the skin and underlying tissue can cause injury to the soft tissues. Patients who are bedridden for prolonged periods, unconscious for hours, or entrapped are at risk. Pressure injuries may also occur when spine boards, splints, or PASGs remain on a patient for an extended period of time.

g. **Associated injuries** p. 105

Patients with crush injuries often have associated trauma due to the mechanism of injury. Fractures or other open or closed wounds may result. Penetrating or blunt objects may cause direct injury. Dust and smoke can cause respiratory and eye problems. Hypothermia or dehydration may result from prolonged entrapment.

h. **Crush syndrome** p. 105

Crush syndrome occurs when body parts are entrapped for 4 hours or longer. Crushed skeletal muscle tissue degenerates (rhabdomyolysis) and releases metabolic toxins into the crushed body part. Upon release of the injured body part, these by-products flood the central circulation. This can lead to renal failure, hypovolemia and shock, cardiac dysrhythmias, and metabolic acidosis.

i. **Injection injuries** pp. 105–106

High-pressure devices may inject fluid through the skin into the subcutaneous tissue, sometimes traveling along the limb. The injected fluid may cause direct damage or chemical damage with subsequent infection. Limb loss or reduced limb function may result.

7. **Given a variety of scenarios, select appropriate dressing and bandaging materials and techniques.** pp. 106–108

a. **Sterile/nonsterile dressing**

Sterile dressings are used for wound care because it is important to reduce the amount of contamination at a wound site to reduce the risk of infection.

b. **Occlusive/nonocclusive dressing**

Most dressings are nonocclusive, which means they permit both blood and air to travel through them in at least a limited way. Occlusive dressings do not permit the flow of either fluid or air and are useful in sealing a chest or neck wound to prevent the aspiration of air or in covering a moist dressing on an abdominal evisceration to prevent its drying.

c. **Adherent/nonadherent dressing**

Adherent dressings support the clotting mechanisms; however, as they are removed they will dislodge the forming clots. Most dressings are specially treated to be nonadherent to reduce reinjury when they are removed from a wound.

d. **Absorbent/nonabsorbent dressing**

Most dressings used to treat wounds are absorbent, and they will soak up blood and other fluids. Nonabsorbent dressings absorb little or no fluid and are used to seal wound sites when a barrier to leaking is desired, for example, the clear membranes that are used to cover venipuncture sites.

e. **Wet/dry dressing**

Wet dressings may provide a medium for the movement of infectious agents into the wound and are not frequently used in prehospital care. They may be used for abdominal eviscerations and burns. Dry dressings are the type most often used in prehospital care for wounds.

©2013 Pearson Education, Inc.
Paramedic Care: Principles & Practice, Vol. 5, 4th Ed.

f. **Hemostatic dressings**

Hemostatic agents are applied directly to a bleeding wound to slow or stop bleeding. Several products are available that work through various mechanisms, but in general, they absorb water, concentrate blood, and promote clot formation.

g. **Self-adherent roller bandage**

The self-adherent roller bandage is soft, gauzelike material that molds to the contours of the body and is effective in holding dressings in place. As its stretch is limited, it does not pose the danger of increasing the bandaging pressure with each wrap, as do some other bandaging materials.

h. **Gauze bandage**

Gauze bandaging is a self-adherent material that does not stretch and may increase the pressure beneath the bandage with consecutive wraps or with edema and swelling from the wound.

i. **Adhesive bandage**

An adhesive bandage is a strong gauze, paper, or plastic material backed with an adhesive. It can effectively secure small dressings to the skin where circumferential wrapping is impractical. It is inelastic and will not accommodate edema or swelling.

j. **Elastic bandage**

An elastic bandage is made of fabric that stretches easily. It conforms well to body contours but will increase the pressure applied with each wrap of the bandage. These bandages are often used to help strengthen a joint or apply pressure to reduce edema but should be used with great care, if at all, in the prehospital setting.

k. **Triangular bandage**

Triangular bandages are strong, inelastic triangles of cotton or linen fabric. They are commonly used for making slings and swathes or to hold splints together. They may also be employed to hold dressings in place although they are not ideal for this purpose, as they do not maintain pressure or immobilize wound dressings well.

8. **Demonstrate the assessment of a variety of soft tissue injuries.**   pp. 108–111

Assessment of patients with soft tissue injuries follows the same assessment process as with other trauma patients. During the scene size-up, look for the mechanism of injury to help determine the nature and extent of each injury. Always manage airway and breathing first, with particular attention in the presence of head or facial wounds. During the rapid trauma assessment, investigate any discolorations, deformities, temperature variations, abnormal muscle tone, or open wounds. Sweep the body with gloved hands to rule out unseen blood loss from hidden injuries. Control moderate to severe hemorrhage immediately. Approximate the amount and relative rate of blood loss. Inspect each body part to determine if discoloration is local, distal, or systemic, and check for circulation compromise, or systemic complications such as shock. Study wounds to determine the depth and evaluate for damage to underlying muscles, nerves, blood vessels, organs, or bones. Ascertain if there are any impaled objects or gross contamination. If extremity wounds are present, check distal pulses, capillary refill, color, and temperature. Palpate the entire body surface for deformity, asymmetry, unexpected masses, or localized loss of skin or muscle tone. Check for evidence of tenderness, swelling, crepitus, and subcutaneous emphysema. If a body part has been amputated, have other responders conduct a brief search for the part. Observe each wound carefully before dressing and bandaging. Be able to describe it (as it will be covered by a dressing and bandaging) to the attending physician upon your arrival at the emergency department.

9. **Given a variety of scenarios, develop management plans for patients with open and closed soft tissue injuries.**   pp. 111–114

Management of soft tissue injuries is a late priority in the care of trauma patients. After stabilizing higher priorities, soft tissue management is directed at controlling hemorrhage, keeping the wound clean (as sterile as possible), and immobilizing the wound site. In most cases, direct pressure is usually effective in controlling hemorrhage. Ensure that bandages and dressings focus pressure directly on the bleeding source. If you cannot control bleeding with direct pressure, immediately apply a tourniquet. Instances in which a tourniquet may be immediately required include severe crush injuries, amputations, and penetrating trauma. Leave tourniquets in place until arrival at the emergency department. After controlling bleeding, keep the wound as clean as possible to reduce the bacterial load and reduce the risk and severity of infection. Generally wounds are not cleansed in the field but in situations of long transport times or gross contamination the wound may be irrigated with normal saline. Immobilization will assist the clotting process and reduce pain and swelling. Immobilize limbs with nonelastic bandaging material to the patient's body or to a rigid padded board or ladder splint. Apply cold packs indirectly to painful injuries or those likely to develop significant edema. Consider use of morphine sulfate, fentanyl, or other analgesics if the patient reports severe pain. Avoid NSAIDs and aspirin, as they interfere with clotting.

Each area of the body requires special considerations for bandaging. Scalp injuries can bleed profusely. To control bleeding apply direct pressure against the skull with a dressing and wrap a bandage around the head. Direct pressure is also effective for bleeding from face wounds. Wrap bandages around the head but do not compromise the airway. Be ready to suction if oral or nasal hemorrhage is present. Wrapping the head circumferentially can be effective treatment for ear injury. In case of fluid leakage from the ear canal, do not attempt to stop the flow. Occlusive dressings may be required for large wounds or severe hemorrhage of the neck. Employ self-adherent roller bandages for shoulder wounds using the axilla, arm, and neck as fixation points. Adhesive tape may be sufficient to hold dressing in place for minor trunk wounds. Larger wounds may require circumferential dressings or the use of ladder splints to secure the bandage. Affix dressings to the groin and hip after positioning the patient for transport so that patient movement does not increase the tightness or pressure of the dressing. Joints should be bandaged with circumferential wraps and splinted. Place the joint in a position of comfort, midway between flexion and extension. Hands and fingers should also be placed in a position of comfort by placing a bulky dressing or roll of gauze in the palm and wrapping around it. Ankle and foot wounds are easily bandaged circumferentially. If strong direct pressure is needed, start wrapping at the toes and move proximally.

10. **Reassess patients with soft tissue injuries for complications of bandaging.**   **pp. 114, 117–118**

Improper application of a dressing may include use of the wrong dressing for the injury or the application of the right dressing in an incorrect manner. Occlusive dressings used for open chest wounds may seal with blood against the chest wall and convert a simple pneumothorax into a tension pneumothorax. Use of a nonocclusive dressing with an open chest wound may permit air to enter the thorax, increasing the severity of a pneumothorax, or use of such a dressing for a neck wound may permit air to enter the jugular vein, creating pulmonary emboli. Use of dry dressings with an abdominal evisceration may permit tissues to dry, adding additional injury, while use of wet dressings in other circumstances provides a route for infection of wounds. Adherent dressings may facilitate natural clotting but may dislodge clots and reinstitute hemorrhage as they are removed. Dressing that are too large may prevent proper inspection of the wound and hide contamination and continued bleeding. They may also not permit application of adequate direct pressure to arrest hemorrhage. If a dressing is too small, it may become lost in the wound and again not provide a focused direct pressure to stop hemorrhage. Bandages and dressings left on too long can become soaked with blood and fluid, serving as incubators for infection.

Improperly applied extremity bandaging may either be insufficient to immobilize the dressing or it may be too tight, restricting swelling and compressing the soft tissues beneath, which can cause reduced or absent blood flow to the distal extremity. On the other hand, a bandage that is too loose may not maintain adequate direct pressure to stop bleeding or may not hold the dressing securely to the injury site. Monitor any limbs bandaged circumferentially to ensure adequate distal pulse, good color, and capillary refill. Circumferential bandages applied to the thorax or abdomen may compromise breathing by directly impeding chest wall excursion or by minimizing movement of abdominal contents during excursion of the diaphragm.

11. **Describe special considerations in the management of the following injuries:**

a. **Amputations**   **p. 114**

Control hemorrhage with direct pressure and tourniquets if necessary. Apply the tourniquet to the area just above the point of severance. Wrap the amputated part in gauze moistened with saline, place in a plastic bag, and immerse the bag in cold water.

©2013 Pearson Education, Inc.
Paramedic Care: Principles & Practice, Vol. 5, 4th Ed.

b. Impaled objects
pp. 114–115

Impaled objects should be immobilized in place by positioning bulky dressings around the object to stabilize it and then securing the dressings in place. Removal of an object in the cheek may be necessary to secure the airway. Objects in the chest of a patient in cardiac arrest need to be removed for cardiopulmonary resuscitation (CPR). If an object is too large to transport or is fixed in place, the object should be cut while minimizing patient movement. Contact medical direction if the patient is impaled on an object that cannot be cut or moved.

c. Crush syndrome
pp. 115–116

Crush syndrome develops as a result of prolonged entrapment. Scene safety and managing immediate life threats take priority. Control any reachable, obvious bleeding. Once extricated, the release of toxic metabolites into the central circulation may cause rapidly progressing shock or death. Fluid resuscitation and administration of alkalizing agents may help correct acidosis, prevent renal failure, and correct hyperkalemia. Consider applying a tourniquet to the injured body part before the entrapping pressure is released if IV access and medications will be delayed. Cardiac monitoring is essential. Sudden cardiac arrest should be treated with defibrillation and appropriate cardiac drugs. Calcium chloride and sodium bicarbonate should be administered in the event of hyperkalemia-induced dysrhythmias.

d. Compartment syndrome
p. 116

The hallmark sign of compartment syndrome is pain out of proportion to the physical findings. Compartment syndrome is most likely to appear 6 to 8 hours after the initial injury. The five P's—pain, paresthesia, paresis, passive stretching pain, and pulselessness—may assist in identifying compartment syndrome. The most effective treatment is elevation of the affected extremity after immobilizing, splinting, and applying cold packs to severe contusions.

e. Injuries to the face and neck
p. 117

Soft tissue injury to the face and neck may present significant challenges because of the potential danger to the airway. Blood and secretions may obstruct the airway, while swelling or traumatic injury may distort anatomical structures. Endotracheal intubation may be difficult due to inadequate visualization of the vocal cords, even with aggressive suctioning. Consider King Airways or LMAs as appropriate alternatives. In the most severe cases, cricothyrotomy (needle or surgical) may be necessary. Use direct pressure to control hemorrhage of facial or neck wounds. Cover open neck wounds with occlusive dressings and bandage firmly in place to prevent the passage of air into the jugular veins. If the wound is to the side of the neck, consider wrapping bandage around the side of the neck through the opposite axilla to hold the dressing in place.

f. Injuries to the thorax
pp. 117–118

Consider all thoracic wounds to be potentially life threatening. Always anticipate internal chest injury associated with superficial soft tissue injuries to the thorax. Never explore a thoracic wound beyond the skin edges, as this may worsen bleeding or convert a minor wound to a pneumothorax. Dress open wounds with occlusive dressings sealed on three sides to prevent converting a simple pneumothorax into a tension pneumothorax. Auscultate the chest frequently to assess respiratory exchange and monitor vitals closely. If a tension pneumothorax develops, unseal the occlusive dressing to allow air to escape.

g. Injuries to the abdomen
p. 118

Consider any soft tissue wound in the abdominal region as potentially damaging to underlying organs. Blunt or penetrating trauma can cause serious internal bleeding or rupture hollow organs, releasing inflammatory contents into the peritoneum. Hemorrhage into the retroperitoneal space may be significant and masked because of reduced pain sensitivity in this region. Cover and dress all open wounds. Cover any abdominal eviscerations with moistened sterile dressings, and then cover with occlusive dressings. Prehospital care is mostly supportive and includes adequate oxygenation, preventing shock, dressing wounds, and rapid transport.

12. Describe considerations in decisions to transport or treat and release patients with soft tissue injuries.
p. 118

Any patient with a wound possibly involving nerves, blood vessels, ligaments, tendons, or muscles needs to be transported. Patients with grossly contaminated wounds, wounds that may result in disfigurement, or wounds involving impaled objects also need to be evaluated in the emergency department.

For patients with minor and superficial injuries treated on scene and not transported, it is critical to instruct the patient in proper wound care, monitoring, protection, dressing change, cleansing, and signs of problems such as infection or hemorrhage. Advise the patient to contact his physician if certain signs and symptoms occur. Patients who have not had a tetanus immunization within 5 years or who do not know their immunization history should be instructed to obtain a tetanus booster with 72 hours.

Case Study Review

Reread the case study on pages 91 and 92 in Paramedic Care: Trauma; *then, read the following discussion.*

This case study depicts a serious injury to the soft tissues and the most common causes for concern with those injuries: serious hemorrhage and underlying structure injury. It gives us the opportunity to examine the assessment and care for this common injury.

Maria and Jon respond to a patient with deep soft tissue injury involving the upper left arm. They wear gloves as part of Standard Precautions but also employ goggles because the wound is bleeding heavily and may involve arterial hemorrhage and the possible danger of splashing blood. Their size-up of the scene reveals no indication of violence or other hazards to themselves or their patient. They recognize no other patients and see no need for additional resources.

During their primary assessment, Maria and Jon form an initial impression of Walter and determine that he is alert, oriented, and otherwise appears healthy. Because he is easily able to articulate in full sentences, they presume his airway is clear and his breathing is adequate. They note that his skin is slightly pale and his pulse is somewhat rapid, due either to excitement and the release of adrenaline or to the early signs of hypovolemia compensation and shock. At the end of the primary assessment, the paramedic team does not consider Walter a candidate for rapid transport. However, they will watch for the early or progressing signs of shock and modify that decision at any time during the remaining assessment and care. They will be especially watchful for an increasing heart rate, a weakening pulse (dropping pulse pressure), or any signs of agitation, nervousness, or combativeness from Walter.

Maria and Jon then perform a focused assessment, looking specifically at the wound to assess its nature, to determine what hemorrhage control techniques are best, and to be able to describe the wound accurately to the attending physician when they arrive at the emergency department. They also examine the distal extremity for loss of nervous control or circulation. They note some patient complaint of tingling and Walter's inability to flex his elbow. They also check both capillary refill time and neurologic function of the injured extremity and compare them against those of the opposite extremity.

As a final assessment step, the paramedics remove the rag applied by Walter, examine the wound carefully, and then cover it with sterile dressings held firmly in place with soft roller bandaging, wrapped tightly to apply direct pressure. They suspect only venous hemorrhage from their examination of the wound and may elevate the extremity once Walter is loaded on the stretcher. This enhances venous return through the injured extremity and will help reduce any continuing blood loss.

Maria and Jon use the AMPLE mnemonic to investigate Walter's medical history and discover that he has not had a recent tetanus booster. This is an important finding, because he will need to receive a booster once at the emergency department. It is also important that they investigate any allergy to the "caine" family of drugs because Walter will likely receive some form of local anesthetic during care. It is also important to investigate any antibiotic and analgesic use.

Finally, the paramedics of Medic 151 provide serial reassessments of Walter and his wound. They reassess the vital signs, Walter's level of consciousness, and the dressing and bandage to ensure that there are no signs of progressing shock or continuing hemorrhage.

©2013 Pearson Education, Inc.
Paramedic Care: Principles & Practice, Vol. 5, 4th Ed.

Content Self-Evaluation

MULTIPLE CHOICE

_____ 1. About what percentage of soft tissue wounds become infected, with a significant resultant morbidity?
- **A.** 2 percent
- **B.** 7 percent
- **C.** 15 percent
- **D.** 50 percent
- **E.** 75 percent

_____ 2. Which of the following glands secrete sweat?
- **A.** Sudoriferous glands
- **B.** Sebaceous glands
- **C.** Subcutaneous glands
- **D.** Adrenal glands
- **E.** None of the above

_____ 3. Which of the following types of cells are found in the dermis?
- **A.** Lymphocytes
- **B.** Macrophages
- **C.** Mast cells
- **D.** Fibroblasts
- **E.** All of the above

_____ 4. The layers of the arteries and veins proceeding in order from exterior to interior are the
- **A.** intima, media, adventitia.
- **B.** media, intima, adventitia.
- **C.** adventitia, intima, media.
- **D.** adventitia, media, intima.
- **E.** intima, adventitia, media.

_____ 5. The blood vessels responsible for distributing blood to the major regions and organs of the body are the
- **A.** arteries.
- **B.** arterioles.
- **C.** capillaries.
- **D.** venules.
- **E.** veins.

_____ 6. The blood vessels able to change their lumen size by a factor of five are the
- **A.** arteries.
- **B.** arterioles.
- **C.** capillaries.
- **D.** venules.
- **E.** veins.

_____ 7. The sheet of thick, fibrous material surrounding muscles is the
- **A.** sebum.
- **B.** fascia.
- **C.** tendon.
- **D.** tension line.
- **E.** tunica.

_____ 8. Lacerations that run parallel to skin tension lines will cause the wound to gape.
- **A.** True
- **B.** False

_____ 9. Which of the following types of wounds are unlikely to heal well?
- **A.** Wounds that gape
- **B.** Wound associated with static tension lines
- **C.** Wounds associated with dynamic tension lines
- **D.** Wounds perpendicular to tension lines
- **E.** All except B

_____ 10. The type of wound characterized by erythema usually seen during the prehospital setting is the
- **A.** abrasion.
- **B.** contusion.
- **C.** laceration.
- **D.** incision.
- **E.** avulsion.

11. Which of the following wounds is not considered open?
   A. Laceration
   B. Abrasion
   C. Contusion
   D. Puncture
   E. Avulsion

12. Which of the following wound types is characterized as a surgically smooth, open wound?
   A. Abrasion
   B. Contusion
   C. Laceration
   D. Incision
   E. Avulsion

13. Crush injuries usually involve injury to
   A. blood vessels.
   B. muscles.
   C. bones.
   D. internal structures.
   E. all of the above.

14. Which of the following is NOT usually considered an open wound?
   A. Abrasion
   B. Crush injury
   C. Incision
   D. Degloving injury
   E. Avulsion

15. The wound that poses the greatest risk for serious infection is the
   A. puncture.
   B. laceration.
   C. contusion.
   D. incision.
   E. hematoma.

16. The injury in which the skin is pulled off a finger, hand, or extremity by farm or industrial machinery is called a(n)
   A. amputation.
   B. incision.
   C. complete laceration.
   D. degloving injury.
   E. transection.

17. Amputations that occur cleanly are likely to be associated with severe hemorrhage.
   A. True
   B. False

18. Vascular, platelet, and coagulation are phases of the process called
   A. hemorrhage.
   B. homeostasis.
   C. hemostasis.
   D. inflammation.
   E. epithelialization.

19. When torn or cut, the muscles in the capillaries constrict, thereby limiting hemorrhage.
   A. True
   B. False

20. The agents that recruit cells responsible for the inflammatory response are called
   A. macrophages.
   B. lymphocytes.
   C. chemotactic factors.
   D. granulocytes.
   E. fibroblasts.

21. The cells that attack invading pathogens directly or through an antibody response include all of the following, EXCEPT
   A. macrophages.
   B. lymphocytes.
   C. white blood cells.
   D. granulocytes.
   E. fibroblasts.

22. The stage of the healing process in which the phagocytes and lymphocytes are most active is
   A. inflammation.
   B. epithelialization.
   C. neovascularization.
   D. collagen synthesis.
   E. none of the above.

©2013 Pearson Education, Inc.
Paramedic Care: Principles & Practice, Vol. 5, 4th Ed.

_____ 23. Regenerated skin, after about four months, is about how strong compared to the original skin?
- A. 20 percent
- B. 30 percent
- C. 40 percent
- D. 50 percent
- E. 60 percent

_____ 24. Infection usually appears how long after the initial wound?
- A. 12 to 24 hours
- B. 1 to 2 days
- C. 2 to 3 days
- D. 4 to 6 days
- E. 7 to 10 days

_____ 25. Which of the following is an infection risk factor with soft tissue wounds?
- A. Advancing age
- B. Crush injury
- C. NSAID use
- D. Cat bites
- E. All of the above

_____ 26. Closing wounds with staples or sutures increases the risk of infection.
- A. True
- B. False

_____ 27. It is common practice to provide tetanus boosters if the patient's last booster was over
- A. one year ago.
- B. two years ago.
- C. three years ago.
- D. four years ago.
- E. five years ago.

_____ 28. Which of the following can interfere with normal clotting?
- A. Aspirin
- B. Warfarin
- C. Streptokinase
- D. TPA
- E. All of the above

_____ 29. The location at greatest risk for compartment syndrome is the
- A. calf.
- B. thigh.
- C. forearm.
- D. arm.
- E. ankle.

_____ 30. The excessive growth of scar tissue within the boundaries of the wound is called
- A. hypertrophic scar formation.
- B. keloid scar formation.
- C. anatropic scar formation.
- D. residual scar formation.
- E. regressive scar formation.

_____ 31. The nature of crush injury produces an injury area that is an excellent growth medium for infection.
- A. True
- B. False

_____ 32. A crush injury that produces crush syndrome usually requires what minimum time of entrapment?
- A. 1 hour
- B. 2 hours
- C. 4 hours
- D. 6 hours
- E. 10 hours

_____ 33. Which of the following is likely with the release of entrapment in the patient suffering crush syndrome?
- A. Kidney failure
- B. Cardiac dysrhythmias
- C. Hypovolemia
- D. Abnormal vascular calcifications
- E. All of the above

_____ 34. The type of dressing that prevents the movement of fluid or air through the dressing is:
- A. sterile.
- B. nonadherent.
- C. absorbent.
- D. occlusive.
- E. nonocclusive.

35. The bandages that increase pressure beneath the bandage with each consecutive wrap are
   A. elastic bandages.
   B. self-adherent roller bandages.
   C. gauze bandages.
   D. adhesive bandages.
   E. triangular bandages.

36. Not only is the skin the first body organ to experience trauma, it is often the only one to display the signs of injury.
   A. True
   B. False

37. Which of the following are important factors to consider in the assessment and management of external hemorrhage?
   A. Type of bleeding
   B. Rate of hemorrhage
   C. Volume of blood lost
   D. Stopping further hemorrhage
   E. All of the above

38. Which of the following is one of the primary objectives of bandaging?
   A. Neat appearance
   B. Hemorrhage control
   C. Allowing easy movement of the wound
   D. Debridement
   E. Aeration

39. Insufficient tourniquet pressure may increase the rate and volume of hemorrhage.
   A. True
   B. False

40. The restoration of circulation once a tourniquet is released may cause which of the following?
   A. Shock
   B. Hypovolemia
   C. Lethal dysrhythmias
   D. Renal failure
   E. All of the above

41. After bandaging a patient's severely hemorrhaging forearm wound, you notice that the limb is cool, capillary refill is slowed, and the radial pulse cannot be found. You should
   A. apply more dressing material and increase the pressure.
   B. leave the bandage as it is.
   C. loosen the bandage.
   D. elevate the extremity and leave the bandage in place.
   E. remove the bandage.

42. Which medication may be administered to help alleviate pain associated with soft tissue injury?
   A. Ibuprofen
   B. Morphine sulfate
   C. Aspirin
   D. Ketorolac
   E. Naproxen

43. With a large and gaping wound to the neck, use a(n)
   A. large absorbent dressing.
   B. large nonadherent dressing.
   C. occlusive dressing.
   D. nonabsorbent dressing.
   E. triangular bandage.

44. The type of dressing recommended for blood and fluid leaking from the auditory canal is a(n)
   A. nonocclusive dressing.
   B. nonadherent dressing.
   C. occlusive dressing.
   D. gauze dressing.
   E. wet dressing.

45. Which of the following is NOT a distal sign that a circumferential bandage is too tight?
   A. Diaphoresis
   B. Pallor
   C. Loss of pulses
   D. Tingling
   E. Swelling

©2013 Pearson Education, Inc.
Paramedic Care: Principles & Practice, Vol. 5, 4th Ed.

46. You find a patient who has suffered a finger amputation. You should keep the amputated part
    A. warm and dry.
    B. warm and moist.
    C. cool and moist.
    D. cool and dry.
    E. packed in ice.

47. If the amputated part cannot be immediately located, wait only a few minutes at the scene because its transport with the patient is extremely important.
    A. True
    B. False

48. In which of the following situations is removal of an impaled object allowed or required?
    A. The object obstructs the airway.
    B. The object prevents performance of CPR.
    C. The object is impaled in the cheek.
    D. The object is impaled in the chest of a trauma patient who needs resuscitation.
    E. All of the above.

49. Care for the patient with crush syndrome includes
    A. rapid transport.
    B. fluid resuscitation.
    C. diuresis.
    D. possibly systemic alkalization.
    E. all of the above.

50. A special fluid need for the resuscitation of the crush syndrome patient is
    A. hetastarch.
    B. heparin.
    C. sodium bicarbonate.
    D. 5 percent dextrose in 1/2 normal saline.
    E. Dextran.

51. It is recommended that you infuse what volume of fluid per hour to the crush syndrome patient?
    A. 10 mL/kg/hr
    B. 20 mL/kg/hr
    C. 30 mL/kg/hr
    D. 50 mL/kg/hr
    E. 100 mL/kg/hr

52. Sudden cardiac arrest care after extrication of the entrapped patient with crush syndrome should include the routine cardiac drugs and
    A. potassium for hypokalemia.
    B. calcium chloride for hyperkalemia.
    C. sodium bicarbonate for hypokalemia.
    D. dopamine for low blood pressure.
    E. none of the above.

53. The most prominent symptom of compartment syndrome is
    A. pain out of proportion to physical findings with the injury.
    B. reduced or absent distal pulses.
    C. increased skin tension in the affected limb.
    D. paresthesia.
    E. paresis.

54. Compartment syndrome is most likely to occur
    A. immediately after injury.
    B. within 2 hours of injury.
    C. within 3 hours of injury.
    D. within 4 hours of injury.
    E. 6 to 8 hours after injury.

55. The most effective treatment in the prehospital setting for compartment syndrome is
    A. a fasciectomy.
    B. the application of cold packs.
    C. elevation of the extremity.
    D. massaging the extremity.
    E. none of the above.

6

Burn Trauma

Review of Chapter Objectives

After reading this chapter, you should be able to:

1. Define key terms introduced in this chapter.

Knowing and being able to apply the key terms in each chapter is critical to understanding chapter concepts. Write the list of key terms. Then write the definition of each one in your own words. Check your understanding by confirming the definitions in the text glossary. Correct any misunderstandings. Create a study aid by writing each key term on the front of an index card and the definition on the back. Use the cards to quiz yourself, or to have someone quiz you.

2. Describe the epidemiology of burn injuries.   **p. 123**

The incidence of burn injury has been declining over the past few decades but still accounts for over 1 million burn injuries and over 45,000 hospitalizations each year. Those at greatest risk are the very young, the elderly, the infirm, and those exposed to occupational risk (firefighters, chemical workers, etc.). Burns are the second leading cause of death in children under 12 and the fourth overall cause of trauma death.

Much of the decline in burn injury and death is attributable to better building codes, improved construction techniques, sprinkler systems, and the use of smoke detectors. Educational programs that teach children not to play with matches or lighters and that instruct the family to turn the water heater down to below 120°F have also helped reduce burn morbidity and mortality.

3. Describe the anatomy and physiology of the skin.   **pp. 123–124**

The skin or integumentary system is the largest organ of the body and consists of three layers, the epidermis, the dermis, and the subcutaneous layer. It functions as the outer barrier of the body and protects it against environmental extremes and pathogens. The outermost layer is the epidermis, a layer of dead or dying cells that provides a barrier to fluid loss, absorption, and the entrance of pathogens. The dermis is the true skin. It houses the sensory nerve endings, many of the specialized skin cells that produce sweat and oil, and the upper-level capillary beds that allow for the conduction of heat to the body's surface. The subcutaneous layer, although not a true part of the skin, works in concert with the skin to insulate the body from heat loss and the effects of trauma.

4. Describe the pathophysiology and complications of: **pp. 124–131**

a. Thermal burns

Thermal burn injury results as the rate of molecular movement in a cell increases, causing the cell membranes and proteins to denature. This causes a progressive injury as the heat penetrates deeper and deeper through the skin and into the body's interior. At the local level, the injury disrupts the envelope of the body, permitting fluid to leak from the capillaries into the tissue and evaporate, resulting in dehydration and cooling. Serious circumferential burns may form an eschar and constrict, compromising ventilation or circulation to a distal extremity.

The systemic effects of serious burns include severe dehydration and infection. Fluid is drawn to the injured tissue as it becomes edematous and then may evaporate in great quantities as the skin loses its ability to contain fluids. Infection can be massive and can quickly and easily overwhelm the body's immune system. The products of cell destruction from the burn process may enter the bloodstream and damage the tubules of the kidneys, resulting in failure. Organ failure due to burn by-products may also affect the liver and the heart's electrical system. Last, the burn injury and the associated evaporation of fluid may cool the body more rapidly than it can create heat. The result is a lowering of body temperature, hypothermia.

b. Electrical burns

Electrical burns result from the flow of electrons from a point of high concentration to one of low concentration. Human tissue varies in conductivity and resistance, with skin being the most resistant and nerve tissue or mucous membranes being the least. The potential for injury increases the longer the duration of contact with the electrical source. Electrical burn damage can be significant as the body heats from the inside out. Internal organs, muscles, nerves, and blood vessels may be severely injured. The muscles of respiration may be immobilized or the patient may experience titanic convulsions or uncontrolled muscle contractions. The heart's electrical system may be disrupted, causing dysrhythmias. Liver and kidney failure may result from tissue degeneration after the initial injury. Flash burns may severely burn or vaporize skin and underlying tissue.

c. Chemical burns

Chemical burns disrupt cell membranes and damage tissue on contact. Generally they are self-limiting as the chemical must destroy tissue progressively. Acids form a thick, insoluble mass at the point of contact called coagulation necrosis. This limits burn depth and causes immediate local pain. Alkalis do not induce pain although they progressively destroy cell membranes in a process called liquefaction necrosis. Deep injury may result.

d. Radiation injury

Radiation changes the structure of molecules through an ionization process and may cause cells to die, become dysfunctional, or reproduce dysfunctional cells. Rapidly dividing cells are most susceptible to damage. There are four types of ionizing radiation. Alpha radiation is weak and cannot penetrate skin. It is a hazard if inhaled or ingested. Beta radiation is stronger and may cause external and internal injury. Gamma rays have significant penetrating power. They may travel through the entire body, causing massive injury and death. Neutron radiation, while strong, is uncommonly encountered. The extent of injury depends on the type of radiation, length of exposure, distance from the radiation source, and protective mechanisms. Additionally, effects will vary, with different tissues impacted to greater or lesser extent. With whole-body exposure, individuals will present with progressive signs of nausea, vomiting, diarrhea, fatigue, confusion, and collapse. Longer-term complications of exposure include infertility and cancer.

e. Inhalation injury

Inhaled gases, heated air, flames, smoke, and steam produce inhalation injuries, with associated airway and respiratory compromise. Entrapped or unconscious victims in enclosed spaces are at greatest risk. Inhalation injury can also involve carbon monoxide poisoning and the absorption of gaseous chemicals through the alveoli. Toxic gases react with lung tissue, causing internal burns, or cross the alveolar-capillary membrane, interfering with delivery and use of oxygen. Signs and symptoms may occur immediately or be delayed. Carbon monoxide (CO) binds with hemoglobin far more readily than oxygen. It also attaches to myoglobin, further reducing oxygen availability. Signs and symptoms are generally related to length of exposure and progress from a mild, general ill feeling with headache, nausea, vomiting, and dizziness to confusion, weakness, tachypnea, chest pain, dysrhythmias, seizures, coma, and cardiac arrest.

5. **Demonstrate the assessment of patients with burn injuries, including particular attention to the patient's airway, and determination of burn depth and extent of body surface area involved.**   pp. 131–133, 135–140, 142–146

Assessment of all burn injuries begins with ensuring the safety of yourself and crew during the scene size-up. Enclosed spaces can harbor intense heat, and toxic gases may represent a significant hazard. If the scene is still hazardous, skilled, properly protected rescuers should bring the patient to you. Then

©2013 Pearson Education, Inc.
Paramedic Care: Principles & Practice, Vol. 5, 4th Ed.

your first priority is to stop the burning process and remove any smoldering clothes or other materials that may produce further thermal injury or restrict swelling and occlude distal circulation.

Airway management is the next priority. When assessing an inhalation injury, you should examine the mechanism of injury to identify any unconsciousness or confinement during the fire or any history of explosive stream expansion and inhalation. Also consider the possibility of toxic inhalation. Study the patient carefully for signs of singed facial or nasal hairs, carbonaceous residue, stridor, coughing, or hoarseness. If you suspect inhalation injury, provide high-concentration oxygen and prepare for early intubation (rapid-sequence intubation [RSI]) as needed. The airway tissues can swell quickly and result in serious airway restriction or complete obstruction. Utilize pulse oximetry and pulse CO-oximetry to evaluate carbon monoxide poisoning. In the presence of CO, pulse oximetry alone may give a falsely high reading. Airway burns may present as supraglottic or infraglottic.

A supraglottic inhalation burn is a thermal injury to the mucosa above the glottic opening. Because of the moist environment and the vascular nature of the tissue, it takes great heat energy to cause burn injury. When such injury occurs, however, the associated swelling can quickly threaten the airway.

Infraglottic (or subglottic) inhalation burns occur much less frequently because the moist supra-glottic tissue absorbs the heat energy and the glottis will likely close to prevent the injury from penetrating more deeply. However, superheated steam, as is produced when a stream of water hits a particularly hot portion of a fire, has the heat energy to carry the burning process to the subglottic region. Lower airway tissue can swell rapidly, reducing the airway lumen. Patients may present with minor hoarseness, progressing to dyspnea and respiratory arrest. Stridor is an ominous sign of impending obstruction and the airway needs to be managed aggressively.

Begin your secondary assessment with either a rapid or focused trauma assessment. Examine the patient's entire body surface to determine the severity of the burn by considering the total body surface area (BSA) burned, the burn injury depth, and the specific body areas involved.

Utilize the "rule of nines" or the "rule of palms" method to determine BSA. The "rule of nines" is most appropriate for determining BSA of large burns while the "rule of palms" is more accurate for smaller burns or scattered burns. The "rule of nines" approximates the body surface area burned by assigning each body region 9 percent of the total. These regions include: each upper extremity, the anterior of each lower extremity, the posterior of each lower extremity, the anterior of the abdomen, the anterior thorax, the upper back, the lower back, and the entire head and neck. The remaining 1 percent is assigned to the genitalia. For children, the head is given 18 percent, and the lower extremities are assigned 13½ percent each. The "rule of palms" method of approximating burn surface area assumes the victim's palm surface is equivalent to 1 percent of the total body surface area. The care provider then estimates the burn surface area by determining the number of palmar surfaces it would take to cover the wound.

Depth of burn damage is classified into three categories. Superficial (first-degree) burns involve only the upper layers of the epidermis and dermis. The effects are limited to an irritation of the upper sensory tissues with some pain, minor edema, and erythema. Partial-thickness (second-degree) burns penetrate slightly deeper than first-degree burns and cause blistering, redness, swelling, and, often, extreme pain. The hallmark characteristic is the development of blisters. Because the cells that reproduce the skin's upper layers are still alive, complete regeneration is expected. Full-thickness (third-degree) burns penetrate the entire dermis, causing extensive destruction to the skin and extending into the subcutaneous tissue or deeper, into muscles, bones, and internal organs. The burned area may display a variety of colors, including white, brown, dark red, or a charred color, and typically have a dry, leather-like appearance. Because nerve endings have been destroyed, these burns may be painless but the burn margins may be partial thickness, involving intense pain.

The third consideration in determining burn severity is the location. Burns to the face, hands, feet, joints, and genitalia, as well as circumferential burns, increase the criticality. Future function may be compromised, while circumferential burns, especially of an extremity, thorax, abdomen, or neck, pose an immediate threat due to swelling and constriction. Carefully assess these burns for compromised distal circulatory status or impedance of chest movement.

Once a transport priority has been established, obtain vitals and continuously monitor for early signs of hypovolemia and airway problems as well as cardiac dysrhythmias often seen with electrical burns.

While the general assessment approach is the same for all burn patients, electrical, chemical, and radiation burns require some additional considerations. Scene safety is always a priority, so be sure that power has been shut off, that chemical spills or toxic fumes have been contained, and that radiation hazards have been isolated. In the event of electrical injury, perform early cardiac monitoring, as electrical current often causes cardiac dysrhythmias or cardiac arrest. Attempt to determine the voltage and current of the source. Look for entrance and exit wounds and remember that external findings may only suggest superficial injury while internal damage is significant. Because electricity produces forceful muscle spasm, consider spinal immobilization and look for other indications of fracture. When responding to chemical burn patients, determine the type of agent, its exact chemical name, the length of the patient's contact time, and the precise body areas affected. Carefully assess airway and monitor the heart for potential cardiac disturbances. For radiation exposures, note the length of exposure, mechanism, and type of radioactive substance involved. Actual patient assessment is simple and usually reveals minimal signs or symptoms of injury. Assess for obvious burns and signs and symptoms of nausea, vomiting, and weakness.

6. **Anticipate and take measures to minimize systemic complications of burns.** pp. 133–134

Typical complications of burns include hypothermia, hypovolemia, eschar formation, and infection.

a. **Hypothermia**

Burns disrupt the body's ability to regulate core temperature. Fluid evaporates at the damaged skin surface as plasma is released into the wound. Blood flow increases to the injured tissue, further enhancing heat loss. Because of the burn, vessels are unable to constrict to conserve heat. Severe hypothermia can rapidly develop. Patients should be covered with a blanket and kept warm by regulating the ambient air temperature in the ambulance.

b. **Hypovolemia**

Damaged blood vessels in the skin cannot contain plasma, while fluids from undamaged tissue cannot be drawn in due to loss of plasma protein. Fluid resuscitation initiated in the field can begin to counteract hypovolemia, which typically occurs hours after the injury. Electrolyte imbalances occur along with these fluid shifts. This is further complicated by the by-products of tissue destruction that are released into the bloodstream. Of particular concern is potassium, which can accumulate, causing life-threatening cardiac dysrhythmias. Patients should be placed on a cardiac monitor and carefully observed.

c. **Eschar formation**

Damaged dermal cells become hard and leathery, producing eschar. This constriction causes a buildup of edematous pressure, which can compromise distal blood flow. Circumferential burns represent the greatest risk, especially if they interfere with chest excursion and respiration. Airway and breathing must be carefully monitored throughout treatment and transport.

d. **Infection**

Skin forms a protective barrier against pathogens. When skin is destroyed in a burn injury, pathogens invade the wound quickly and continue to multiply and spread. Although this process takes days to weeks to become life threatening, efforts to minimize exposure should be initiated in the field. Use Standard Precautions, clean and sterile dressings, and clean equipment, and avoid contamination of the burn injury.

7. **Recognize indications that burns may have resulted from abuse.** p. 135

Burns associated with child abuse often result from scalding water immersion, open flame burns, or cigarette-type injuries. The child presents with a history of a burn that does not make sense, such as stove burns when he cannot yet reach the stove, multiple circular burns (cigarettes), or burns isolated to the buttocks, which occur as the child lifts his legs during attempts at immersion in hot water. "Stocking" burns may be evident if the child's feet and legs have been dipped in scalding water.

©2013 Pearson Education, Inc.
Paramedic Care: Principles & Practice, Vol. 5, 4th Ed.

8. **Identify patients whose burns are considered critical.** pp. 138–139

Critical burns are those partial-thickness burns covering more than 30 percent of the BSA, full-thickness burns over 10 percent of the BSA, and any significant inhalation injury. Critical burns also include any burn that involves any partial- or full-thickness burn to the hands, feet, genitalia, joints, or face. Circumferential burns should also be deemed critical, as the area underneath the burn may be drastically compressed as an eschar forms, hindering respiration, restricting distal blood flow, or causing hypoxia of underlying tissue. Burn patients who are very young, very old, or have a significant preexisting disease and those with coincident trauma are at increased risk for the systemic problems associated with burn injury. They cannot tolerate the massive fluid losses often associated with burns because they have smaller fluid reserves, and they cannot effectively fight the ensuing massive infection commonly associated with large burns. They should be considered one step closer to critical than consideration of their burn type and BSA would normally place them.

9. **Given a variety of scenarios, develop management plans for patients with:** pp. 136–137, 140–146

a. **Thermal burn** management focuses on preventing shock, hypothermia, and minimizing further wound contamination after managing life-threats, especially the airway. Protect the airway early with placement of an endotracheal tube or RSI if the patient is conscious or has a gag reflex. Further treatment will then depend on whether the burn is a minor, local burn or a more extensive moderate to severe injury.

Local cooling is used to treat minor soft tissue burns involving only a partial-thickness injury and a small BSA proportion. Remove any smoldering or restricting clothing or jewelry. Cover burns with a clean, nonadherent dressing or sheet and elevate the injury. Do not apply ointments or other substances to the burned tissue. If clothing is adhered to the injury, cut around it. Pulling it away may cause further damage. Offer the patient comfort and support. Consider morphine sulfate or fentanyl for pain. Obtain the patient's tetanus immunization history.

Moderate to severe burns require additional attention. Do not use cooling, as this may induce hypothermia. Cover the burns with dry, clean nonadherent dressings or a clean sheet. If the patient has sustained full-thickness burns to the fingers, toes, or other locations where burned surfaces may contact each other, place soft, nonadherent dressings between the burned skin areas. Because serious burns lead to significant fluid loss, early and aggressive fluid therapy is indicated. Attempt to place an IV in a non-burned area. If this is not possible, place the catheter through tissue with partial-thickness burns proximal to more serious damage. Secure the IV with gentle, circumferential bandaging using nonadherent gauze instead of tape. Infuse normal saline or lactated Ringer's according to the Parkland formula or local protocol. Frequently recheck airway to ensure that swelling and edema have not worsened. Provide patients with narcotic analgesia administered intravenously in 2-mg increments every 5 minutes until pain is controlled, provided there is no hypotension or respiratory depression. Although unlikely, if transport is long, medical direction may request you to perform an emergency escharotomy to counteract constriction that may reduce or halt distal circulation or restrict respiration.

Maintain the patient's body temperature by covering with a blanket and ensuring a warm environment. Any burn patient with serious injury should be transported to a burn center to receive specialized treatment. Ensure that the burn patient receives therapeutic communication while you are at the scene and during transport. Burn injuries may be very painful and the appearance can be quite frightening. Constantly talk with the patient. Try to distract him from the injury, and monitor level of consciousness and anxiety level throughout your care and transport.

b. **Inhalation injuries** are commonly associated with burn injuries. Swelling can develop rapidly, occluding the airway and progressing to respiratory arrest if not promptly managed. Early intubation by the most experienced provider can be lifesaving. If the patient is conscious, nasotracheal or RSI may be required. In patients with severe burns, avoid using succinylcholine, as it may worsen hyperkalemia. In extreme cases, needle cricothyrostomy may be a lifesaving necessity. Confirm tube placement with three methods and provide positive pressure ventilation (PPV) using the reservoir and high-concentration oxygen.

When carbon monoxide poisoning is suspected, administer 100 percent oxygen regardless of the pulse oximetry reading. If available, confirm with a pulse CO-oximeter. Apply continuous positive airway pressure (CPAP), which forces more oxygen into the bloodstream, displacing carbon monoxide more quickly. Under some protocols patients should be transported to a facility with hyperbaric oxygen therapy capability.

Cyanide frequently coexists with carbon monoxide. Antidotal treatment must be initiated early in patients presenting with cyanide toxicity—severe dyspnea, chest pain, altered mental status, seizures, and unconsciousness. Two cyanide antidote regimens are available: the older cyanide kit containing amyl nitrite, sodium nitrite, and sodium thiosulfate and the newer Cyanokit, which contains hydroxocobalamin. The latter is a safer alternative administered intravenously. The older cyanide kit is administered in a two-stage process. In either case, aggressively manage the airway and provide ventilatory support prior to implementing antidotal therapy.

c. **Electrical burn** injuries are caused by the passage of electrical current through the body. Suspect spinal injury in any patient sustaining significant electrical contact and provide appropriate spinal precautions. Victims of lightning lightening strikes may sustain extensive internal injury, or limited damage if the current passes over the exterior of the body. Remove smoldering clothing and shoes as well as any constrictive items from the fingers, limbs and neck. Aggressively manage airway if the patient presents in respiratory arrest. Perform electrocardiogram (ECG) monitoring for cardiac dysrhythmias. Treat visible burns ("entrance" and "exit" wounds) with cooling and the application of dry, clean dressings. For serious electrical burn injuries initiate at least a large-bore IVs and administer 1,000 mL of fluid per hour in 20-mL/kg boluses. Consider administering sodium bicarbonate and mannitol per local protocol. Immobilize fractures secondary to managing life-threatening problems. Remember that widespread internal injury to vessels, nerves, and other structures is likely, so rapid transport is indicated. If electrical burn patients present in cardiac arrest, prolonged resuscitation may permit survival. Follow the usual resuscitative cardiac arrest algorithms.

d. **Chemical burn** injury is most frequently found in the industrial setting and is often associated with the effects of strong acids or alkalis. Management begins with having contaminated clothing removed and isolated. If airway involvement compromises breathing, consider early intubation and ventilation. Monitor heart rate and rhythm with ECG monitoring. Further treatment typically involves copious irrigation. If you suspect phenol, dry lime, sodium, or riot agents, treat as follows: Use alcohol to dissolve phenol and irrigate using large volumes of cool water. Brush dry lime off the patient and rinse the contaminated area with large volumes of cool to cold water. Remove sodium contamination by gentle brushing and cover the wound with oil used to store the substance. Treat eye exposures with mace and pepper spray by irrigation with normal saline. Additional treatment is supportive. For extensive chemical contamination, deliver large volumes of water with a garden hose or other low-pressure source. Remove remaining clothing and gently wash the burn with a mild soap. Then continue to irrigate with a constant flow of water until arrival at the emergency department. Avoid use of neutralizing agents. For chemical splashes involving the eyes, irrigation with water or normal saline is indicated. Be careful to avoid cross-contamination of the opposite eye. Irrigate acid burns for at least 5 minutes and alkali burns for 15 minutes.

e. **Radiation** exposure is a relatively rare injury but poses serious risks to the victim and responders. The objective of rescue and care is to limit the exposure for both the patient and rescuer. Because radiation exposure is cumulative, removal of the victim from the source is a priority. Treatment should be initiated by properly trained and protected personnel if the victim is contaminated. Patients should be disrobed and rinsed with large volumes of water, then washed with a soft brush and rinsed again. Ordinary dish detergent is an effective cleansing agent. Once decontaminated, treat as you would any other patient. Make the patient comfortable, treat symptomatically, and provide psychological support. Cover burns with sterile dressings, provide oxygen, and initiate an IV. Maintain body temperature and transport.

©2013 Pearson Education, Inc.
Paramedic Care: Principles & Practice, Vol. 5, 4th Ed.

Case Study Review

Reread the case study on pages 122 and 123 in Paramedic Care: Trauma; *then, read the following discussion.*
The scenario presented in this case study illustrates the dangers associated with the fire-ground and with inhalation injuries. It also identifies the difficulty you might have in recognizing respiratory injury and the importance of treating it early.

The scene observed by Ben and Ronny demonstrates the dangers associated with a working fire and a real-time assessment of the mechanism of injury. As fire rescue paramedics, they are wearing turnout gear, boots, and heavy gloves as they approach the injured firefighter. They ensure that the scene is safe and recognize that hazards can include debris, still-energized electrical lines, leaking gas, further structural collapse, and much more. They will work quickly to move their fellow firefighter to a safe location and continue care. Once at a safe location, Ben and Ronny remove the firefighter's clothing as they begin their primary assessment. They replace their work gloves with sterile latex or plastic ones because they know that infection is a common and serious consequence of the types of burns this patient received. They will do all they can to protect the wounds from further contamination by quickly covering them with dry sterile dressings.

The firefighter they assess in this incident experiences the classic evolution of the burn and inhalation injury. He was initially found to be stable, with signs, symptoms, and vital signs suggestive of minor injury. The major concern for this patient might well be the fractured forearm. However, the paramedics are wary because of the significant area burned and the patient's history, hoarseness, and the sooty sputum. They anticipate serious fluid loss through the burn and infection risk, as well as airway injury that will likely worsen during their care.

Ben must be careful regarding any articles of clothing or jewelry that could continue to burn or contain the swelling that often accompanies burn injury. His initial action should be to stop any further burning. This calls for complete inspection of the burn area and the surrounding clothing. Once the burn area is exposed, the depth and area involved can be assessed. In this case, the patient has a fracture, possible inhalation injury, and a serious burn. The area burned, the posterior chest and abdomen and the upper left extremity, represents a body surface area of about 22½ percent. The combination of traumatic injury, burn, and inhalation injury are reasons to consider the patient to have critical injuries.

The paramedics initiate an IV with a large-bore catheter and begin running normal saline. A 1,000-mL bag is hung with a non-flow-restrictive (trauma or blood tubing) administration set just in case the signs of shock appear. Fluids are run rapidly in 250- to 500-mL boluses to get ahead of the loss normally associated with severe burns. If this were a 125-kg man with the burns identified (22½ percent by the rule of nines), the needed fluid would be 4 mL × 22½ (percent of burn area) × 125 kg, or a total of 11,250 mL in the first 24 hours (Parkland formula). Half of this is needed in the first 8 hours. That is more than 700 mL per hour.

The signs of respiratory involvement, though subtle, are even more significant than the burn or fracture. Inhalation injury is likely due either to the chemical burning caused by the products of combustion reacting with the soft tissue of the respiratory tract or to thermal burns caused by superheated steam created when the water extinguished the flames. In either case, respiratory damage can be extensive. Patients with respiratory burns usually display progressive dyspnea, as in this case. The only effective way to treat this problem is to anticipate that progression and be aggressive in airway care. Intubation equipment should be readied and used when any sign of developing airway compromise appears. With inhalation injury it might be prudent to consider rapid sequence intubation to allow the passage of the endotracheal tube before the airway swells and makes the procedure very difficult. Ken should also be considered for immediate transport because of the difficulty in managing the airway.

Ben and Ronny must also be prepared for the worst. If the firefighter had experienced severe dyspnea and airway restriction while 20 to 30 minutes from the hospital, a needle or surgical cricothyrotomy might have been necessary. Likewise, had they waited on the scene to splint, bandage, and care for the patient, the time spent on those tasks would have permitted the airway and patient to deteriorate. This case study clearly identifies the need for rapid recognition and transport of the patient with developing airway compromise.

Content Self-Evaluation

MULTIPLE CHOICE

_____ 1. The incidence of burn injury has been on the decline over the past decade.
   A. True
   B. False

_____ 2. A preventive action that will reduce the incidence of scalding injuries is
   A. use of childproof faucets.
   B. education of children on the dangers of hot water.
   C. placing caution stickers on water faucets.
   D. lowering the water heater temperature to 120°F.
   E. none of the above.

_____ 3. The layer of skin that is made up of mostly dead cells and provides the waterproof envelope that contains the body is the
   A. dermis.   D. sebum.
   B. subcutaneous layer.   E. corium.
   C. epidermis.

_____ 4. Which of the following is NOT a function of the skin?
   A. Protecting the body from bacterial infection
   B. Protecting the body from excessive fluid loss
   C. Allowing for joint movement
   D. Preventing all heat loss
   E. Insulating from trauma

_____ 5. Burns result from the disruption of the proteins found in cell membranes.
   A. True
   B. False

_____ 6. The area of a burn that suffers the most damage is generally the
   A. zone of hyperemia.   D. zone of coagulation.
   B. zone of denaturing.   E. zone of most resistance.
   C. zone of stasis.

_____ 7. The theory of burns that explains the burning process is
   A. the thermal hypothesis.   D. the hypermetabolism dynamic.
   B. Jackson's theory of thermal wounds. E. none of the above.
   C. the Phaseal discussion of burns.

_____ 8. The order in which the phases of the body's response to a burn would normally be expected to occur is
   A. emergent, fluid shift, hypermetabolic.
   B. fluid shift, hypermetabolic, emergent.
   C. fluid shift, emergent, hypermetabolic.
   D. hypermetabolic, fluid shift, emergent.
   E. emergent, hypermetabolic, fluid shift.

_____ 9. Which of the following skin types has the greatest resistance to the passage of electrical current?
   A. Mucous membranes   D. The skin on the inside of the arm
   B. Wet skin   E. The skin on the inside of the thigh
   C. Calluses

©2013 Pearson Education, Inc.
Paramedic Care: Principles & Practice, Vol. 5, 4th Ed.

10. Electrical injury is likely to cause which of the following?
    A. Serious injury in which the electricity enters the body
    B. Serious injury in which the electricity exits the body
    C. Damage to nerves
    D. Damage to blood vessels
    E. All of the above

11. Prolonged contact with alternating current may result in respiratory paralysis.
    A. True
    B. False

12. Chemical burns involving strong alkalis are likely to be deep because of coagulation necrosis.
    A. True
    B. False

13. Which of the following radiation types is the most powerful type of ionizing radiation?
    A. Lambda
    B. Alpha
    C. Gamma
    D. Beta
    E. Delta

14. Which of the following is a type of radiation present only inside nuclear reactors and bombs?
    A. Neutron
    B. Alpha
    C. Gamma
    D. Beta
    E. Delta

15. To protect themselves from radiation exposure, EMS personnel should
    A. limit the duration of exposure.
    B. increase the shielding from exposure.
    C. increase the distance from the source.
    D. ensure that the patient is decontaminated.
    E. all of the above.

16. The radiation dose that is lethal to about 50 percent of those exposed is
    A. 0.2 Gray.
    B. 100 rads.
    C. 1 Gray.
    D. 4.5 Grays.
    E. 200 rads.

17. As radiation exposure increases, the signs of exposure become less evident and only reappear later in the course of the disease.
    A. True
    B. False

18. Which of the following is commonly associated with inhalation injury?
    A. Carbon monoxide poisoning
    B. Toxic inhalation
    C. Supraglottic injury
    D. Subglottic injury
    E. All of the above

19. Which type of circumstance is most likely to cause subglottic thermal burn injury?
    A. Inhalation of hot air
    B. Inhalation of flame
    C. Inhalation of superheated steam
    D. Standing in a burn environment
    E. Inhalation of toxic substances

20. What percentage of burn patients who die have associated airway burn injury?
    A. 20 percent
    B. 35 percent
    C. 50 percent
    D. 60 percent
    E. 85 percent

21. The burn characterized by erythema, pain, and blistering is the
    A. superficial burn.
    B. partial-thickness burn.
    C. full-thickness burn.
    D. electrical burn.
    E. chemical burn.

22. The burn characterized by discoloration and lack of pain is the
    A. superficial burn.
    B. partial-thickness burn.
    C. full-thickness burn.
    D. electrical burn.
    E. chemical burn.

23. An adult has received burns to the entire anterior chest and to the entire left upper extremity, circumferentially. Using the rule of nines, the percentage of body surface area (BSA) involved is
    A. 9 percent.
    B. 18 percent.
    C. 27 percent.
    D. 36 percent.
    E. 48 percent.

24. A child has received burns to the entire left lower extremity and the genitals. Using the rule of nines, the percentage of the body surface area involved is
    A. 9 percent.
    B. 10 percent.
    C. 14 ½ percent.
    D. 19 percent.
    E. 21½ percent.

25. An adult has received burns to the entire left lower extremity and the genitals. Using the rule of nines, the percentage of the body surface area involved is
    A. 9 percent.
    B. 10 percent.
    C. 18 percent.
    D. 19 percent.
    E. 21 percent.

26. A child receives burns to his entire head and neck and upper back. What percentage of body surface area is involved?
    A. 9 percent
    B. 10 percent
    C. 18 percent
    D. 19 percent
    E. 27 percent

27. Which of the following systemic complications should you suspect with all serious burns?
    A. Hypothermia
    B. Hypovolemia
    C. Infection
    D. Eschar formation
    E. All of the above

28. Which of the following conditions would increase the impact a burn has on a patient?
    A. Being very young
    B. Being very old
    C. Having the flu
    D. Emphysema
    E. All of the above

29. Which of the following should NOT be removed from any burned area of a patient?
    A. Nylon clothing such as a windbreaker
    B. Small pieces of burned fabric lodged in the wound
    C. Shoes and socks
    D. Rings, watches, and other articles of jewelry
    E. Leather belts

30. When considering intubation of the patient with suspected airway injury due to inhalation of the by-products of combustion, you should have several smaller-than-normal endotracheal tubes ready.
    A. True
    B. False

31. In severe inhalation injury due to airway burns, it may be necessary to perform a cricothyrotomy to secure an adequate airway.
    A. True
    B. False

©2013 Pearson Education, Inc.
Paramedic Care: Principles & Practice, Vol. 5, 4th Ed.

_____ 32. High-concentration oxygen therapy is very helpful in cases of carbon monoxide poisoning because it will then be carried in sufficient quantities in the plasma to maintain life.
  A. True
  B. False

_____ 33. Your assessment reveals an area of burn that is reddened, painful, and just beginning to display blisters. What burn classification would you give this burn?
  A. Superficial burn
  B. Partial-thickness burn
  C. Full-thickness burn
  D. First-degree burn
  E. A or D

_____ 34. The patient you are attending has her entire left upper extremity seriously burned. The forearm and hand are very painful and reddened, while the upper arm is relatively painless and a dark red color. What percentage of the BSA and burn depth would you assign this patient?
  A. 9 percent full-thickness burn
  B. 9 percent partial-thickness burn
  C. 4½ percent full-thickness burn
  D. 4½ percent partial-thickness burn
  E. 4½ percent partial-thickness and 4½ percent full-thickness burn

_____ 35. Your assessment reveals a burn patient with superficial burns to 27 percent of the body. What classification of burn severity would you assign her?
  A. Minor
  B. Moderate
  C. Serious
  D. Critical
  E. None of the above

_____ 36. Your assessment reveals a burn patient with full-thickness burns to the entire left thigh and calf. What classification of burn severity would you assign him?
  A. Minor
  B. Moderate
  C. Serious
  D. Critical
  E. None of the above

_____ 37. Your assessment reveals a burn patient with partial-thickness burns to all of both lower extremities. What classification of burn severity would you assign her?
  A. Minor
  B. Moderate
  C. Serious
  D. Critical
  E. None of the above

_____ 38. Your assessment reveals a burn patient with partial-thickness burns to her entire lower extremities and a suspected femur fracture. What classification of burn severity would you assign her?
  A. Minor
  B. Moderate
  C. Serious
  D. Critical
  E. None of the above

_____ 39. Cool water immersion may reduce the depth and significance of small burns if applied within
  A. 1 to 2 minutes.
  B. 2 to 4 minutes.
  C. 4 to 5 minutes.
  D. 10 minutes.
  E. 20 minutes.

_____ 40. The patient with any full-thickness burn should be considered for administration of tetanus toxoid because the wound is an open one.
  A. True
  B. False

41. In general, moderate to severe burns should be covered with
   A. moist occlusive dressings.
   B. dry, sterile dressings.
   C. cool water immersion.
   D. plastic wrap covered by a soft dressing.
   E. warm water immersion.

42. Adjacent full-thickness burns, such as those affecting the fingers and toes, should be held together without dressings to ensure rapid healing.
   A. True
   B. False

43. The Parkland formula for fluid administration calls for administration of 4 mL of fluid to a patient multiplied by the patient's BSA involved. What other factor(s) determines the total fluid administered in the first 24 hours?
   A. Patient's age
   B. Patient's weight
   C. Depth of burns
   D. Age of the patient
   E. All of the above

44. Which of the following is the preferred fluid for resuscitation of the severely burned patient?
   A. Lactated Ringer's solution
   B. ½ normal saline
   C. Dextrose 5 percent in water
   D. Normal saline
   E. Dextrose 5 percent in normal saline

45. Which of the following drugs may be given to the patient with severe burns in the prehospital setting?
   A. Ipratropium
   B. Fentanyl
   C. Epinephrine
   D. Furosemide
   E. Haloperidol

46. Which of the following may be appropriate when a forming eschar is restricting distal blood flow to an extremity?
   A. Elevating the extremity
   B. Incising the eschar to relieve the pressure
   C. Wrapping the extremity in dry sterile dressings
   D. Administering morphine
   E. Immersing the limb in cold water

47. A patient was found unconscious in a burning mobile home. Your assessment discovers severe dyspnea, no airway restriction, chest pain, altered mental status, and some seizure activity. What condition would you suspect?
   A. Carbon monoxide poisoning
   B. Cyanide poisoning
   C. Chemical burns to the lungs
   D. Hypoxia due to inhalation of oxygen-deprived air
   E. Superheated steam inhalation

48. If an IV line is not yet established in a patient with suspected cyanide poisoning, you should administer which of the following?
   A. Amyl nitrite
   B. Sodium nitrite
   C. Sodium thiosulfide
   D. Haloperidol
   E. Ipratropium

©2013 Pearson Education, Inc.
Paramedic Care: Principles & Practice, Vol. 5, 4th Ed.

_____ **49.** In addition to the entrance and exit wounds normally expected with the passage of electrical current through the human body, the paramedic should expect
A. ventricular fibrillation.
B. cardiac irritability.
C. internal damage.
D. smoldering clothing.
E. all of the above.

_____ **50.** In the United States, lightning strikes hit about how many people per year?
A. 25
B. 50
C. 100
D. 300
E. 500

_____ **51.** The patient who is unresponsive, apneic, and pulseless due to a lightning strike is not a likely candidate for successful resuscitation.
A. True
B. False

_____ **52.** In general, caustic chemical contamination should be cared for by
A. dry, sterile dressings.
B. chemical antidotes.
C. rigorous scrubbing.
D. cool water irrigation.
E. rapid transport.

_____ **53.** The chemical phenol is soluble in
A. water.
B. dry lime.
C. normal saline.
D. ammonia.
E. alcohol.

_____ **54.** Which chemical agent reacts vigorously with water?
A. Phenol
B. Bleach
C. Sodium
D. Riot control agents
E. Ammonia

_____ **55.** Known antidotes and neutralizers for chemical contamination and burns will reduce the injury caused by the agent if administered immediately.
A. True
B. False

_____ **56.** How long should you irrigate a patient's eye contaminated with chemicals of an unknown nature?
A. Less than 2 minutes
B. Up to 5 minutes
C. Up to 15 minutes
D. Up to 20 minutes
E. None of the above

_____ **57.** When chemicals are splashed into the eye of the patient wearing contact lenses, the contacts should be removed to ensure irrigation will remove all of the agent.
A. True
B. False

_____ **58.** If the source of radiation cannot be contained or moved away from the patient, then
A. the patient should be brought to you.
B. care should be offered by you in protective gear.
C. care should be offered by specialists in protective gear.
D. care should be offered by the highest-ranking officer.
E. A or C.

_____ **59.** Which action can be used to reduce rescuer exposure to a radiation source?
A. Increase the distance from the source
B. Decrease the time exposed to the source
C. Increase the shielding between the rescuer and source
D. Protect against inhalation of contaminated dust
E. All of the above

60. Once exposed to a significant radiation source, the patient will become a source of radiation that the rescuer must then protect himself against. No amount of decontamination will reduce this danger.

    A. True

    B. False

Special Project

Drip Math Worksheet 2

Formulas

Rate = Volume/Time   mL/min = drops per min/drops per mL

Volume = Rate × Time   drops/min = mL per min × drops per mL

Time = Volume/Rate   mL = drops/drops per mL

Please complete the following drip math problems:

1. You are asked to administer a 250-mL solution to a patient over 2 hours. What drip rate would you use with a:

    A. 10-drops-per-mL administration set

    B. 15-drops-per-mL administration set

    C. 60-drops-per-mL administration set

2. Your protocol directs that an IV drip is to be run at 30 drops per minute with a 60-drops-per-mL administration set. How long will it take to infuse:

    A. 200 mL

    B. 350 mL

3. How much fluid would you administer to a patient over 15 minutes with a macrodrip (15-drops/mL) administration set, running at 1 drop per second?

4. Your protocol requires you to administer a drug at 15 drops per minute with a 60-drops-per-mL administration set. You only have a 45-drops-per-mL set available. At what drip rate would you run it?

©2013 Pearson Education, Inc.
Paramedic Care: Principles & Practice, Vol. 5, 4th Ed.

7

Orthopedic Trauma

Review of Chapter Objectives

After reading this chapter, you should be able to:

1. Define key terms introduced in this chapter.

Knowing and being able to apply the key terms in each chapter is critical to understanding chapter concepts. Write the list of key terms. Then write the definition of each one in your own words. Check your understanding by confirming the definitions in the text glossary. Correct any misunderstandings. Create a study aid by writing each key term on the front of an index card and the definition on the back. Use the cards to quiz yourself, or to have someone quiz you.

2. Describe the considerations in preventing orthopedic injuries. **pp. 151–152**

Prevention of musculoskeletal injuries relies on engineering controls, better awareness and education, as well as an emphasis on physical conditioning. Modern vehicle design, restraint systems, and highway safety have reduced injuries secondary to automobile crashes. Workplace safety laws and standards have reduced on-the-job injuries. By their nature, sports injuries will occur; however, better protective gear, improved equipment design, and athlete conditioning can lessen their incidence. Public education on safety practices in the home, including installation of railings and grab bars, proper step-ladder use, removal of throw rugs and proper footwear, can help minimize occurrences, especially among the elderly.

3. Describe the anatomy and physiology of the musculoskeletal system. **pp. 152–161**

The skeletal system is a living body system that protects vital organs, acts as a storehouse for body salts and other materials needed for metabolism, produces erythrocytes, permits us to have an upright stature, and allows for efficient movement. The skeletal system is comprised of approximately 206 bones forming two major divisions, the axial and appendicular skeletons. The axial skeleton consists of the bones of the head, thorax, and spine. The appendicular skeleton consists of the upper and lower extremity bones, including the shoulder girdle and the pelvis. The upper and lower extremities are affixed to the axial skeleton and articulate with multiple joints. Bones are classified according to shape and are labeled long, short, flat, irregular, or sesamoid.

Bones contain living cells called osteocytes, osteoblasts, and osteoclasts. These cells are involved in maintaining, building, and dissolving salt deposits and protein fibers as necessary. Bones have a constant supply of blood, which brings oxygen and removes carbon dioxide. Blood vessels enter and exit the bone through perforating canals, then travel lengthwise along the bone through small tubes called haversian canals. When blood supply is reduced, bone tissue will become ischemic and die.

The common long bone consists of a diaphysis, metaphysis, and epiphysis. The diaphysis is the hollow skeletal shaft of the long bone. It is covered by the periosteum, which contains sensory nerve fibers and initiates the bone repair cycle. The metaphysis is the transitional region between the diaphysis and the epiphysis. In this region, the thin layer of compact bone of the diaphysis shaft becomes the honeycomb of the weight-bearing epiphyseal region. The epiphysis is the articular end of the bone. Through the widening of the metaphysis and the cancellous bone underneath, the weight-bearing, articular surface distributes support over a large surface area. Within the diaphysis and epiphysis is a chamber called the medullary canal that is filled with yellow bone marrow. This area stores fat for energy. The larger long bones, pelvis, and sternum contain red bone marrow where erythrocytes are produced.

Bones join at an area called a joint, where they move together to permit articulation. Joints are classified according to the degree of movement they permit. Synarthroses are immovable joints. Amphiarthroses are joints that allow limited movement. Diarthroses permit relatively free movement and are further classified by the range of movement they allow. Ligaments are bands of connective tissue that attach bones to each other and surround a joint to form the joint capsule. Synovial fluid in the joint capsule and bursae lubricate the joint to reduce friction. The actual surface of movement is the articular surface. Cartilage, a smooth, shock-absorbing sponge, on the joint surface allows free movement between the two ends of the adjoining bones. Cartilage, unlike bone, cannot repair itself in the event of injury.

Muscles make up most of the body's mass, are the driving power behind body motion, and also produce most of the body's heat energy. There are three types of muscle tissue in the body—cardiac, smooth, and skeletal. The myocardium is composed of cardiac tissue. Smooth muscle is involuntary, controlled by the autonomic nervous system. Skeletal muscle is under somatic control. This type is most commonly injured in trauma. Skeletal muscles lie beneath the skin and subcutaneous fat. They are attached to bones in two locations by strong connective tissue called tendons. The point of attachment that remains stationary with muscle contraction is the origin, while the point of attachment that moves is the insertion. Because muscles can only contract, not lengthen, they are usually paired on each side of a joint. This arrangement, with one opposing the motion of the other, allows for flexion and extension. Even when at rest, muscles remain in a condition of slight contraction known as muscle tone. Muscle tone varies among individuals based on physical fitness, age, disease states, and other variables.

4. **Discuss the effects of aging on the musculoskeletal system.**   p. 157

Bones initially form in the embryo as loose cartilaginous tissue. This makes them extremely flexible but not self-supporting. Gradually, bones ossify and become firm and strong. Bones lengthen from the epiphyseal plate near the bone ends, an area where fracture may disrupt the growth process. With increasing age, children's bones become more rigid, but they are prone to fractures such as the greenstick, breaking and splintering on one side but not breaking completely. By the late teen years, the bone tissue reaches its maximum strength. The epiphyseal plates narrow and cartilage production ceases. As an adult reaches 40 years of age, bone degeneration begins. The bones become less flexible and more prone to fracture. They also heal more slowly. There may be progressive loss of body height and curvature of the spine. With advancing age and continuing bone degeneration, fractures may occur with normal stresses, especially at the high-stress points of the lumbar spine and the neck of the femur. The elderly are at higher risk for fracture from falls. Aging also results in degeneration of the cartilage between the ribs, causing shallower, more energy-consuming respiration. Degeneration of the intravertebral disks in the spine may result in herniation and shortening or stiffening of the trunk.

5. **Describe the pathophysiology of the following injury types:**   pp. 161–164

   a. **Muscular**—Muscular injury can be caused by blunt or penetrating mechanisms, overexertion, or decreased oxygen supply. Blunt trauma crushes muscle, damaging both muscle cells and their blood supply. Blood and fluid accumulate, causing swelling, pain, and erythema. If the tissue is compressed for an extended period of time, compartment syndrome may develop. Penetrating injuries may disrupt tendons and ligaments along with the muscle mass. This limits movement, requiring surgical intervention. Muscle fatigue and cramps occur as muscles use up available oxygen and

©2013 Pearson Education, Inc.
Paramedic Care: Principles & Practice, Vol. 5, 4th Ed.

energy reserves. Metabolic waste products build up, causing diminished strength and muscle contraction or spasm. Strains occur when muscle fibers are overstretched by forces exceeding their strength. Fibers are damaged and the injury is painful, but bleeding and edema are minimal.

    b. **Joint**—Joint injuries include sprain, subluxation, and dislocation. Sprains are caused by a tearing of the ligaments attached to a joint capsule. The joint is weakened and presents with inflammation and swelling. Sprains are classified according to the degree of tearing. A subluxation occurs when a bone end partially displaces from the joint during stress. This stretches the ligaments and reduces the joint's stability and mobility. When bones completely displace from the joint capsule the injury is termed a dislocation. Dislocations have associated ligament damage with potential joint capsule and articular cartilage injury as well. Nerves and blood vessels may also be damaged.

    c. **Bone**—A fracture is a break in the continuity of the bone. These may occur from direct or indirect injury. During indirect injury, the kinetic forces are transmitted away from the impact point, causing proximal damage. Fractures disrupt bone cells, collagen, blood vessels, and nerves along with the bone's inner (endosteum) and outer lining (periosteum). If the broken bone ends displace, additional injury may occur to muscles, tendons, and ligaments. Nonpenetrating fractures with intact skin are called closed fractures. If the outer skin surface is breached, the break is termed an open fracture. Open fractures carry a higher risk for infection. Hairline or impacted fractures may be relatively stable. Small cracks or compression weakens the bone but the bone remains in position and maintains some integrity. Further movement or stress, however, may fracture the remaining bone or displace bone ends. The exact nature of a fracture is determined by x-ray. Fractures may be straight, angulated, curved, or splintered. Prolonged or repeated stress may produce stress fractures. These are often seen in runners or those engaging in vigorous aerobic activity. The bone weakens and fractures from the repetitive application of modest forces. A rare, but severe, complication of bone injury is fat embolism. If the medullary canal is injured, fat may enter the venous system and travel to the heart and then into the pulmonary circulation, where it causes a pulmonary embolism.

6. **Describe special considerations in pediatric, geriatric, and sports-related orthopedic injuries.**
                                                      pp. 165, 170–171

Pediatric bones contain a greater percentage of cartilage than those of adults and are still growing from the epiphyseal plate. Due to the flexible nature of their bones, children are prone to partial fractures called greenstick or buckle fractures. In both types only one side of the bone is disrupted. Care must be taken in repairing the bone in a manner that minimizes growth asymmetry as the bone heals. Fractures of the growth plates can reduce or halt bone growth in that area. Due to increased metabolism and bone tissue replacement, fractures in children generally stabilize more quickly than in adults.

    Geriatric patients have bones that are less flexible, more brittle, and more easily fractured due to the aging process that decreases bone mass and collagen. Bones heal more slowly. Elderly patients are at risk for skeletal injury due to decreased muscle mass and coordination. Bones may also fracture in the absence of significant trauma. Osteoporosis and osteopenia both involve bone deterioration, with the former being more serious. These conditions may lead to spinal curvature and higher incidences of fracture.

    Athletes are prone to musculoskeletal injury often involving major body joints such as the shoulder, elbow, wrist, knee, and ankle. Injuries to tendons and ligaments can be serious enough to require surgery and may result in permanent limitations in sports participation or even limb mobility. Injured athletes should refrain from playing until they have been examined by a physician.

7. **Discuss the impact of inflammatory and degenerative conditions on the musculoskeletal system.**
                                                      pp. 166–167

Inflammatory and degenerative conditions may limit mobility and cause joint pain, tenderness, and fatigue. Common inflammatory diseases include bursitis, tendonitis, and arthritis. Bursitis is an inflammation of the synovial sacs (bursae), which reduce friction and cushion ligaments and tendons. The elbow, shoulder, and knee are most commonly affected. Tendonitis occurs from inflammation of the tendon and its protective sheath, typically from repetitive trauma. Upper and lower extremities are most commonly affected. Arthritis is joint inflammation caused by damage or destruction to the cartilage. Most forms result in varying degrees of pain, swelling, stiffness, joint immobility, and deformity. Osteoarthritis results from general degeneration of connective tissue, typically attributed to aging, and is the most common type. Rheumatoid arthritis is a chronic, systemic, and progressive disease of peripheral joint connective tissue. Septic arthritis occurs as a result of joint capsule infection. Gout and Lyme disease also cause joint inflammation. Gout results from an accumulation of uric acid crystals, whereas joint inflammation from Lyme disease is the result of an infectious agent that stimulates inflammatory agents.

8. **Given a variety of scenarios, demonstrate the assessment of musculoskeletal injuries.**   pp. 167–170

Musculoskeletal injuries are usually not life threatening or associated with the development of shock. They are usually evaluated during the rapid or focused trauma assessment. However, musculoskeletal injuries are common…in patients who have…other serious traumatic injury. They should not distract you from identifying and caring for life-threatening findings first. Follow the standard assessment process for all trauma patients. Consider mechanism of injury during the scene size-up to anticipate the nature and severity. Evaluate mental status, airway, and breathing first and look for evidence of hemorrhage. Consider spinal precautions and remember that musculoskeletal injuries can mask symptoms of spinal injury. Perform a rapid trauma assessment for patients with serious injury. Pay close attention to possible pelvic or femur fracture, as these may contribute to significant blood loss. Look for signs of tissue swelling and deformity. Palpate for crepitus, pain, and instability. Extremity fractures may disrupt blood vessels and nerves, compromising future use of a limb. Vascular damage may restrict distal blood flow to the limb, increasing capillary refill time, diminishing pulse strength and limb temperature, and causing discoloration and a "pins-and-needles" sensation. Nerve injury may result in paresthesia, loss of sensation, weakness, and loss of muscle control. Muscle or tendon damage may restrict limb mobility. Compartment syndrome may develop if muscle tissue is badly damaged and swells within the fascia. Use a four-pronged approach during your evaluation: expose, observe, question about, and palpate the injury. Expose the site by removing clothing and restrictive jewelry. Look for deformities, discolorations, soft tissue damage, and asymmetry or inequality in limb length. Observe for contamination or protruding bone. Palpate the bone for crepitus, instability, deformity, unusual motion, muscle tone, and areas of coolness or warmth. Check distal pulses, capillary refill, sensation, and movement. If distal circulation or innervation is interrupted by the injury, immediate intervention and rapid transport may be indicated. Question the patient about pain, pain with movement or touch, discomfort, or unusual feelings or sensations. Consider the "six Ps" when evaluating an extremity:

Pain. The patient with musculoskeletal injury may report pain, pain on touch (tenderness), or pain on movement of the injured limb.
Pallor. The skin at the injury site and distal to it may be pale or flushed and capillary refill may be delayed.
Paralysis. The patient may have inability to, or difficulty in, moving the limb
Paresthesia. The patient may report numbness or tingling in the affected extremity.
Pressure. The patient may experience a feeling of tension within the extremity.
Pulses. The distal pulses may be diminished or absent distal to the injury site.
A seventh P sometimes considered is poikilothermia, in which the limb may be cool to the touch.

Suspect compartment syndrome is any patient who has any paraesthesia; firm masses or increased skin tension at the injury site; who has pain out of proportion to the injury; or who has pain that increases when you move the limb.

During the exam, question the patient about any abnormal sounds or feelings they experienced during the injury, such as popping, tearing, or snapping. Evaluate pain severity on the 0–10 scale. Conclude your focused trauma assessment by identifying all injuries, prioritizing them, and establishing an order of management. Reassess musculoskeletal injuries frequently by monitoring distal sensation, motor function, capillary refill, and pulses.

©2013 Pearson Education, Inc.
Paramedic Care: Principles & Practice, Vol. 5, 4th Ed.

9. Adhere to the general principles of musculoskeletal injury management. pp. 171–173

The primary goals of musculoskeletal injury management are to prevent further injury and reduce patient discomfort. Open wounds should be covered with sterile dressings and bandaged. Proper limb alignment will increase circulation, minimize further damage, and enhance patient comfort. Extremity fractures can be gently aligned by applying axial traction to the distal limb while holding the proximal limb in position. Position the injured extremity in a position of function (halfway between flexion and extension) for splinting. This places the least stress on the joint ligaments and the muscles and tendons surrounding the injury. Dislocations or fractures within 3 inches of a joint should not be aligned unless distal circulation is compromised or transport is lengthy. Immobilizing musculoskeletal injuries prevents further injury, by restricting fractured bones ends from lacerating soft tissues, blood vessels, and nerves or dislodging clots. Immobilize the joint above and below the injury for both joint and midshaft fractures. If using circumferential wrapping to secure the splint, wrap from the distal point to a proximal one. Apply firm pressure when wrapping. Both prior to and following splinting, evaluate distal circulation, motor function, and sensation. Compare findings to the opposite limb. Frequently reassess neurovascular status. Apply local cooling to the injury using a cold pack wrapped in a towel. This helps to reduce local pain, inflammation, and swelling.

10. Given a variety of musculoskeletal injury scenarios, select and apply an appropriate splinting device. pp. 173–175

There are numerous devices available to immobilize musculoskeletal injuries. A splint should be chosen for ease in application, ability to immobilize the fracture or dislocation site (and the joint above and below), and patient comfort. Rigid splints are firm supports with padding built in or affixed. They are secured to the injury using tape, cravats, or bandaging circumferentially wrapped. Formable splints are constructed of malleable material that can be shaped to the contour of the injury and secured by wrapping circumferentially. Vacuum splints are employed for long-bone fractures. They are comprised of an airtight fabric bag filled with small plastic particles. The splint is applied to the injury and air is extracted, creating a firmly fixed shape around the injury. Soft splints use padding or air pressure and include devices such as air splints, pelvic slings, and pillows. Air splints are appropriate for extremity injuries; however, they should not be used for injuries at or above the knee or elbow, as they cannot immobilize the proximal limb joint. Pelvic slings are wrapped around the pelvis to contain, compress, and immobilize the injury. Pillow splints are used to enfold an ankle or foot, then wrapped circumferentially to secure. A traction splint is a frame that applies traction to a fractured femur. The splint prevents bone ends from overriding secondary to muscle spasm and reduces patient pain. Two primary types include the bipolar frame device (Hare, Fernotrac) and the unipolar (Sager) splint. In cases of multisystem trauma, splinting may be more rapidly accomplished by splinting limbs to the body or by simply immobilizing the patient on a spine board. For isolated injuries, slings and swaths can further limit motion after the injury is splinted. The following devices should be utilized only if they can accomplish the goals of splinting effectively:

Pelvis sling—long spine board with pelvic sling
Hip—long spine board, orthopedic stretcher
Femur—traction splint
Knee—padded board splints, ladder, vacuum, or other malleable splint
Tibia and fibula—padded board splints, air splint
Ankle—pillow splint, padded board splint, air splint
Foot—pillow splint, padded board splint, air splint, conforming splint
Shoulder—sling and swathe, ladder splint
Humerus—cuff and collar sling and swathe
Elbow—padded board splint, ladder, vacuum, or other malleable splint
Radius and ulna—padded board splint, air splint
Wrist—padded board splint, air splint
Hand—padded board splint, conforming splint, air splint
Finger—conforming splint, padded board splint

11. Describe special considerations in the management of fractures, joint injuries, and injuries of muscle and connective tissue. pp. 175–176

Fractures that occur near joints are likely to involve blood vessels, nerves, and joint capsules. Any fractures that occur within 3 inches of a joint should be treated as joint injuries. The limb should be immobilized in the position found unless there are circulatory or nerve deficits. In the latter case, attempt to correct the problem with gently repositioning. After one attempt, splint and transport the patient. Be sure to immobilize both the fracture site and adjacent joints. Upper extremities may be secured to the body and lower extremities to the opposite limb.

Joints should also be immobilized in the position found. Use a ladder, vacuum, or other malleable splint. Immobilize the injured joint and both the joint above and below the injury. You may also secure the limb to the body. In some cases reduction is appropriate. Be sure the injury is a dislocation. If transport is delayed or lengthy or neurovascular status distal to the injury is comprised, attempt reduction. This moves the displaced joint ends to their anatomical position. Consider analgesics before attempting the maneuver. If the reduction is successful you should hear a "pop" as the joint moves back into position and the patient should report reduced pain. The joint should become mobile shortly thereafter.

Musculoskeletal soft tissue injuries may be quite painful although they are rarely life threatening. Compartment syndrome, however, can produce severe disability. Deep contusions and hematomas can cause significant blood loss. Managing muscle, tendon, and ligament injuries requires immobilizing the surrounding region. Gentle circumferential bandaging can reduce hemorrhage, edema, and pain. Local cooling should be applied by wrapping a cold pack in a dressing or towel and applying to the injury. This reduces edema and patient discomfort. Place the limb in a position of function and elevate the extremity. Monitor distal neurovascular function.

12. Describe the special considerations in management of the following fractures: pp. 177–179

Pelvis. The pelvis is a large, strong, important supporting structure. Significant force is required to fracture this bone. Fractures may involve either the iliac crest or pelvic ring. Crest fractures are generally isolated and stable. Ring fractures are considered a high priority/critical injury. Injury to this area may result in significant hemorrhage, with potential for losses exceeding 2 liters. Circulation to one or both lower extremities may also be compromised. Suspect other internal or musculoskeletal injuries with pelvic fractures. Care is focused on stabilizing the pelvis and supporting the patient hemodynamically by administering normal saline to maintain a blood pressure of at least 80 mmHg.

Femur. The femur is the largest long bone of the body, and its fracture requires great energy, resulting in a serious and very traumatic injury. The injury is generally very painful, causing the large muscles of the thigh to contract and naturally splint the site. This action pushes the broken femur ends into the muscles of the thigh, increasing the pain and causing further muscle spasm. The patient may present with limb shortening and external rotation. Gentle traction can prevent further damage and pain from the femur movement and then relax the muscle masses, allowing the femur ends to move back to a more anatomical position. This enhances blood flow through the limb and reduces soft tissue injury caused by the overriding bones. Gentle traction is applied manually and then is maintained by a traction splint device. The traction splint should not be used if the patient has concurrent pelvic, knee, tibia, or foot injuries. Likewise, proximal fractures of the femur are considered hip fractures and traction splints are not indicated. If other injuries or the need for rapid transport preclude using a traction splint, immobilize the patient on a long spine board and consider using long padded rigid splints to secure the limb and tie that limb to the uninjured extremity.

Tibia/Fibula. The tibia is the most commonly injured leg bone, often causing an open wound. Fibular fractures frequently involve the knee or ankle. These often occur together. Compartment syndrome is a serious potential consequence. Immobilize the limb while applying gentle traction and frequently reassess circulation, sensation, and motor function.

Clavicle. The clavicle is the most frequently fractured bone in the body. Due to its proximity to the lungs and upper vasculature, serious internal injury may result. Patients may present with pain, a palpable deformity, and the shoulder shifted anteriorly. Immobilize with a sling and swathe or use a figure-eight dressing around the chest to gently pull the shoulders back.

©2013 Pearson Education, Inc.
Paramedic Care: Principles & Practice, Vol. 5, 4th Ed.

Humerus. Humerus fractures may be difficult to immobilize, as the proximal end is buried within the arm and shoulder muscles. Mechanical traction may disrupt blood flow through the axillary artery. Utilize a sling and swathe to immobilize the limb against the chest, ideally using a "cuff-and-collar" technique. Alternatively, apply a long, padded, rigid splint to the medial aspect of the upper extremity and secure it with circumferential wrapping.

Radius/Ulna. Fractures may occur anywhere along the length of the forearm and may involve both the radius and ulna. A fracture at the distal end of the radius is known as Colles' fracture, with the wrist turned up at an angle. The major concern is compromised distal circulation and nervous function. Splint forearm fractures with a padded, rigid splint supporting the hand and the arm. Place a large dressing in the palm to maintain it in a position of function. Bend the elbow across the chest and secure it with a sling and swathe.

13. **Describe the special considerations in management of the following joint injuries:**
pp. 179–182

Hip. Hip dislocations may dislocate anteriorly or posteriorly. An anterior dislocation presents with the foot turned out. The femur head may be palpable in the groin area. Posterior dislocations present with the knee flexed and foot rotated internally. The femur head is displaced into the buttocks. Posterior dislocations may be reduced in the field, whereas anterior dislocations generally require hospital management. Reductions should never be attempted if there are concomitant serious injuries such as pelvic fracture. Immobilize patients with hip dislocations to a long spine board and use padding to maintain patient comfort.

Knee. Knee injuries are serious and may compromise the ability to walk. Injuries may include fractures of the femur or tibia, patellar dislocations, or frank dislocation of the knee. Blood vessels may also be disrupted, interfering with distal circulation. Knee injuries should be immobilized in the position found using rigid or malleable splints. If distal circulation, sensation, or motor function is disrupted or transport time will exceed 2 hours, a reduction may be attempted. Success is noted by feeling the bone ends "pop" into place, allowing freer movement and a reduction in patient discomfort.

Ankle. Ankle injuries may present with gross deformity due to malleolar fracture or dislocation. Dislocations may occur anteriorly, posteriorly, or laterally, which is the most common. Sprains will not present with deformity. Attempt reduction if neurovascular compromise is evident. Otherwise, immobilize using air splints, rigid splints, or pillow splints. Apply cooling to ease pain and reduce swelling.

Foot. Foot injuries include fractures of the heel and toes or dislocations. Heel (calcanei) fractures typically result from falls. Maintain a high index of suspicion for bilateral foot injury and lumbar spine injury. Immobilize foot injuries with pillow, vacuum, ladder, or air splints. Monitor distal circulation, skin temperature, and color.

Shoulder. Shoulder injuries are often quite painful and may be difficult to immobilize. Fractures commonly involve the proximal humerus, lateral scapula, or distant clavicle. Dislocations may be anterior, in which the humeral head displaces forward, creating a "hollow" or "squared off" appearance. Posterior dislocations rotate the arm internally. The patient will generally hold the elbow and forearm away from the chest. Inferior dislocations present with the patient's arm locked above the head. Immobilize shoulder injuries in position found using splints, slings, swathes, and pillows for support as needed. Ladder or malleable splints are often a good choice. Only attempt reduction if pulse, sensation, or motor function distal to the injury is absent.

Elbow. Elbow injuries include fractures and dislocations. Neurovascular compromise is frequently associated with these injuries, as many nerves and vessels traverse this region. If neurovascular compromise is noted, the joint should be moved very gently and minimally to restore circulation. Immobilize with appropriate splinting and secure the limb to the chest, keeping the wrist slightly elevated to encourage venous return and reduce swelling and pain.

Wrist/Hand. Hand and wrist fractures usually result from direct trauma. Deformities may be quite obvious. Colles' fractures are common among athletes and children and will present with a "silver fork" appearance. Handle wrist and hand injuries gently to prevent or minimize vascular and neural damage.

Immobilize using rigid, vacuum, or air splints after placing a roll of dressing in the hand to maintain position of function. Elevate the wrist above the elbow to maximize venous return and reduce swelling.

Fingers/Toes. Fingers and toes may dislocate or fracture. Dislocations typically occur between phalanges or between the proximal phalanx and metacarpal. Although these injuries may be quite painful, they are generally not serious. Splint finger fractures using small tongue blades or malleable material or tape the finger to an adjoining finger (buddy taping). Toes can be effectively immobilized by buddy taping. Reductions are not generally indicated.

14. **Discuss considerations in pain management in the care of musculoskeletal injuries.** pp. 182–183

Musculoskeletal injuries can be extremely painful, with pain exacerbated by movement during splinting. Medications are frequently administered to reduce pain and anxiety. Diazepam, while not an analgesic, reduces patient perception and memory of pain. It may be used to premedicate prior to dislocation reduction. Administer 5–15 mg slow IV push into a large vein. Onset of action is rapid. Morphine is an opium alkaloid that reduces pain and anxiety. Because morphine is a vasodilator, it should not be used in patients who are hypotensive or hypovolemic. Side effects may include respiratory depression, nausea/vomiting, and a mild, red, itchy rash. Administer a 2-mg bolus slow IV push and repeat every few minutes as needed. Fentanyl is a potent opiate narcotic that has a very rapid onset of action. A benefit in trauma patients is that it does not cause hypotension to the same degree as morphine. The typical loading dose of fentanyl is 25 to 50 mcg IV. Repeat doses of 25 mcg may be provided as needed to control pain.

15. **Describe considerations for patients with musculoskeletal injuries who refuse treatment or transport.** p. 184

Patients with isolated sprain or strain injuries may refuse treatment and/or transport. In these instances, carefully assess the patient to ensure there are no other injury signs, symptoms, or complaints. Evaluate neurovascular status of the limb to confirm positive distal pulses, sensation, and motor function. Consider immobilizing the injury and referring the patient for x-rays and appropriate follow-up care. Document referrals to personal physicians and refusals carefully, ensuring that follow-up care is clearly communicated.

Case Study Review

Reread the case study on pages 150 and 151 in Paramedic Care: Trauma; *then, read the following discussion.*

This case identifies some of the important aspects of skeletal injury assessment and care. It also presents an elderly patient; elderly patients are common victims of long-bone injuries because of skeletal degeneration associated with advancing age.

The description of the events surrounding the injury of this 91-year-old patient is typical of the geriatric hip injury. Weakened with age, the femur can no longer withstand the stresses of articulation and it fractures. (These types of fractures frequently occur on steps, where stresses on the bone are somewhat increased.) As the bone gives way, the patient usually feels it snap and then falls. Because the injury is not of traumatic origin, the internal soft tissue damage is generally limited, and the patient may be relatively comfortable with the injury.

The primary assessment of Mary Herman reveals a hemodynamically stable elderly woman but an otherwise healthy patient with less pain than expected from a femur fracture. Because she is oriented and can speak well, Mark and Steffany feel that her airway and respirations are adequate. They quickly check her pulse rate and strength and move quickly to the focused trauma assessment. The assessment reveals an extremity that is aligned, but unstable, and only slightly painful. Further assessment reveals that the lower extremities have bilaterally equal distal pulses, color, temperature, sensation, and capillary refill times. This suggests that both innervation and circulation to the distal extremity are not compromised. Based on these findings, this patient is not a candidate for rapid transport and trauma center care. However, Mark and Steffany carefully monitor Mrs. Herman's extremity to detect any early signs of distal neurologic or vascular

©2013 Pearson Education, Inc.
Paramedic Care: Principles & Practice, Vol. 5, 4th Ed.

compromise. They also monitor her vital signs to track any early signs of shock because Mrs. Herman's age suggests she is not as able to compensate for blood loss as a younger adult might be. As a precaution, they initiate an IV line running "to keep open" but are ready to infuse a significant volume of fluid should the signs of shock appear.

Mark applies oxygen to ensure efficient respirations and the oximeter to ensure adequate oxygen delivery to the body cells. He also frequently auscultates the lung fields and evaluates respiration because emboli from the fracture site may travel there. The team also places an ECG on Mrs. Herman, as her age predisposes her to cardiac problems that may be exacerbated by this injury.

In the field of emergency care, this call might seem routine and anything but exciting. Care of minor "emergencies," especially those dealing with the elderly, are common. While to the paramedic there may be a desire to consider this call a "taxi ride," to the patient the injury threatens lifestyle and is an important life event. Mark and Steffany realize their responsibility to make Mary Herman as comfortable as possible, to provide the appropriate assessment and care, and to place emphasis on the patient's emotional support during care, packaging, and transport. She is treated with respect and consideration.

Content Self-Evaluation

MULTIPLE CHOICE

_____ 1. Musculoskeletal injuries can include injury to
  A. bones.
  B. tendons.
  C. ligaments.
  D. muscles.
  E. all of the above.

_____ 2. Which of the following is NOT a function performed by the musculoskeletal system?
  A. Vital organ protection
  B. A portion of the immune response
  C. Storage of material necessary for metabolism
  D. Hemopoietic activities
  E. Efficient movement against gravity

_____ 3. The bone cell responsible for maintaining bone tissue is the
  A. osteoblast.
  B. osteoclast.
  C. osteocyte.
  D. osteocrit.
  E. none of the above.

_____ 4. The bone cell responsible for dissolving bone tissue is the
  A. osteoblast.
  B. osteoclast.
  C. osteocyte.
  D. osteocrit.
  E. none of the above.

_____ 5. The central portion of a long bone is called the
  A. diaphysis.
  B. epiphysis.
  C. metaphysis.
  D. cancellous bone.
  E. compact bone.

_____ 6. The transitional area between the end and central portion of the long bone is called the
  A. diaphysis.
  B. epiphysis.
  C. metaphysis.
  D. cancellous bone.
  E. compact bone.

_____ 7. The type of bone tissue filling the end of the long bone is called the
  A. diaphysis.
  B. epiphysis.
  C. metaphysis.
  D. cancellous bone.
  E. compact bone.

8. The covering of the shaft of the long bones that initiates the bone repair cycle is the
    A. periosteum.
    B. peritoneum.
    C. perforating canal.
    D. osteocyte.
    E. epiphysis.

9. Immovable joints such as those of the skull are termed
    A. synovial.
    B. synarthroses.
    C. amphiarthroses.
    D. diarthroses.
    E. A or D.

10. The smooth, flexible structures that act as the actual articular surface of joints are the
    A. bursae.
    B. tendons.
    C. ligaments.
    D. cartilages.
    E. synovials.

11. The elbow is an example of which type of joint?
    A. Monaxial
    B. Biaxial
    C. Triaxial
    D. Synarthrosis
    E. Amphiarthrosis

12. Bands of strong material that stretch and hold the joint together while permitting movement are the
    A. bursae.
    B. tendons.
    C. ligaments.
    D. cartilage.
    E. metaphyses.

13. The small sacs filled with synovial fluid that reduce friction and absorb shock are the
    A. bursae.
    B. tendons.
    C. ligaments.
    D. cartilage.
    E. metaphyses.

14. The most commonly fractured bone in the body is the
    A. femur.
    B. pelvis.
    C. clavicle.
    D. humerus.
    E. scapula.

15. Which of the following is a bone of the upper arm?
    A. Humerus
    B. Radius
    C. Olecranon
    D. Phalanges
    E. Carpal

16. Which of the following is a bone of the palm of the hand?
    A. Humerus
    B. Radius
    C. Olecranon
    D. Phalanges
    E. Metacarpal

17. Which of the following is the bone of the thigh?
    A. Tarsal
    B. Tibia
    C. Fibula
    D. Femur
    E. Phalanges

18. Skeletal maturity is reached by age
    A. 6.
    B. 10.
    C. 20.
    D. 40.
    E. 45.

19. The muscular system consists of about how many muscle groups?
    A. 100
    B. 200
    C. 300
    D. 500
    E. 600

©2013 Pearson Education, Inc.
Paramedic Care: Principles & Practice, Vol. 5, 4th Ed.

_____ **20.** The muscle attachment to the bone that moves when the muscle mass contracts is the
  A. flexor.
  B. extensor.
  C. origin.
  D. insertion.
  E. articulation.

_____ **21.** More than half the energy created by muscle motion is in the form of heat energy.
  A. True
  B. False

_____ **22.** Contusion can account for significant fluid loss into the more massive muscles of the body.
  A. True
  B. False

_____ **23.** A specific sign associated with compartment syndrome is
  A. deep pain.
  B. absent distal pulses.
  C. pain when flexing the foot.
  D. absent distal sensation.
  E. diaphoresis.

_____ **24.** The condition in which exercise draws down the supply of oxygen and energy reserves and metabolic waste products accumulate, limiting the ability of a muscle group to perform is called
  A. cramp.
  B. fatigue.
  C. strain.
  D. sprain.
  E. spasm.

_____ **25.** The tissue that is normally damaged in a sprain is the
  A. tendon.
  B. ligament.
  C. muscle.
  D. articular cartilage.
  E. epiphyseal plate.

_____ **26.** The overstretching of a muscle that presents with pain is a
  A. strain.
  B. sprain.
  C. cramp.
  D. spasm.
  E. subluxation.

_____ **27.** Which of the following fractures is relatively stable?
  A. Hairline
  B. Impacted
  C. Transverse
  D. Comminuted
  E. Both A and B

_____ **28.** Which of the following fractures is most likely to be open?
  A. Fibula
  B. Tibia
  C. Femur
  D. Humerus
  E. Ulna

_____ **29.** In serious long-bone fractures, especially those that are manipulated after injury, there is the possibility of fat embolizing and becoming lodged in the lungs.
  A. True
  B. False

_____ **30.** Which of the following types of fractures is likely to occur only in the pediatric patient?
  A. Greenstick
  B. Oblique
  C. Transverse
  D. Comminuted
  E. Spiral

_____ **31.** The bones of the elderly are likely to be
  A. less flexible.
  B. more brittle.
  C. more easily fractured.
  D. more slow to heal.
  E. all of the above.

32. The dislocation, or fracture, in the area of a joint is generally less significant than the long-bone shaft fracture because it does not have as high an incidence of vascular and nervous injury.
   A. True
   B. False

33. The energy and degree of manipulation needed to cause further injury after a bone has broken are much less than was initially needed to cause the fracture.
   A. True
   B. False

34. The growth of bone that comes after a fracture and encapsulates the fracture site is called the
   A. epiphyseal outgrowth.
   B. periosteum.
   C. callus.
   D. natural splinting.
   E. comminution.

35. Which of the following is caused by a buildup of uric acid crystals in the joints?
   A. Gout
   B. Rheumatoid arthritis
   C. Osteoarthritis
   D. Bursitis
   E. Tendinitis

36. An inflammation of the small synovial sacs that reduces friction and cushions tendons from trauma is
   A. gout.
   B. rheumatoid arthritis.
   C. osteoarthritis.
   D. bursitis.
   E. tendinitis.

37. Which of the following is an indication for fluid resuscitation in the patient with skeletal injury?
   A. Pelvic fracture
   B. Serious tibial fracture
   C. Femur fracture
   D. Hip dislocation
   E. Both A and C

38. With which of these fractures should you consider immediate transport of the patient because of possible internal blood loss?
   A. Humerus
   B. Femur
   C. Tibia
   D. Pelvis
   E. Both B and D

39. When assessing a limb for possible fracture, you should examine distally for
   A. sensation.
   B. motor strength.
   C. circulation.
   D. crepitus.
   E. all of the above.

40. A patient complains of a deep burning pain out of proportion with the apparent injury, and a serious crushing-type mechanism has caused his calf to feel "almost board hard." What injury would you suspect?
   A. Tibial fracture
   B. Muscular contusion
   C. Compartment syndrome
   D. Tendinitis
   E. Subluxation

41. An elderly patient who has suffered a fracture because of bone degeneration is expected to experience what level of pain when compared to a traumatic fracture?
   A. About the same
   B. More pain
   C. Less pain
   D. No pain at all
   E. Extreme pain

©2013 Pearson Education, Inc.
Paramedic Care: Principles & Practice, Vol. 5, 4th Ed.

_____ 42. As the effects of the fight-or-flight response wear off, the symptoms of fracture will become less evident.
A. True
B. False

_____ 43. It is essential to tell the patient that limb alignment will cause some increased pain because this will help maintain his confidence in you.
A. True
B. False

_____ 44. In general, long-bone shaft fractures should be splinted
A. aligned, except if resistance is experienced.
B. as found.
C. extended, except if resistance is experienced.
D. flexed, except if resistance is experienced.
E. none of the above.

_____ 45. Any fracture within 3 inches of the joint should be treated the same way as a dislocation.
A. True
B. False

_____ 46. Which of the following limb positions is ideal for the immobilization of most extremity injuries?
A. Extended
B. Flexed
C. Hyperextended
D. Hyperflexed
E. Neutral

_____ 47. Ascending to altitude in a helicopter will cause the pressure in the air splint to
A. increase.
B. decrease.
C. remain the same.
D. become less uniform.
E. become more uniform.

_____ 48. The traction splint is designed to splint which musculoskeletal injury?
A. Knee dislocation
B. Hip dislocation
C. Pelvic fracture
D. Midshaft femur fracture
E. All of the above

_____ 49. Which of the following is a disadvantage of the vacuum splint when applying it to splint fractures?
A. It is difficult to apply.
B. It is bulky and heavy.
C. It shrinks slightly during application.
D. It takes more than two rescuers to apply.
E. All of the above.

_____ 50. Align a seriously angulated long-bone fracture unless
A. there is an absent distal pulse.
B. there is absent sensation.
C. both sensation and pulses are intact.
D. you meet with resistance.
E. you feel crepitus.

_____ 51. If after moving a limb to alignment you notice the distal pulse is absent, you should
A. splint the limb as is.
B. gently move the limb to restore the pulse.
C. return the limb to the original position.
D. elevate the limb and then splint it.
E. splint and apply an ice pack.

52. With joint injury you should not move the limb, even to restore circulation or sensation.
    A. True
    B. False

53. Early reduction of a dislocation usually results in which of the following?
    A. Less stress on the ligaments
    B. Less stress on the joint structure
    C. Better distal circulation
    D. Better distal sensation
    E. All of the above

54. Signs that a reduction of a dislocation has been effective include
    A. feeling a "pop."
    B. patient reports of less pain.
    C. greater mobility in the joint.
    D. less deformity of the joint.
    E. all of the above.

55. Heat may be applied to a muscular injury
    A. immediately.
    B. after 1 hour.
    C. after 24 hours.
    D. after 48 hours.
    E. not at all.

56. The splinting device recommended for a painful and isolated fracture of the femur is
    A. the vacuum splint.
    B. the ladder splint.
    C. the spine board and padding.
    D. long padded board splints.
    E. none of the above.

57. The splinting device recommended for a painful and isolated fracture of the tibia is the
    A. traction splint.
    B. malleable splint.
    C. long spine board and padding.
    D. padded board splint.
    E. sling and swathe.

58. The splinting device(s) recommended for an isolated fracture of the humerus is (are) the
    A. traction splint.
    B. sling and swathe.
    C. air splint.
    D. padded board splint.
    E. both B and D.

59. The fracture of the forearm close to the wrist that presents with the "silver fork" deformity is called:
    A. Richardson's fracture.
    B. Colles' fracture.
    C. Volkman's contracture.
    D. Blundot's inversion.
    E. none of the above.

60. An anterior hip dislocation normally presents with the
    A. foot turned outward.
    B. foot turned inward.
    C. knee flexed.
    D. knee turned outward.
    E. knee turned inward.

61. In general, anterior dislocations of the hip can be reduced in the prehospital setting.
    A. True
    B. False

62. Which of the following is NOT a sign of patellar dislocation?
    A. Knee in the flexed position
    B. Significant joint deformity
    C. Extremity drops at the knee
    D. Lateral displacement of the patella
    E. None of the above

63. If a patient presents with an ankle deformed with the foot turned to the side, you would suspect which type of ankle dislocation?
    A. Anterior
    B. Posterior
    C. Lateral
    D. Medial
    E. Inferior

©2013 Pearson Education, Inc.
Paramedic Care: Principles & Practice, Vol. 5, 4th Ed.

_____ **64.** If a patient presents with an ankle deformed with the foot pointing upward, you should suspect which type of ankle dislocation?
  A. Anterior
  B. Posterior
  C. Lateral
  D. Medial
  E. Inferior

_____ **65.** When a patient's shoulder appears "squared-off," the patient complains of severe pain, and she cannot move her arm, you should suspect what type of shoulder dislocation?
  A. Anterior
  B. Inferior
  C. Superior
  D. Posterior
  E. Lateral

_____ **66.** The elbow dislocation is a simple injury but one that is essential to reduce in the field.
  A. True
  B. False

_____ **67.** Which of the following injuries can be adequately splinted by using the short padded board splint, placing the hand in the position of function, and slinging and swathing the extremity?
  A. Radial fractures
  B. Ulnar fractures
  C. Wrist fractures
  D. Finger fractures
  E. All of the above

_____ **68.** Morphine in the prehospital setting
  A. reduces anxiety.
  B. reduces the perception of pain.
  C. sedates the patient.
  D. may cause respiratory depression.
  E. all of the above.

_____ **69.** Which of the following is NOT an analgesic that is used to control the pain of musculoskeletal injuries?
  A. Meperidine
  B. Morphine
  C. Nalbuphine
  D. Diazepam
  E. Astramorph

_____ **70.** The "I" within the acronym RICE used by athletic trainers stands for
  A. immobilization.
  B. ice for the first 48 hours.
  C. instability.
  D. intensity of pain.
  E. both A and B.

Special Projects

Recognizing Bones and Bone Injuries

I. Write the names of the bones marked with letters on the accompanying diagram of the human skeleton.

A. _____

B. _____

C. _____

D. _____

E. _____

F. _____

G. _____

H. _____

I. _____

J. _____

AXIAL SKELETON

APPENDICULAR SKELETON

Skull
- Cranium
- Face

A

Ribs

Vertebral
column

B

G

Clavicle

C

D

E

F

Pelvis

Carpals

H

Phalanges

Femur

Patella

I

J

Tarsals

Metatarsals

Phalanges

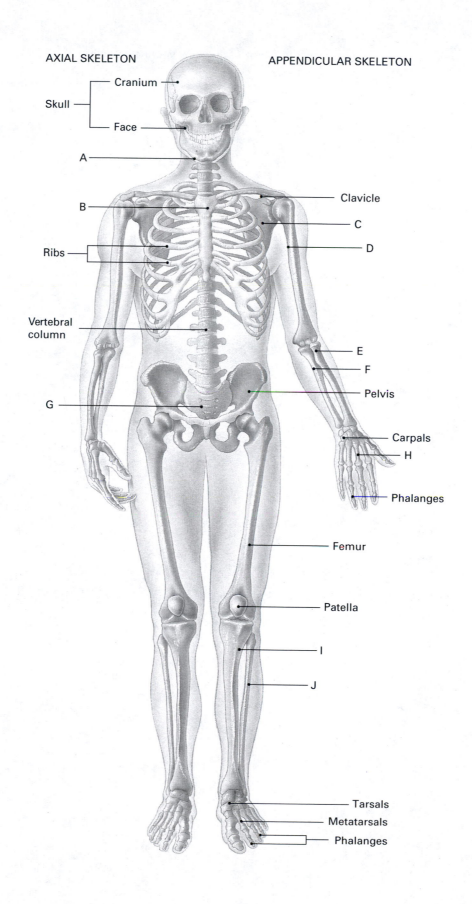

II. Write the names of the types of fractures illustrated in the accompanying pictures.

A. _____

B. _____

C. _____

D. _____

E. _____

F. _____

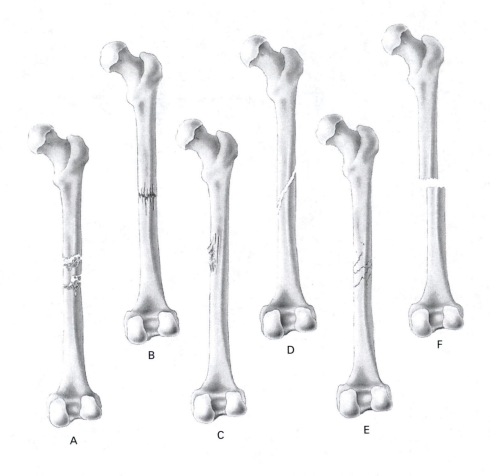

Drugs Used for Musculoskeletal Injuries

Emergency management for musculoskeletal injuries utilizes many of the pharmacological agents that are available to the paramedic. Please review and memorize the various names/classes, descriptions, indications, contraindications, precautions, and dosages/routes for the following, with special attention to those used in your system. Use the drug flash cards found at the back of the Workbook for Volume 1.

Diazepam

Morphine

Fentanyl

Nalbuphine

8

Thoracic Trauma

Review of Chapter Objectives

After reading this chapter, you should be able to:

1. Define key terms introduced in this chapter.

Knowing and being able to apply the key terms in each chapter is critical to understanding chapter concepts. Write the list of key terms. Then write the definition of each one in your own words. Check your understanding by confirming the definitions in the text glossary. Correct any misunderstandings. Create a study aid by writing each key term on the front of an index card and the definition on the back. Use the cards to quiz yourself, or to have someone quiz you.

2. Discuss the anatomy and physiology of the thorax and the structures within it.

pp. 189–192

The ribs, thoracic spine, sternum, and diaphragm define the structure of the thoracic cage. The skeletal components allow the cage to expand as the ribs are lifted upward and outward by contraction of the intercostal muscles, and the intrathoracic volume further expands as the diaphragm contracts and moves downward. The net action of this muscle movement is to increase the volume of the thoracic cage and to reduce its internal pressure. Air from the environment moves through the airway into the alveoli to equalize this pressure, and inspiration occurs. The intercostal muscles relax and the thorax settles, while the diaphragm rises back into the thorax and the volume of the cavity decreases. This increases the intrathoracic pressure, and air rushes out to equalize with the environment. This is expiration. The pleura, two serous membranes, seal the lungs to the interior of the thoracic cage during this action and ensure that the lungs expand and contract with the changing volume of the thoracic cavity. The lungs have exceptional circulation, with capillary beds surrounding the alveoli to ensure a free exchange of oxygen and carbon dioxide between the alveolar air and the bloodstream.

The lungs fill all but the central portion of the chest cavity and are found on either side of the central structure, called the mediastinum. The mediastinum contains the heart, trachea, esophagus, major blood vessels, and several nerve pathways. The heart is located in the left central chest and is the major pumping element of the cardiovascular system. The inferior and superior vena cavae collect blood from the lower extremities and abdomen and the upper extremities, head, and neck, respectively, and return it to the heart. The pulmonary arteries and veins carry blood to and from the lungs, respectively, and the aorta distributes the cardiac output to the systemic circulation. The trachea enters the mediastinum just beneath the manubrium and bifurcates at the carina into the left and right mainstem bronchi. The esophagus enters the mediastinum just behind the trachea and exits through the diaphragm.

3. **Describe the pathophysiology of blunt and penetrating thoracic trauma.** pp. 192–193

As in other regions of the body, thoracic trauma results from either blunt or penetrating mechanisms of injury. Blunt trauma may result from deceleration (as in an auto crash), crushing mechanism (as in a building collapse), or blast injury (as with an explosion). Blast injuries result from pressure waves traveling through the body. This pressure can be especially damaging to air-filled structures. Mechanisms may cause respiratory system injuries or vascular tears leading to hemorrhage, pneumothoraces, and air embolism. When the body is compressed between an object and a hard surface, a crush injury may occur. Crushing mechanisms may cause damage to the chest wall, diaphragm, heart, or tracheobronchial tree. Deceleration injuries occur when the body is in motion and impacts a fixed object. Injury occurs from the direct force as well as organs striking the internal thoracic cavity. Shear forces may cause organs to rip from their points of fixation. Deceleration mechanisms can disrupt the myocardium, great vessels, and tracheobronchial tree. Rapid chest compression against a closed glottis may cause the "paper-bag" syndrome,

Penetrating trauma results in direct injury as well as secondary injury from the cavitational wave forces of a projectile. Any structure within the thorax may be damaged, with injury to the heart and great vessels most likely to be lethal. Lung tissue is rather resilient and suffers limited injury with a high-energy projectile, while the heart and great vessels may rupture because fluid transmits kinetic energy better than air. Slower-velocity penetrating objects result in damage that is limited to the actual pathway of the object. Penetrating trauma often leads to pneumothorax, which may be bilateral depending on the track of the object.

4. **Describe the pathophysiology, assessment, and management of the following types of thoracic injuries:**

a. **Chest Wall Injuries** pp. 194–196

Blunt chest trauma commonly results in closed chest wall injury, while penetrating mechanisms cause open wounds with damage to underlying structures. An intact chest wall is necessary to create the positive and negative pressure necessary for effective ventilation. Chest wall contusions involve damaged soft tissue covering the thoracic cage. Patients typically present with pain, worsened by deep breathing, and limited chest expansion. Auscultation may reveal limited breath sounds. Redness and bruising may be apparent with tenderness noted on palpation. Rib fractures are found in over half of patients sustaining serious blunt trauma. Ribs may fracture in multiple places. As the ribs compress and flex they are subject to break at the weakest points. Fractures may also be evident at the point of impact or at a point remote from the injury site. Patients generally present with significant pain and limited chest wall excursion, which leads to hypoxia, hypoventilation, and muscle spasms at the fracture site. Fractures of the sternum result from significant impact. Often, underlying cardiac injury is present, including cardiac rupture, pericardial tamponade, and pulmonary contusion.

A flail chest occurs when three or more adjacent ribs fracture in two or more places. Respirations cause the bones to move, causing further muscle and soft tissue damage. In this injury the flail segment will move in the opposite direction of the rest of the chest, compromising ventilation, increasing respiratory effort, and displacing the mediastinum away from the injury. Flail chest is often associated with severe underlying pulmonary or other internal injury. Assessment may reveal crepitus with chest wall movement or palpation. Deformity may be noticeable. Care is directed at maintaining respiratory status by providing high-concentration oxygen and administering positive-pressure ventilation or intubation as needed.

b. **Pulmonary Injuries** pp. 196–200

Pulmonary injuries are caused by blunt or penetrating mechanisms that injure lung tissue or the system that holds the lung to the thoracic cavity. Injuries include simple, open, and tension pneumothorax, hemothorax, and pulmonary contusion. Simple pneumothorax occurs when air escapes into the pleural cavity through ruptured airways. A rib fracture may puncture a lung or the alveoli may rupture from chest impact. In a small, simple pneumothorax, the pressure within the chest cavity does not build up enough to collapse the lung or cause a mediastinal shift. The patient may present with no apparent signs or symptoms. An increasingly larger pneumothorax will present along a continuum from mild dyspnea to severe dyspnea and hypoxia if the lung collapses. Tachypnea, local chest pain, and diminished lung sounds may also be present. Open pneumothorax

©2013 Pearson Education, Inc.
Paramedic Care: Principles & Practice, Vol. 5, 4th Ed.

is like simple pneumothorax, though in this case the injury penetrates the thoracic wall. High-velocity bullets or shotgun blasts at close range are often responsible. The injury must be significantly large in order for air to move into and out of the wound during inspiration and expiration. This causes the characteristic "sucking" sound. Air passage and hemorrhage may produce frothy blood around the opening. The patient typically presents with tachypnea and hypoxia. Any simple or open pneumothorax may develop into a tension pneumothorax if the pressure in the thorax exceeds the atmospheric pressure. The increasing pressure prevents air from escaping during exhalation. Eventually, the lung on the side of the injury collapses, causing intercostal and suprasternal bulging. Pressure on the mediastinum causes a shift away from the injured lung. The uninjured lung and vena cava become compressed, reducing cardiac output. At this stage the patient will present with jugular venous distention, a narrowed pulse pressure, possible tracheal deviation, and severe hypoxia.

A hemothorax is a collection of blood in the pleural space. It may occur with or without pneumothorax. It is frequently associated with rib fractures and other blunt or penetrating trauma mechanisms. Hemothorax generally becomes a hypovolemic problem before it seriously endangers respiration. The patient may experience dyspnea or even respiratory failure along with the signs and symptoms of hypovolemic shock. A pulmonary contusion is soft tissue damage to the lungs resulting from deceleration with blunt chest impact and pressure waves from an explosion or bullet. Both cause alveolar/capillary membrane disruption, leading to microhemorrhage and edema. Pulmonary contusions may range from minor to life threatening depending on the degree of compression, stretch, and shear of tissue. The lungs become less compliant, making ventilation more difficult. The increasing thickness of the alveolar wall raises pulmonary pressure, increasing cardiac workload. These factors in combination can lead to atelectasis, hypovolemia, hypoxemia, hypotension, and possibly respiratory failure and shock. Signs and symptoms may be slow to appear. The patient may present with increasing shortness of breath, increased respiratory effort, and gradually progressing hypoxia. Auscultation may reveal diminished breath sounds with crackles. Oxygen saturation may fall and the patient may cough up blood. Care for pulmonary injuries is aimed at managing oxygenation and ventilation. If tension pneumothorax develops, chest needle decompression is required.

c. **Cardiovascular Injuries**   pp. 200–203

Cardiovascular injuries secondary to chests lead to the greatest mortality. They generally involve blunt cardiac injury causing cardiac contusion or vascular trauma resulting in significant hemorrhage or cardiac collapse. Blunt cardiac injury occurs most commonly from severe anterior chest trauma. Blunt forces cause the heart to become compressed between the sternum and thoracic spine, resulting in muscle tearing, stretching, hemorrhage, and edema. Cardiac output may be reduced and arrhythmias may be present. Patients may complain of chest pain. Pericardial tamponade restricts cardiac filling due to pressure produced by blood in the pericardial sac. It is generally the result of penetrating injury. Accumulating blood puts pressure on the heart, limiting chamber filling. This leads to decreased cardiac output and systemic hypotension. Pulse strength will diminish, pulse pressure will narrow, and jugular venous distention may be apparent. Heart tones may be muffled or distant. Myocardial aneurysm or rupture occurs almost exclusively with blunt trauma. Any part of the heart may be damaged. Patients may present with pericardial tamponade or heart failure if the valves are involved. Rupture is usually fatal. Aortic dissection or rupture is usually associated with high-speed automobile crashes. Shear forces cause the arterial layers of the aorta to separate, typically at its fixation points. Blood, under high pressure, begins dissecting the vessel causing rupture. Once ruptured, the patient will by severely hypotensive. The patient may complain of severe, tearing chest pain and present with pulse deficits between the left and right upper extremities. Care is aimed at supporting circulation by administering IV fluids to maintain a systolic blood pressure of 80 mmHg.

d. **Injuries to the diaphragm, esophagus, and tracheobronchial tree**   pp. 203–204

Diaphragmatic injury is usually due to severe compression of the abdomen during blunt abdominal trauma or penetrating trauma along the border of the rib cage. With penetrating trauma to the lower chest the diaphragm is at risk because it moves up and down with respiration. Injury may result in herniation of abdominal organs into the chest cavity, most commonly the bowel. Misplaced abdominal contents place pressure on the lung and mediastinal structures, moving them toward the opposite side of the injury. The injury may present similarly to tension pneumothorax as the abdominal contents displace the lung tissue, and patients may present with dyspnea, hypoxia, hypotension, and jugular venous distension (JVD). Esophageal injury does not usually present with acute symptoms other than a history of penetrating trauma to the central chest. Perforation may permit food, drink, or gastric contents to enter the mediastinum, where it either forms an excellent medium for infection (with gastric contents) or damages some of the structures within. The patient may complain of difficulty swallowing, chest pain with respiration, and pain radiating to the midback. Tracheobronchial injuries are usually related to penetrating trauma to the upper mediastinum. The injuries permit air to enter the mediastinum and possibly the neck. The patient will have dyspnea (possibly severe) and may have subcutaneous emphysema. Positive pressure ventilation may make matters worse because air is then actively "pushed" into the mediastinal space. The patient may also experience pneumothorax and tension pneumothorax. General care for patients with diaphragmatic, esophageal, or tracheobronchial injury requires surgical intervention. Priority care entails airway management along with ensuring removal of blood and fluids to avoid aspiration. Patients should be carefully monitored for development of tension pneumothorax and decompressed if necessary. Positive pressure ventilation should be done carefully so as not to worsen the condition.

e. Traumatic asphyxia pp. 204–205

Traumatic asphyxia is a crushing-type injury in which the crushing mechanism remains in place and restricts both respiration and venous return to the central circulation. The patient may display bulging eyes, petechial hemorrhage, and red or blue skin above the level of compression. The injury may damage many internal blood vessels but tamponades hemorrhage because of the continuing compression. Once the compression is released, accumulated toxins return to central circulation. In conjunction with profound hypovolemia the patient may rapidly deteriorate. Fluid resuscitation and possible administration of sodium bicarbonate are mainstays of treatment.

5. **Given a variety of scenarios, demonstrate the assessment and management of patients with thoracic injuries, including specific management of the following:** pp. 194–212

Assessment of patients with chest injury follows the standard assessment process. Careful primary assessment, however, is crucial, as chest injury often rapidly results in life-threatening airway and circulatory conditions. Serious signs and symptoms must be immediately managed as they become apparent. Carefully assess patients for dyspnea, asymmetrical, paradoxical, exaggerated, or limited chest movement or hyperinflation. Check for retractions, accessory muscle use, and tracheal deviation. Subcutaneous emphysema may be evident in the face or neck. Examine skin color for cyanosis, ashen, or dark red or blue discoloration. Monitor pulse oximetry and capnography. Maintain a high index of suspicion for internal injury and hemorrhage.

Chest injury may induce cardiac arrhythmias so attach the electrocardiogram (ECG) electrodes and monitor carefully. Use techniques of palpation, auscultation, and percussion while performing the rapid trauma assessment. Feel for swelling, deformity, crepitus, or crackling. Listen for lung sounds and adequacy of air movement. Auscultate the heart, noting distant or muffled sounds. Percuss the chest to assess for air and/or fluid accumulation. Remember that blunt or penetrating trauma manifests in different signs and symptoms. Vital signs must be frequently reassessed to ensure early recognition of shock. General management focuses on ensuring good oxygenation, adequate ventilation, and cardiovascular support. Be alert to the possibility of problems related to interventions. Positive pressure ventilation may induce tension pneumothorax. Aggressive fluid resuscitation may worsen hemorrhage or cause pulmonary edema.

a. Rib fracture pp. 194–195, 209

Pain induced by rib fractures may limit respiratory effort and lead to hypoventilation. Atelectasis may occur as the patient hypoventilates, further reducing gas exchange. Assessment may reveal overlying chest wall contusions with crepitus noted on palpation. Be alert for internal injuries caused by jagged rib ends. The liver or spleen may be injured, with serious hemorrhage. Laceration of the intercostal artery can result in hemothorax, while intercostal nerve damage may cause focal neurologic deficits of the affected muscle. Ensure oxygenation and ventilation as needed. Consider administering analgesics to improve chest excursion.

©2013 Pearson Education, Inc.
Paramedic Care: Principles & Practice, Vol. 5, 4th Ed.

b. **Sternoclavicular dislocation**   pp. 195, 209

Although dislocation at the sternoclavicular joint is uncommon, lateral compression mechanisms may cause this injury. The clavicle may dislocate anteriorly or posteriorly. Protruding or depressed deformities may be evident. These injuries may compress or lacerate underlying vessels or damage the trachea or esophagus. The patient will have a history of blunt chest trauma and may complain of chest pain similar to that of a myocardial infarction. Administer oxygen, monitor the heart with an ECG, and watch the patient very carefully. If the patient is in significant respiratory distress despite supportive oxygen therapy, consider dislocation reduction.

c. **Flail chest**   pp. 195–196, 209

Patients will typically experience significant pain from multiple rib fractures and may present with chest wall splinting. Stabilize the injury with a large, bulky dressing with bandaging. Provide high-concentration oxygen and monitor pulse oximetry and end-tidal carbon dioxide (CO_2). Positive pressure ventilation or endotracheal intubation may be necessary. Monitor cardiac activity with ECG. Consider the flail chest patient a candidate for rapid transport.

d. **Open pneumothorax**   pp. 197, 209–210

Patients may present with dyspnea and a "sucking" sound or frothy blood around the opening as air moves into and out of the chest. Cover the wound with an occlusive dressing taped on three sides to prevent further progress of the pneumothorax. Provide high-concentration oxygen and monitor the patient for the development of tension pneumothorax. If the patient's respiratory status declines, remove the occlusive dressing to allow air to escape, then reseal the wound.

e. **Tension pneumothorax**   pp. 197–199, 210

The side of the chest with the injury becomes hyperinflated, hyperresonant to percussion, with bulging intercostal tissue. Lung sounds will be diminished progressing to absent. The patient may be cyanotic, diaphoretic, and hypotensive with JVD. Perform a chest needle decompression by inserting a 14-gauge catheter into the 2nd intercostal space. Provide oxygen with a nonrebreather mask or bag-valve mask (BVM) and intubate if needed. Monitor the patient closely for a recurring tension pneumothorax. Without intervention this will be fatal.

f. **Hemothorax**   pp. 199, 210

Lung sounds will be normal except directly over the accumulating fluid. Lung percussion over the area filled with fluid will be dull with muffled, distant breath sounds. Administer fluid to maintain a systolic blood pressure of 80 mmHg. Consider positive pressure ventilation or continuous positive airway pressure (CPAP) if the patient's respiratory status worsens.

g. **Blunt cardiac injury**   pp. 200–201, 211

Patients will likely present with a complaint of chest or retrosternal pain. The cardiac electrical system may be disturbed, presenting with a variety of atrial or ventricular arrhythmias. There may be other serious sequelae, such as pericardial tamponade, congestive heart failure, cardiogenic shock, or myocardial rupture. Initiate cardiac monitoring, provide oxygen therapy, and treat with cardiac medications per advanced cardiac life support protocol. Rapidly transport.

h. **Pericardial tamponade**   pp. 201–202, 211

As the pericardial sac fills with blood, pulse strength diminishes, pulse pressure decreases, and jugular veins become distended. The patient will be agitated, tachycardic, diaphoretic, and ashen in appearance. Cyanosis may be noted along with Beck's triad. Pulsus paradoxus or pulsus alternans may be noticed. In extreme cases the patient may be in pulseless electrical activity (PEA). Provide oxygen and IV fluid. Definitive, life-saving care is insertion of a needle into the pericardial sac and the withdrawal of fluid, so any patient suspected of this injury requires immediate transport to the closest hospital.

i. **Aortic dissection**   pp. 203, 211

Aortic dissection is an extremely life-threatening injury. Because a dissection may imminently rupture, rapid, gentle handling and transport is indicated. Patients may complain of severe tearing chest pain radiating to the back. A pulse deficit between the left and right upper extremities and/or reduced pulse strength in the lower extremities may be apparent. Blood pressure may by high or low. Conservatively administer IV fluid to maintain a systolic blood pressure of 80 mmHg. Provide aggressive fluid and cardiac resuscitation in the event of rupture. Calm and reassure the patient.

j. Tracheobronchial injury   pp. 204, 212

Tracheobronchial injury is a rare, but often fatal condition. Patients may present with severe respiratory distress, cyanosis, hemoptysis, and occasionally massive subcutaneous emphysema. Care includes provision of high-concentration oxygen and suctioning of blood and secretions. If intubation is required, monitor carefully for development of tension pneumothorax while providing positive pressure ventilation. Rapidly transport the patient for surgical intervention.

k. Traumatic asphyxia   pp. 204–205, 212

Severe thoracic compression engorges veins and capillaries of the head and neck, causing classical discoloration. The patient's face may appear swollen and deep red or purple. The eyes may bulge, with noticeable conjunctival hemorrhages. Assess for severe dyspnea, hypovolemia, hypotension, and shock. Administer oxygen and consider positive pressure ventilation to ensure adequate ventilation. Provide aggressive fluid resuscitation and monitor the ECG for arrhythmias. If the patient has been entrapped for more than 20 minutes, consider administration of sodium bicarbonate.

Case Study Review

Reread the case study on pages 188 and 189 in Paramedic Care: Trauma; *then, read the following discussion.*

This case study presents many of the important elements of assessment and care for the patient who has suffered penetrating injury to the chest. It identifies the need to recognize and aggressively manage the patient. It also highlights the value of rapid transport, when called for.

The paramedics on Medic 101, Victoria and Christian, use the time during their response to identify their duties, the equipment that will likely be needed, and procedures they may perform. Of primary concern is scene safety for the paramedics, fellow rescuers, bystanders, and the patient, especially because shots have been fired. The paramedics are also concerned about the severity of the injuries that may have resulted. They mentally review the steps of assessment and management of both chest and abdominal injuries. As the rescue unit arrives, it is apparent that the police have secured the scene and concern can be directed to the patient.

The primary assessment of the patient presents only minor signs of injury. The wounds are small and not bleeding severely. The patient does not appear to be in much pain. Victoria and Christian do notice that the patient's level of consciousness and color suggest shock, as do the labored, rapid, and shallow breathing and the patient's ability to speak only in short phrases. Their quick primary assessment reveals reasons to be concerned about the airway (reduced level of consciousness) and breathing (speaking in short phrases and poor color). Circulation is deficient, as the paramedics note the distal pulses are absent and the carotid pulse is rapid and weak. This patient is clearly one who merits a rapid trauma assessment and rapid transport to the trauma center.

The rapid trauma assessment reveals that the patient was struck by four bullets, increasing the likelihood that critical structures were injured. Even though the wounds are small, the paramedics remember the severe injuries a bullet can produce. They also note powder burns and residue on Conrad's shirt due to the proximity of the gun barrel to his chest when it was fired. They carefully remove the shirt without cutting it. (If cutting was required, they would have cut without cutting through the bullet holes.) Their actions help maintain the integrity of the evidence, as it may be used in court.

Victoria and Christian quickly cover each wound with an occlusive dressing, sealed on three sides to prevent entry of air into the chest and to permit any air under pressure to escape (as with the development of tension pneumothorax). Their assessment finds full jugular veins, a normal finding in a normovolemic patient in the supine position. The slightly diminished breath sounds on the right side suggest some pneumothorax and reason to perform frequent reassessments evaluating the right side for breath sounds.

Conrad receives care in anticipation of shock, including high-concentration oxygen and IVs started in each upper extremity with large-bore catheters and macrodrip or trauma tubing. The paramedics also employ spinal precautions with him, just in case one of the bullets has damaged the vertebral column and endangered the spinal cord.

©2013 Pearson Education, Inc.
Paramedic Care: Principles & Practice, Vol. 5, 4th Ed.

Careful reassessments reveal a continuing degeneration in the patient's condition. This prompts Victoria and Christian to search for a possible cause of the deterioration. Increasingly quieter breath sounds on the right side, hyperinflation of the right side, tracheal deviation (a late and infrequent sign of tension pneumothorax), increasing dyspnea, and overall patient degeneration together suggest a developing pneumothorax, possibly a tension pneumothorax. The team first tries to relieve the condition by unsealing the dressings covering the wound sites. These actions are unsuccessful, so medical direction is contacted and the paramedics receive authorization to perform a needle decompression of the thorax at the 2nd intercostal space, midclavicular line. Victoria places a large-bore (14-gauge) catheter just above the third rib (into the 2nd intercostal space) until she feels a "pop" and hears air rush out. The attempt is successful, as demonstrated by the escaping air. The bullet wound dressings are reapplied and a valve assembly (a cut glove finger) is applied to the needle hub. Then Christian and Victoria watch their patient very carefully during transport for the redevelopment of the tension pneumothorax because they know that the catheter inserted in the chest may kink or clog with blood or other fluid.

Content Self-Evaluation

MULTIPLE CHOICE

_____ 1. About what percentage of vehicle deaths are attributable to thoracic injuries?
    A. 10   D. 45
    B. 25   E. 65
    C. 35

_____ 2. Which of the following is located within the thorax?
    A. The heart   D. The trachea
    B. Both lungs   E. All of the above
    C. The esophagus

_____ 3. How many rib pairs are floating ribs?
    A. 1   D. 6
    B. 2   E. 8
    C. 3

_____ 4. Which of the following lines is used to describe position on the chest wall?
    A. Posterior axillary line   D. Midclavicular line
    B. Anterior axillary line   E. All of the above
    C. Medial axillary line

_____ 5. How high does the diaphragm rise in the chest during a maximum expiration?
    A. To the 2nd intercostal space posteriorly
    B. To the 4th intercostal space posteriorly
    C. To the 6th intercostal space posteriorly
    D. To the 8th intercostal space posteriorly
    E. To the manubrium anteriorly

_____ 6. The muscle(s) of respiration responsible for reducing the distance between ribs and helping lift the thorax is (are) the
    A. intercostal muscles.   D. scalene.
    B. diaphragm.   E. rectus abdominis.
    C. sternocleidomastoid muscles.

_____ 7. The structure that separates the chest cavity from the abdominal cavity is the
    A. mediastinum.   D. diaphragm.
    B. peritoneum.   E. vena cava.
    C. perineum.

8. At the beginning of and during most of expiration, the pressure within the thorax is
   A. less than the atmospheric pressure.
   B. more than the atmospheric pressure.
   C. equal to the atmospheric pressure.
   D. first lower than and then higher than the atmospheric pressure.
   E. first higher than and then lower than the atmospheric pressure.

9. Which structure(s) enter(s) or exit(s) the lungs at the pulmonary hilum?
   A. Right mainstem bronchus   D. Pulmonary veins
   B. Thoracic duct   E. All except B
   C. Pulmonary artery

10. The right lung has only two lobes because the heart's greatest mass is on the right.
   A. True
   B. False

11. The serous structure that ensures the lungs expand with the thoracic cage wall and diaphragm is the
   A. pleura.   D. lobular attachment.
   B. hilum.   E. mediastinum.
   C. ligamentum arteriosum.

12. Which of the following act(s) as a shut-off switch for respiration?
   A. Chemoreceptors in the carotid bodies
   B. Chemoreceptors in the medulla oblongata
   C. The apneustic center
   D. Chemoreceptors in the aortic bodies
   E. Both A and D

13. Which of the following structures is NOT located within the mediastinum?
   A. Thoracic duct   D. Vagus nerve
   B. Phrenic nerve   E. Esophagus
   C. Pulmonary hilum

14. Which of the following statements is NOT true regarding the pericardium?
   A. The pericardial fluid is straw colored.
   B. The pericardial fluid acts as a lubricant.
   C. The pericardium normally contains no more than 5 mL of fluid.
   D. The epicardium and visceral pericardium are one and the same.
   E. The fibrous pericardium is not the parietal pericardium.

15. The outer layer of the heart is the
   A. fibrous pericardium.   D. endocardium.
   B. epicardium.   E. myocardium.
   C. pericardium.

16. The intercostal arteries and nerves run
   A. behind the ribs.
   B. above the ribs.
   C. in front of the ribs.
   D. below the ribs.
   E. both A and D.

©2013 Pearson Education, Inc.
Paramedic Care: Principles & Practice, Vol. 5, 4th Ed.

_____ 17. Which of the following is NOT likely to be associated with blunt trauma?
  A. Pericardial tamponade
  B. Pneumothorax (paper bag syndrome)
  C. Traumatic asphyxia
  D. Aortic dissection
  E. Blunt cardiac injury

_____ 18. Which of the following is NOT likely to be associated with penetrating trauma?
  A. Open pneumothorax   D. Cavitational lung injury
  B. Esophageal disruption   E. Comminuted fracture of the ribs
  C. Traumatic asphyxia

_____ 19. Rib fracture is found in about what percent of significant chest trauma?
  A. 10 percent   D. 50 percent
  B. 25 percent   E. 65 percent
  C. 35 percent

_____ 20. Which ribs are fractured the most frequently?
  A. 1 and 3   D. 8 through 11
  B. 4 through 8   E. 9 through 12
  C. 7 through 9

_____ 21. Which rib group, when fractured, is most frequently associated with aortic rupture?
  A. 1 and 3   D. 9 through 12
  B. 4 through 8   E. both A and D
  C. 7 through 9

_____ 22. Which of the following groups is more likely to experience internal injury without rib fracture?
  A. Pediatric patients   D. Elderly female patients
  B. Adult male patients   E. Elderly male patients
  C. Adult female patients

_____ 23. Which of the following are associated with a rib fracture?
  A. Local pain   D. Hemothorax
  B. Crepitus   E. All of the above
  C. Limited chest excursion

_____ 24. Which of the following is most frequently associated with sternal fracture?
  A. Hemothorax   D. Simple pneumothorax
  B. Blunt cardiac injury   E. Open pneumothorax
  C. Esophageal injury

_____ 25. Air from under the flail segment in flail chest does which of the following?
  A. Moves out from under the segment during expiration
  B. Moves toward the mediastinum during expiration
  C. Does not move with the segment
  D. Moves out from under the segment during inspiration
  E. None of the above

_____ 26. As the pain of the flail chest increases with time, the amount of paradoxical movement will decrease due to muscular splinting.
  A. True
  B. False

27. Simple pneumothorax is associated with what percent of serious thoracic trauma?
   A. 5 percent
   B. 15 to 50 percent
   C. 25 to 50 percent
   D. 60 percent
   E. more than 75 percent

28. The condition in which a part of the chest wall moves in opposition to the rest of the chest due to numerous rib fractures is called
   A. pneumothorax.
   B. tension pneumothorax.
   C. hemothorax.
   D. atelectasis.
   E. none of the above.

29. The chest injury that causes the patient to experience increasing dyspnea because of an open or closed pneumothorax that has a valve-like function and allows intrathoracic pressure to increase is referred to as
   A. subcutaneous emphysema.
   B. traumatic asphyxia.
   C. hyperbaric mediastinal displacement.
   D. tension pneumothorax.
   E. flail chest.

30. For a significant amount of air to move through an open wound to create an open pneumothorax, the wound opening must be
   A. just large enough to permit air passage.
   B. two-thirds the size of the tracheal opening.
   C. the size of the trachea.
   D. about the size of a hunting rifle bullet.
   E. larger than the trachea.

31. Which of the following is a very late sign of tension pneumothorax?
   A. Head and neck petechiae
   B. Intercostal bulging
   C. A narrowing pulse pressure
   D. Tracheal deviation away from the injury
   E. Distended jugular veins

32. Each hemithorax can hold up to what volume of blood from a hemothorax?
   A. 500 mL
   B. 750 mL
   C. 1,500 mL
   D. 3,000 mL
   E. 4,500 mL

33. Which of the following statements is NOT true regarding hemothorax?
   A. Hemorrhage into the thorax is more severe due to decreased pressure there.
   B. Serious hemothorax may displace an entire lung and has a 75 percent mortality rate.
   C. Hemothorax often occurs with pneumothorax.
   D. Hemothorax rarely occurs with simple rib fractures.
   E. None of the above.

34. Distant or absent breath sounds heard during auscultation of the chest and the signs of shock are suggestive of which pathology?
   A. Pneumothorax
   B. Tension pneumothorax
   C. Aortic dissection
   D. Pulmonary contusion
   E. Hemothorax

35. Which of the following problems would most likely result in a chest area that is dull to percussion?
   A. Pneumothorax
   B. Tension pneumothorax
   C. Hemothorax
   D. Subcutaneous pneumothorax
   E. Pericardial tamponade

©2013 Pearson Education, Inc.
Paramedic Care: Principles & Practice, Vol. 5, 4th Ed.

36. Your patient has received chest trauma yet did not initially present with crackles. However, as the assessment continues, they are heard in both the lower lung fields. This condition is most likely a result of which of the following?
   A. Pulmonary contusion
   B. Hemothorax
   C. Pneumothorax
   D. Aortic dissection
   E. Pericardial tamponade

37. Extensive pulmonary contusions may account for blood losses up to 1,500 mL.
   A. True
   B. False

38. The most common cause of blunt cardiac injury is
   A. blunt anterior chest trauma.
   B. blunt lateral chest trauma.
   C. penetrating anterior chest trauma.
   D. blunt posterior chest trauma.
   E. the pressure wave of an explosion.

39. A patient presents with the signs of shock, jugular vein distention, distant heart sounds, and a narrowing pulse pressure. The lung fields are clear. Which condition is most likely the cause?
   A. Tension pneumothorax
   B. Hemothorax
   C. Traumatic asphyxia
   D. Pericardial tamponade
   E. Atelectasis

40. Pericardial tamponade occurs with what frequency in serious chest trauma patients?
   A. Less than 2 percent of the time
   B. 10 percent of the time
   C. 20 percent of the time
   D. 25 percent of the time
   E. 30 to 45 percent of the time

41. Which of the following is a sign of pericardial tamponade?
   A. Pulsus paradoxus
   B. A narrowing pulse pressure
   C. Distended jugular veins
   D. Hypotension
   E. All of the above

42. The patient with pericardial tamponade may be in hypovolemic shock due to the volume of blood lost into the pericardial sac.
   A. True
   B. False

43. A decrease in jugular vein distention during inspiration is known as
   A. Beck's triad.
   B. pulsus paradoxus.
   C. Cushing's reflex.
   D. Kussmaul's sign.
   E. electrical alternans.

44. A blood pressure drop of more than 10 mmHg with inspiration is known as
   A. Beck's triad.
   B. pulsus paradoxus.
   C. Cushing's reflex.
   D. Kussmaul's sign.
   E. electrical alternans.

45. If the chamber of the heart is significantly damaged yet does not rupture immediately, it is likely to rupture in around two weeks.
   A. True
   B. False

46. Your patient was involved in a lateral-impact auto collision. The car is greatly deformed, though the patient does not have many signs of injury. During your assessment, he complains of a tearing sensation in his central chest and numbness in his left upper extremity. Your highest index of suspicion of injury is for
   A. traumatic asphyxia.
   B. pulmonary contusion.
   C. aortic dissection.
   D. blunt cardiac injury.
   E. pericardial tamponade.

47. What percentage of patients with traumatic aortic dissection will survive the initial impact and injury?
   A. As high as 5 percent
   B. As high as 20 percent
   C. 50 percent
   D. 70 percent
   E. 73 percent

48. In a patient with a history of blunt lateral trauma and a suspected traumatic aortic dissection, which signs or symptoms would you expect to find?
   A. Severe, tearing chest pain
   B. Pulse deficit between extremities
   C. Reduced pulse strength in the lower extremities
   D. Hypertension
   E. All of the above

49. A harsh systolic murmur is heard over the central chest. This is suggestive of which pathology?
   A. Pneumothorax
   B. Tension pneumothorax
   C. Traumatic aortic dissection
   D. Pulmonary contusion
   E. Hemothorax

50. The right side is the site of most diaphragmatic ruptures because most assailants are right-handed.
   A. True
   B. False

51. The traumatic diaphragmatic rupture is likely to present like which of the following thoracic injuries?
   A. Tension pneumothorax
   B. Pulmonary contusion
   C. Aortic dissection
   D. Pericardial tamponade
   E. Esophageal injury

52. The two major problems associated with traumatic asphyxia are restriction of chest excursion and
   A. distortion of the airway.
   B. restriction of venous return.
   C. atelectasis.
   D. hemorrhage during the compression.
   E. massive strokes.

53. The classic signs of traumatic asphyxia include which of the following?
   A. Bulging eyes
   B. Conjunctival hemorrhage
   C. Petechiae of the head and neck
   D. Dark red or purple appearance of the head and neck
   E. All of the above

54. Serious penetrating trauma will likely require which of the following Standard Precaution procedures?
   A. Gloves
   B. Face shield
   C. Gown
   D. Mask
   E. All of the above

55. During your assessment of a supine patient with blunt chest trauma, you notice slight jugular vein distention. With no other signs of injury, this suggests which of the following?
   A. A normal patient
   B. Pericardial tamponade
   C. Tension pneumothorax
   D. Traumatic asphyxia
   E. B, C, and D

©2013 Pearson Education, Inc.
Paramedic Care: Principles & Practice, Vol. 5, 4th Ed.

56. Crackles heard during auscultation of the chest are suggestive of which pathology?
   A. Pneumothorax
   B. Tension pneumothorax
   C. Aortic aneurysm
   D. Pulmonary contusion
   E. Hemothorax

57. Hyperresonance heard during percussion of the chest is suggestive of which pathology?
   A. Pneumothorax
   B. Tension pneumothorax
   C. Hemothorax
   D. Pulmonary contusion
   E. Both A and B

58. Which of the following thoracic structures takes the least energy to fracture and often results as a more common, yet less serious, thoracic injury?
   A. Ribs 1 through 3
   B. Ribs 4 through 8
   C. Ribs 9 through 12
   D. The sternum
   E. The manubrium

59. A patient who displays subcutaneous emphysema is most likely to have which of the following conditions?
   A. Traumatic asphyxia
   B. Tension pneumothorax
   C. Paper-bag syndrome
   D. Pulmonary contusion
   E. Cardiac contusion

60. Overdrive ventilation (bag-valve masking) of the patient with flail chest will cause the flail segment to move with, rather than in opposition to, the chest wall.
   A. True
   B. False

61. Which of the following is an indication for the use of IV infusion?
   A. Diaphragmatic rupture
   B. Penetrating chest injury
   C. Chest trauma with a blood pressure below 80
   D. Chest trauma with a blood pressure below 50
   E. Suspected pericardial tamponade

62. Meperidine, diazepam, or morphine may be given to the minor rib fracture patient to reduce pain and increase respiratory excursion.
   A. True
   B. False

63. The patient who is suspected of a flail chest or other thoracic cage injury, without suspected spine injury, should be positioned
   A. on the uninjured side.
   B. on the injured side.
   C. supine with legs elevated.
   D. on the left lateral side.
   E. on the right lateral side.

64. The open pneumothorax should be cared for using which of the following techniques?
   A. Pack the wound with a sterile dressing.
   B. Cover the wound with an occlusive dressing and tape securely.
   C. Cover the wound with an occlusive dressing, taped on three sides.
   D. Attempt to close the wound with a hemostat and then cover with a sterile dressing.
   E. Cover the wound loosely with a sterile dressing.

65. Which location is recommended for prehospital pleural decompression?
   A. 2nd intercostal space, midclavicular line
   B. 5th intercostal space, midclavicular line
   C. 5th intercostal space, midaxillary line
   D. A and B
   E. A and C

66. A few minutes after you have inserted a needle and decompressed a tension pneumothorax, you notice that a patient's dyspnea is getting worse and breath sounds on the injured side are becoming diminished. Which action would you take?
    A. Insert a second needle.
    B. Remove the dressing.
    C. Provide overdrive ventilation.
    D. Consider nitrous oxide administration.
    E. All of the above.

67. A patient is trapped in a wrecked auto for about half an hour and is suspected of having traumatic asphyxia. Care should include which of the following?
    A. Two large-bore IVs
    B. Normal saline or lactated Ringer's solution
    C. Fluids run rapidly
    D. Consideration of sodium bicarbonate
    E. All of the above

©2013 Pearson Education, Inc.
Paramedic Care: Principles & Practice, Vol. 5, 4th Ed.

Special Projects

Labeling Diagrams

I. Write the names of the organs and structures of the thorax marked A, B, C, D, E, F, G, and H in the following figure.

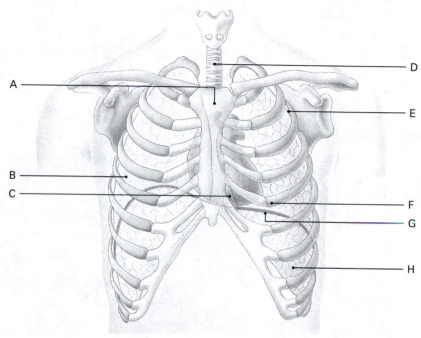

A. _____

B. _____

C. _____

D. _____

E. _____

F. _____

G. _____

H. _____

II. Match the labels A through K on the accompanying diagram to the following respiration volumes.

_____   **1.** Inspiratory reserve

_____   **2.** Expiratory reserve

_____   **3.** Residual volume

_____   **4.** Vital capacity

_____   **5.** Tidal volume

_____   **6.** Total lung capacity

_____   **7.** Inspiratory capacity

_____   **8.** Functional reserve capacity

_____   **9.** Normal respiration

_____   **10.** Maximum inspiration

_____   **11.** Maximum expiration

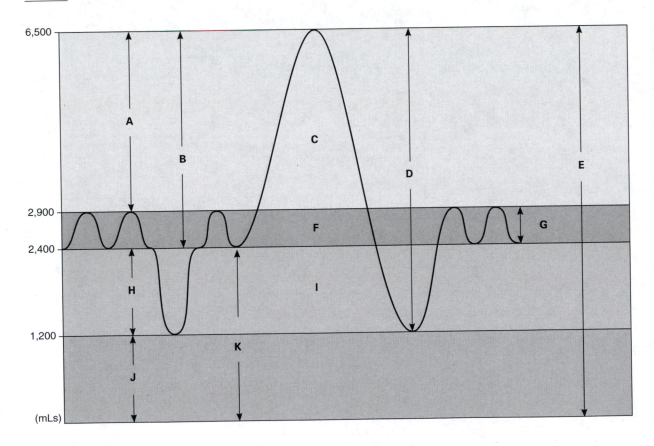

©2013 Pearson Education, Inc.
Paramedic Care: Principles & Practice, Vol. 5, 4th Ed.

Problem Solving—Chest Injury

One of the more serious respiratory-related emergencies is the tension pneumothorax. Identify the signs and symptoms you would expect to find in a patient with this pathology and its increasing intrathoracic pressure.

_____

_____

_____

_____

_____

_____

Give a patient report to medical direction based upon the signs and symptoms identified above. Use only that information you feel is important for the medical direction physician. (You are attempting to receive permission to provide pleural decompression.)

_____

_____

_____

_____

_____

_____

Identify the exact location of your decompression attempt.

_____

_____

_____

_____

_____

_____

Abdominal Trauma

Review of Chapter Objectives

After reading this chapter, you should be able to:

1. **Define key terms introduced in this chapter.**

   Knowing and being able to apply the key terms in each chapter is critical to understanding chapter concepts. Write the list of key terms. Then write the definition of each one in your own words. Check your understanding by confirming the definitions in the text glossary. Correct any misunderstandings. Create a study aid by writing each key term on the front of an index card and the definition on the back. Use the cards to quiz yourself, or to have someone quiz you.

2. **Describe the anatomy and physiology of the abdominal cavity and its contents.**

   pp. 217–223

   The abdomen is one of the body's largest cavities, bounded superiorly by the diaphragm, laterally by the flank muscles, inferiorly by the pelvis, posteriorly by the spine and back muscles, and anteriorly by the abdominal muscles. Because most of its border is soft tissue, it is rather unprotected from injury. The abdomen contains the continuous, muscular tube of digestion, the alimentary canal. It enters the abdomen through the hiatus of the diaphragm as the esophagus. It joins the stomach, an organ that physically mixes the food with gastric juices, and then sends it out and into the small bowel. The first portion of the bowel, the duodenum, mixes the digesting food with bile (a by-product of the liver) and pancreatic juices and then begins the process of absorption. The remainder of the small bowel draws the nutrients from the food.

   As the digesting food enters the large bowel it is mixed with bacteria, releasing water and any remaining nutrients. The large bowel ascends superiorly along the right side of the abdomen, crossing over just below the liver and stomach before descending down the left lateral abdomen. Nutrients are absorbed, and the material is pushed by peristalsis to the rectum, awaiting defecation. The bowel is a thin and vascular tube that drains its blood supply through the liver for detoxification, where some nutrients are stored and others added to the circulation.

   The liver is a large, vascular, solid organ found in the right upper quadrant, just below the diaphragm. It is responsible for detoxification of blood and digestive materials in addition to functioning as a storage site for glycogen, protein synthesis, and fluid regulation. It is held firmly in place by several ligaments. Behind and beneath the liver is the gall bladder. It stores and releases bile for fatty food digestion. The pancreas is a delicate organ found in the lower aspect of the upper left quadrant with a portion of it extending into the right upper quadrant. In addition to digestive juices, it manufactures insulin and glucagon. The kidneys are found deep within the flanks and filter blood to remove excess water and electrolytes. They are very vascular organs that excrete urine into the ureters, through which the urine then travels to the bladder. The bladder (in the central pelvic space) rids the body of urine through the urethra. The spleen is an organ of the immune system and is very delicate and vascular, residing in the left upper quadrant behind the stomach. It stores a large volume of blood.

The abdominal organs receive blood through the large abdominal aorta and its many branches. At the inferior margin of the abdominal cavity the iliac arteries bifurcate to become the femoral arteries, which travel through the pelvis. They are firmly attached to the pelvis and may tear if the pelvis is fractured. The inferior vena cava runs along the spinal column, collecting venous blood for return to the heart. Additionally, the abdomen houses the portal system, which collects venous blood, fluids, and nutrients absorbed by the bowel for transport to the liver.

The abdominal cavity is lined with a serous membrane, the peritoneum. It covers the anterior abdominal organs and a double-layer sheath of it forms the omentum, which covers the anterior surface of the abdomen. The bowel is slung from the posterior wall of the abdomen by connective tissue called the mesentery that also provides perfusion to the bowel. Not all abdominal organs are covered by the peritoneum. The kidneys, spleen, duodenum, pancreas, and bladder as well as most major vascular structures are considered retroperitoneal. This is significant in abdominal trauma, as hemorrhage within the peritoneal space is more likely to present with overt signs and symptoms than fluid collecting in the retroperitoneal area.

3. **Describe the changes in anatomy and physiology associated with pregnancy.**   pp. 221–222

The gravid uterus progressively enlarges during pregnancy, ultimately filling the abdominal cavity to the level of the lower rib margin. As it grows, intra-abdominal pressure increases and the diaphragm is displaced upward. This reduces lung capacity, while the pregnancy itself requires an increase in tidal volume. Circulatory volume also increases, with a resulting rise in heart rate and increase in cardiac output. Although blood volume increases, red blood cells do not keep pace, causing a relative anemia. During the last trimester, the weight of the uterus may compress the vena cava, reducing cardiac preload and causing temporary hypotension in the supine patient

4. **Discuss the pathophysiology of blunt and penetrating mechanisms of abdominal trauma.**   pp. 223–224

Because the abdomen is bound by muscles rather than skeletal structures, blunt and penetrating trauma transmit greater energy to internal organs and structures. Overt signs of injury are often limited or delayed.

Blunt trauma compresses, shears, or decelerates the various organs and structures within the abdomen, resulting in rupture of the hollow organs, fracture or tearing of the solid organs, or tearing or severance of the abdominal vasculature. The spleen is the most frequently injured organ; the liver is the second most commonly injured structure, followed by the bowel and kidneys. Severe abdominal compression may rupture the diaphragm and push abdominal organs into the thorax. Contusions or organ rupture may result. Abdominal injury, however, is a secondary concern with blast injuries.

Penetrating injury to the abdomen may involve low- and high-velocity objects. Bullets disrupt tissue beyond their direct path through cavitation and are especially damaging to hollow organs filled with fluid and to the extremely dense and delicate solid organs (liver, spleen, kidneys, pancreas) of the abdomen. Additionally, debris and contaminants may be drawn into the wound, causing infection or poor healing. Mortality is about 10 times greater with high-energy bullets than with stab-type wounds. Penetrating mechanisms may cause uncontrolled hemorrhage, direct organ damage, spillage of hollow organ contents, and peritoneal irritation. The liver is affected more frequently than the bowel, with the spleen, kidneys, and pancreas injured in descending order of frequency. A special category of penetrating injury is the shotgun blast. At short range (under 3 yards), the projectiles have tremendous energy and create numerous tracts of serious injury.

Paramedic Care: Principles & Practice, Vol. 5, 4th Ed.

5. **Describe the pathophysiology of the following types of abdominal injuries.**

pp. 224–228

a. **Abdominal wall injuries**

The abdominal wall is composed of tough skin and muscle, making it more resistant to injury than the internal organs. No obvious signs may be present initially from blunt trauma. Penetrating wounds may also be concealed as the muscles and skin tension close the wound opening. Large, deep lacerations may cause an evisceration injury, where abdominal contents, frequently the bowel, protrude. The tissue is then at risk for compromised circulation, bowel obstruction, and dehydration. Infectious material may be introduced into peritoneum. The flank, back, and buttock muscles are thick and resist penetrating trauma. However, deep wounds may penetrate into the abdominal cavity with resulting organ damage. Injury to the lower chest may lacerate the diaphragm, impairing ventilation and allowing abdominal contents to enter the thoracic cavity.

b. **Hollow organ**

Hollow organs include the stomach, small and large bowel, rectum, gallbladder, urinary bladder, and pregnant uterus. Compression may contuse them or cause them to rupture, especially if the organ is full and distended. Penetrating injury may perforate them. The gallbladder, stomach, and first part of the small bowel may release digestive juices that will chemically irritate and damage the abdominal structures. Injury can cause the rest of the bowel to release material high in bacterial load that can induce infection. The rupture of the urinary bladder will release blood and urine into the abdomen. Injury to the abdomen may cause blood in emesis (hematemesis), blood in the stool (hematochezia), or blood in the urine (hematuria).

c. **Solid organ**

The spleen is well protected, although it is very delicate and not contained within a strong capsule. It frequently ruptures and bleeds heavily. The pancreas is located deep within the central upper abdomen. When injured, it may hemorrhage and release pancreatic enzymes into the abdomen, causing severe internal damage. The kidneys are well protected both by their location deep within the flank and by strong capsules. Injury may present with hematuria. The liver is the largest abdominal organ. It is a very dense and vascular structure protected by the lower thoracic border. Although it is contained within a strong capsule, it may be lacerated during severe deceleration as it moves against its restraining ligament (the ligamentum teres). Severe hemorrhage may result.

d. **Vascular structure**

The major vascular structures of the abdomen include the abdominal aorta, the inferior and superior vena cava, the renal and hepatic arteries, and other arteries branching to the abdominal organs. These vessels may be injured by blunt trauma as deceleration causes the organs to pull against their vascular attachments. If penetrating trauma strikes a major artery, severe internal hemorrhage occurs. The abdomen does not develop internal pressure against hemorrhage, as do the muscles and other solid regions of the body, so bleeding may continue unabated. Due to its large size, the accumulation of blood in the abdomen can be significant before swelling becomes apparent.

e. **Mesentery and bowel injury**

The mesentery supports the bowel and may be injured as it stretches, most commonly at points of fixation such as the ileocecal or duodenal/jejunal junctures. Blood vessels may be damaged, causing ischemia, necrosis, and possibly rupture. Bleeding is usually contained by the peritoneum and is limited. In the presence of penetrating trauma, tears may occur anywhere along the length of the bowel. Contents are released into the peritoneal space but signs and symptoms are typically delayed. The small bowel is most commonly affected because of its central location. Lateral penetrations are more likely to affect the large bowel.

f. **Peritoneal Injury**

The peritoneum is the delicate and sensitive lining of the anterior abdominal cavity. Peritoneal injury is generally related to irritation either by chemical action (most rapid) or by bacterial contamination (12 to 24 hours). Bacterial contamination results from spillage of bowel contents into the abdomen or open wounds. Chemical peritonitis occurs quickly when digestive enzymes, acids, or urine are released. Blood alone does not typically produce the signs and symptoms of peritonitis.

g. **Pelvic fracture**

Pelvic fractures and crushing mechanisms can cause injury to the bladder, urethra, ureters, genitalia, rectum, and some very large blood vessels, with serious associated hemorrhage. Trauma and sexual assault may cause direct injury to the genitalia, with resulting pain and bleeding.

h. **Injury in pregnancy**

Numerous physiological changes during pregnancy have consequences for both blunt and penetrating trauma. Structurally, the abdominal organs are displaced superiorly. Blunt or penetrating trauma to the lower abdomen may protect these organs while the fetus and uterus are endangered. The uterus may rupture or tear, causing severe hemorrhage, disruption of the blood supply to the fetus, and release of amniotic fluid into the abdomen. If the amniotic sac ruptures, labor may be induced. The placenta may also be torn from the uterine wall because of its relative inelasticity, with a high incidence of fetal mortality. The size and weight of the fetus and uterus may further complicate traumatic injury. Hypotension, secondary to hemorrhage, is further exacerbated by compression of the vena cava with associated hypotension. Venous hemorrhage from pelvic fractures or lower extremity wounds may be more severe due to increased intra-abdominal pressure. Pregnant women have increased vascular volume, which masks shock, allowing the mother to compensate while reduced placental circulation endangers the fetus.

i. **Abdominal injuries in pediatric patients**

Pediatric patients are more prone to abdominal organ injury than adults due to their poorly developed abdominal musculature and their reduced anterior/posterior diameter. Additionally, the rib cage is more flexible, allowing forces to be transmitted internally. The liver, spleen, and kidneys are at greatest risk. Hemorrhage may be obscured, as children compensate longer for blood loss.

6. **Given a variety of scenarios, demonstrate assessment of patients with abdominal injuries.**   pp. 228–232

Assessment of injury to the abdominal contents is limited because it is often difficult to ascertain, and definitive care is usually surgical intervention. More than 30 percent of patients with serious abdominal injury have no clear signs or symptoms of injury; thus, developing an index of suspicion based on mechanism of injury is critical. Many others present with diffuse signs and symptoms, making it very hard to differentiate among the different abdominal pathologies. Try to relate the mechanism of injury or any patient complaints to the anatomical region involved and the specific organs found there. With blunt trauma, determine the strength and direction of forces and where the body may have been impacted. For vehicular injury, determine if seat belts were worn properly and if other safety devices deployed. Look for intrusion into the vehicle or interior deformity. The type of vehicular impact should guide your thinking on possible injuries. With penetrating trauma, ascertain the type of object and its insertion angle and depth. For gunshot injuries, determine the number of shots fired, the gun's caliber, and the distance and angle from which it was fired. Suspect internal hemorrhage and be alert for signs and symptoms of shock, including altered mental status, increasing anxiety, thirst, tachycardia, decreasing pulse pressure, and increasing capillary refill time. Remember that low blood pressure is a late sign of shock.

During the primary assessment, note the patient's level of consciousness and orientation. Determine whether alcohol, drugs, or head injury may be involved. These factors may limit the patient's ability to reliably report signs and symptoms of abdominal trauma. Evaluate airway, breathing, and circulation, especially noting any signs or symptoms suggesting hypovolemia. Rapid, shallow respirations accompanied by a rapid pulse rate and diminished pulse pressure warn of hypoperfusion. Peritonitis or blood irritating the diaphragm may present with limited chest movement. A ruptured diaphragm may cause shallow respirations due to herniation of abdominal contents in the thorax. Abdominal trauma patients are likely to vomit, so monitor the airway closely.

Abdominal trauma may or may not be evident during the rapid trauma exam. Examine the anterior abdominal surface, the flanks, and the back. You may note a slight reddening of the skin or minor abrasions on the abdominal surface. Look for bruising, contusions, open wounds, eviscerations, and impaled objects. Significant discoloration is usually absent in the prehospital setting, as it takes time to develop. Examine the abdomen's general shape and note any signs of distention. Due to the size of the abdominal cavity, significant blood loss will occur before distention is apparent. Inspect the pelvis. Signs such as crepitus or instability suggest pelvic fracture, with a high likelihood of lower abdominal organ injury.

©2013 Pearson Education, Inc.
Paramedic Care: Principles & Practice, Vol. 5, 4th Ed.

Pay attention to pain, tenderness, and rebound tenderness as you palpate each quadrant. Listen to any voiced complaints. Spleen injuries may present with referred pain to the left shoulder region. If the pancreas is damaged the patient may complain of upper abdominal pain that radiates to the back. Renal injury may result in back or flank pain and hematuria. If the liver has been injured the patient may present with tenderness along the right lower thoracic border. The patient may also complain of pain the upper right shoulder as blood accumulates against the diaphragm. Feel for spasm and guarding. A board-hard abdomen may indicate injury to the pancreas, duodenum, or stomach. If you note any pulsating masses in the abdomen, suspect arterial injury.

Check for entrance and exit wounds in cases of gunshot injury. Look for powder debris and subcutaneous emphysema. Count the number of entry and exit wounds. Consider that a bullet may fragment or deflect within the body and cause damage at multiple sites away from the entry point. For penetrating objects such as knives or arrows, visualize the entry wound for depth and hemorrhage but do not pry open the wound or remove impaled objects during assessment.

While obtaining a history, question the patient about last oral intake. Remember that a full or distended bladder, bowel, or stomach are more likely to rupture. Obtain vital signs and assess for signs of shock. With a high index of suspicion for abdominal injury, do not depend on overt signs and symptoms to assign a priority transport. Reassess frequently and monitor for changes in blood pressure, pulse, capillary refill time, oxygen saturation, appearance, and level of consciousness and orientation. Signs and symptoms of progressing abdominal injury or continuing hemorrhage may manifest as the patient compensates for progressive shock. Increase your suspicion for intractable hemorrhage if fluid resuscitation appears ineffective.

7. **Given a variety of scenarios, develop a management plan for patients with abdominal injuries.**
pp. 232–234

The management of the patient with suspected abdominal trauma is basically supportive, with airway maintenance, oxygen, ventilation as needed, fluid resuscitation, and care for specific injuries such as open wounds or eviscerations. Place the patient in a position of comfort with the knees flexed or in the left lateral recumbent position if spinal immobilization is not indicated. Control any external hemorrhage with direct pressure and bandaging. Consider pain management. If abdominal organs are exposed, cover the evisceration with a sterile dressing soaked in normal saline, then apply a sterile, occlusive dressing to the area to prevent evaporation. Keep the region clean and do not attempt to replace exposed organs. If an object is impaled, place bulky dressings around the area and secure in place. Do not remove the object but secure it firmly enough to limit movement. For large wounds that may have penetrated the thoracic cavity, seal the wound with an occlusive dressing taped on three sides to prevent development of a tension pneumothorax. Establish a large-bore IV but do not run fluids aggressively unless the blood pressure drops below 80 mmHg. Use of the pneumatic antishock garment (PASG) may be helpful, especially if the blood pressure drops below 50 mmHg. As with all hypovolemia patients, keep the patient warm and provide rapid transport.

Case Study Review

Reread the case study on pages 216 in Paramedic Care: Trauma; *then, read the following discussion.*
This case study permits us to examine the relevant components of the assessment and care of a patient who has sustained a penetrating injury to the abdomen.

Doug and Janice respond to a domestic disturbance with "shots fired." They appreciate the danger associated with this scene and approach with caution. Only after they are told by police that the scene is safe do they enter and begin their assessment and care. They don gloves and prepare to attend penetrating wounds. When they perform their primary assessment, they note that Marty is conscious, alert, and fully oriented. He is speaking in full sentences and appears in no serious or immediate distress. From this, they determine that he has a patent airway and breathing is adequate. They quickly check his pulse and find it strong and regular at 80. Janice quickly visualizes the wound and determines that there is no serious external hemorrhage, though she appreciates the likelihood of serious continuing internal blood loss. Doug quickly looks for an expected exit wound in the flanks or back but finds none. They apply oxygen via nonrebreather mask and apply a pulse oximeter that immediately reveals a saturation of 99 percent. They plan for rapid transport to the hospital (a trauma center) as they begin their focused assessment.

Marty's description of his pain is classic for an abdominal injury. The expanding "burning" pain and the tenderness are suggestive of peritonitis caused as bowel or gastric contents spread into the peritoneal space. Janice covers the small wound with a dressing and prepares Marty for rapid transport. En route, Janice auscultates the abdomen (though she knows she is unlikely to hear bowel sounds) and does likewise to the lower chest because she wishes to rule out chest penetration. Remember that the diaphragm moves up and down in the region of the thoracic border and that bullets frequently deflect from a straight path.

Once the rapid trauma assessment is complete, Janice initiates an IV line with a large catheter and trauma tubing and runs lactated Ringer's solution at a to-keep-open rate. If Marty begins to show signs of hypovolemia and vascular compromise, she will administer a fluid bolus of normal saline. Reassessments begin to suggest shock compensation, with the pulse rate rising from 80 to 86 to 88 (though it remains strong). The systolic blood pressure remains at 112, but the diastolic is rising from 86 to 96 (a decreasing pulse pressure), suggesting increasing peripheral vasoconstriction and shock compensation. Marty's shallow respirations also suggest continuing blood loss and developing shock. As this team arrives at the emergency department, it will be very important for them to report these findings and describe both the shooting scene (including the weapon caliber) and wound appearance to the attending physician.

Content Self-Evaluation

MULTIPLE CHOICE

_____ 1. Due to the anatomy of the abdomen, injury to its contents often presents with limited signs and symptoms.
   A. True
   B. False

_____ 2. Which of the following abdominal organs is found in the left upper quadrant?
   A. Spleen
   B. Gallbladder
   C. Appendix
   D. Sigmoid colon
   E. Ascending colon

_____ 3. Which of the following abdominal organs is found in the right lower quadrant?
   A. Spleen
   B. Gallbladder
   C. Appendix
   D. Sigmoid colon
   E. Liver

_____ 4. Which of the following abdominal organs is found in all of the abdominal quadrants?
   A. Pancreas
   B. Gallbladder
   C. Appendix
   D. Sigmoid colon
   E. Small bowel

_____ 5. Which of the following statements is TRUE regarding the digestive tract?
   A. It is a 25-foot-long hollow tube.
   B. It churns food.
   C. It introduces digestive juices.
   D. It moves food via peristalsis.
   E. All of the above.

_____ 6. In what order does digesting food pass through the digestive tract?
   A. Duodenum, ileum, jejunum, colon
   B. Duodenum, jejunum, ileum, colon
   C. Jejunum, ileum, colon, duodenum
   D. Ileum, jejunum, colon, duodenum
   E. Colon, jejunum, ileum, duodenum

©2013 Pearson Education, Inc.
Paramedic Care: Principles & Practice, Vol. 5, 4th Ed.

_____ 7. The movement of digesting material through the digestive system occurs through a process called
   A. peristalsis.
   B. chyme.
   C. peritonitis.
   D. emulsification.
   E. evisceration.

_____ 8. The largest solid organ of the abdomen is the
   A. spleen.
   B. small bowel.
   C. pancreas.
   D. gallbladder.
   E. liver.

_____ 9. The delicate vascular organ that performs some immune functions is the
   A. spleen.
   B. small bowel.
   C. pancreas.
   D. gallbladder.
   E. liver.

_____ 10. The solid organ that produces insulin, glucagon, and some digestive juices is the
   A. spleen.
   B. small bowel.
   C. pancreas.
   D. gallbladder.
   E. liver.

_____ 11. The urinary bladder may contain as little as 100 mL of fluid or as much as 2,000 mL of fluid.
   A. True
   B. False

_____ 12. The genital structure that contains the developing fetus during gestation is the
   A. vagina.
   B. uterus.
   C. fallopian tube.
   D. ovary.
   E. cervix.

_____ 13. The genital structure that releases an egg every 28 days is the
   A. vagina.
   B. uterus.
   C. fallopian tube.
   D. ovary.
   E. cervix.

_____ 14. At what point does the uterus and developing fetus fill the abdominal cavity to the lower rib margin?
   A. 12 weeks
   B. 20 weeks
   C. 32 weeks
   D. 40 weeks
   E. 52 weeks

_____ 15. Pregnancy causes what change in the maternal blood volume?
   A. 10 percent decrease
   B. 25 percent decrease
   C. 25 percent increase
   D. 45 percent increase
   E. 65 percent increase

_____ 16. The abdominal aorta divides into what arteries as it enters the pelvic cavity?
   A. Femoral arteries
   B. Innominate arteries
   C. Iliac arteries
   D. Phrenic arteries
   E. Renal arteries

_____ 17. The serous lining of the abdominal cavity is the
   A. perineum.
   B. mesentery.
   C. peritoneum.
   D. retroperitoneum.
   E. ileum.

_____ 18. Which of the following is a retroperitoneal organ?
   A. Duodenum
   B. Spleen
   C. Urinary bladder
   D. Kidneys
   E. All of the above

_____ 19. Bullets cause an abdominal wound mortality rate that is about equal to that caused by slow-moving penetrating objects.
   A. True
   B. False

_____ 20. What percentage of the time does a penetrating mechanism injure the liver?
   A. 50 percent
   B. 40 percent
   C. 30 percent
   D. 20 percent
   E. 10 percent

_____ 21. What percentage of the time does a penetrating mechanism injure the large bowel?
   A. 50 percent
   B. 40 percent
   C. 30 percent
   D. 20 percent
   E. 10 percent

_____ 22. Which of the following organs is most frequently damaged during blunt abdominal trauma?
   A. Small bowel
   B. Liver
   C. Spleen
   D. Kidneys
   E. Pancreas

_____ 23. Solid and hollow organs respond similarly to trauma.
   A. True
   B. False

_____ 24. Penetration of the abdominal wall resulting in protrusion of the abdominal contents is called
   A. peristalsis.
   B. chyme.
   C. peritonitis.
   D. emulsification.
   E. evisceration.

_____ 25. The abdominal organs, with deep expiration, move as far up into the thorax as
   A. the xiphoid process.
   B. the tips of the floating ribs.
   C. the nipple line.
   D. the 7th intercostal space.
   E. none of the above.

_____ 26. The term describing frank blood in the stool is
   A. hematochezia.
   B. hematemesis.
   C. hemoptysis.
   D. hematuria.
   E. hematocrit.

_____ 27. The organ most likely to be injured by left-flank blunt trauma is the
   A. small bowel.
   B. liver.
   C. spleen.
   D. kidney.
   E. pancreas.

_____ 28. The organ that is likely to be injured in severe deceleration as its ligament restrains, then lacerates it, is the
   A. small bowel.
   B. liver.
   C. spleen.
   D. kidney.
   E. pancreas.

_____ 29. Blunt injury to the right-flank region is likely to cause which of the following?
   A. Spleen injury
   B. Kidney injury
   C. Bowel injury
   D. Bladder injury
   E. Colon injury

©2013 Pearson Education, Inc.
Paramedic Care: Principles & Practice, Vol. 5, 4th Ed.

30. Penetrating injury to the central anterior abdomen is likely to cause which of the following?
   A. Liver injury
   B. Spleen injury
   C. Bowel injury
   D. Bladder injury
   E. None of the above

31. Most abdominal vascular injuries are associated with penetrating trauma.
   A. True
   B. False

32. Hemorrhage into the abdomen is of serious concern because it
   A. quickly puts pressure on internal organs.
   B. limits respirations.
   C. rapidly affects the heart.
   D. may trigger a vagal response, slowing the heart.
   E. none of the above.

33. Blunt injury to the mesentery often occurs at
   A. the gastric-duodenal juncture.
   B. the duodenal-jejunal juncture.
   C. the jejunal-ileal juncture.
   D. the ileocecal juncture.
   E. both B and D.

34. How long does it take bacteria to grow in sufficient numbers to irritate the peritoneum?
   A. 2 to 4 hours
   B. 4 to 6 hours
   C. 6 to 8 hours
   D. 8 to 10 hours
   E. over 12 hours

35. The number-one killer of pregnant females is
   A. heart attack.
   B. ectopic pregnancy.
   C. allergic reactions.
   D. trauma.
   E. stroke.

36. Unrestrained pregnant occupants in vehicles are how many more times likely to suffer fetal mortality in an auto collision than their belted counterparts?
   A. Two
   B. Three
   C. Four
   D. Five
   E. Six

37. The late-term pregnant female is at increased risk for vomiting and aspiration.
   A. True
   B. False

38. Supine positioning of the mother may cause hypotension due to
   A. compression of the inferior vena cava.
   B. increased circulation to the uterus.
   C. increased intra-abdominal pressure.
   D. decreased intra-abdominal pressure.
   E. Kussmaul's respirations.

39. It may take a maternal blood loss of what percentage before the heart rate begins to increase in the late-term pregnancy?
   A. 10 to 15 percent
   B. 15 to 20 percent
   C. 20 to 25 percent
   D. 25 to 30 percent
   E. 30 to 35 percent

©2013 Pearson Education, Inc.
Paramedic Care: Principles & Practice, Vol. 5, 4th Ed.

CHAPTER 9 *Abdominal Trauma* 119

40. Due to the flexibility of the pediatric thorax, which injury is more likely to occur with blunt trauma?
   A. Liver injury
   B. Splenic injury
   C. Kidney injury
   D. All of the above
   E. None of the above

41. Children may not show signs of blood loss until they have lost what percentage of their volume?
   A. 25 percent
   B. 35 percent
   C. 45 percent
   D. 50 percent
   E. 65 percent

42. What percentage of patients with abdominal injury do not present with any signs or symptoms?
   A. 10 percent
   B. 20 percent
   C. 30 percent
   D. 40 percent
   E. 50 percent

43. Hemorrhage into the abdomen may account for how much blood loss before it becomes noticeable?
   A. 500 mL
   B. 750 mL
   C. 1,000 mL
   D. 1,500 mL
   E. 2,500 mL

44. Prehospital administration of IV fluid should be limited to
   A. 1,000 mL.
   B. 2,000 mL.
   C. 3,000 mL.
   D. 4,000 mL.
   E. 5,000 mL.

45. Care for the abdominal evisceration includes use of which of the following?
   A. A dry adherent dressing
   B. A dry nonadherent dressing
   C. A sterile dressing moistened with normal saline
   D. An occlusive dressing
   E. A sterile cotton gauze dressing

46. At what blood pressure would you consider applying the PASG in the presence of an abdominal evisceration?
   A. 120 mmHg
   B. 100 mmHg
   C. 90 mmHg
   D. 50 mmHg
   E. 30 mmHg

47. Which position is indicated for the late-pregnancy patient?
   A. Supine
   B. Left lateral recumbent
   C. Right lateral recumbent
   D. Trendelenburg
   E. With the head elevated 30°

48. Unless the blood pressure is less than 50 mmHg, use of the PASG is contraindicated in
   A. geriatric patients.
   B. patients with low blood pressure.
   C. tuberculosis patients.
   D. abdominal evisceration patients.
   E. diabetic patients.

©2013 Pearson Education, Inc.
Paramedic Care: Principles & Practice, Vol. 5, 4th Ed.

_____ **49.** Aggressive fluid resuscitation may aggravate the relative anemia associated with late-term pregnancy.
A. True
B. False

_____ **50.** Tilting the spine board 15 degrees for the immobilized, late-term mother may be beneficial.
A. True
B. False

Special Project

Writing a Run Report

Writing the run report is one the most important tasks you will perform as a paramedic. Reread the case study on page 216 of Paramedic Care: Trauma; _then, read the following additional information about the call. From this information complete the run report for this call._

The 911 center dispatches Unit 95 to the Harborview Apartments, apartment 112, at 3:25 A.M. Janice and Doug arrive on scene at 3:32 and finish their first set of vitals at 3:35 as oxygen is applied. Marty is moved to the stretcher a minute later and then to the ambulance. The team departs the scene at 3:38 and is diverted to St. Joseph's Hospital. Janice starts an IV en route with a 14-gauge angiocatheter in the right antecubital fossa, running a bolus of 250 mL. A second set of vitals is taken at 3:42 and finds Marty still fully oriented. Janice questions Marty to find he has a history of seizures but is taking his Dilantin and phenobarbital. He has no allergies and his most recent tetanus shot was three years ago. Janice finishes her last set of vitals as they back into St. Joseph's Emergency Department at 3:47. The team fills out its report and radios "back in service" at 4:00.

Date	Emergency Medical Services Run Report	Run # 914

Patient Information | Service Information | Times

Name:	Agency:	Rcvd :
Address:	Location:	Enrt :
City:　　　　St:　　Zip:	Call Origin:	Scne :
Age:　　Birth: / / 　　Sex: [M][F]	Type: Emrg[ ] Non[ ] Trnsfr[ ]	LvSn :
Nature of Call:		ArHsp :
Chief Complaint:		InSv :

Description of Current Problem:

Medical Problems

Past		Present
[ ]	Cardiac	[ ]
[ ]	Stroke	[ ]
[ ]	Acute Abdomen	[ ]
[ ]	Diabetes	[ ]
[ ]	Psychiatric	[ ]
[ ]	Epilepsy	[ ]
[ ]	Drug/Alcohol	[ ]
[ ]	Poisoning	[ ]
[ ]	Allergy/Asthma	[ ]
[ ]	Syncope	[ ]
[ ]	Obstetrical	[ ]
[ ]	GYN	[ ]

Other:

Trauma Scr:　　　Glasgow:

On-Scene Care:	First Aid:
	By Whom?

O₂ @ 　L : 　Via	C-Collar :	S-Immob. :	Stretcher :

Allergies/Meds:	Past Med Hx:

Time	Pulse		Resp.		BP S/D	LOC	ECG
:	R:	[r][i]	R:	[s][l]	/	[a][v][p][u]	
Care/Comments:							
:	R:	[r][i]	R:	[s][l]	/	[a][v][p][u]	
Care/Comments:							
:	R:	[r][i]	R:	[s][l]	/	[a][v][p][u]	
Care/Comments:							
:	R:	[r][i]	R:	[s][l]	/	[a][v][p][u]	
Care/Comments:							

Destination:	Personnel:	Certification
Reason:[ ]pt　[ ]Closest　[ ]M.D.　[ ]Other	1.	[P][E][O]
Contacted:　　[ ]Radio　[ ]Tele　[ ]Direct	2.	[P][E][O]
Ar Status:　　[ ]Better　[ ]UnC　[ ]Worse	3.	[P][E][O]

10

Head, Face, Neck, and Spinal Trauma

Review of Chapter Objectives

After reading this chapter, you should be able to:

1. Define key terms introduced in this chapter.

Knowing and being able to apply the key terms in each chapter is critical to understanding chapter concepts. Write the list of key terms. Then write the definition of each one in your own words. Check your understanding by confirming the definitions in the text glossary. Correct any misunderstandings. Create a study aid by writing each key term on the front of an index card and the definition on the back. Use the cards to quiz yourself, or to have someone quiz you.

2. Describe the epidemiology of injuries to the head, face, neck, and spinal column.

p. 239

Approximately 1.54 million people experience significant head trauma each year, with 1 in 5 requiring hospitalization. Severe head trauma is the most common cause of trauma death, being especially lethal in auto collisions. Gunshot wounds to the head are less frequent but have a mortality of 75 to 80 percent. The populations most at risk for head injury are males between 15 and 24 years of age, infants and young children, and the elderly. Sports injuries and falls, especially in the elderly, account for a significant number of head, face, neck, and spinal column injuries.

3. Describe the anatomy and physiology of:

pp. 239–250

a. The structures that make up the head

pp. 239–241

Several layers of soft, connective, and skeletal tissues protect the brain. These include the scalp, the cranium, and the meninges. The scalp is a thick and vascular layer of tissue loosely connected to the skull. It is comprised of skin, muscle, and connective tissues that are strong and flexible and able to absorb tremendous kinetic energy. Beneath the skin are several layers of connective and muscular fascia that further protect the skull and its contents.

The skull consists of numerous bones, fused together at pseudo joints called sutures. These bones form a container for the brain called the cranium. The cranium is made up of three layers of bone, two thin layers of compact bone separated by a layer of cancellous bone. This construction makes the cranium both light and very strong. This vault for the brain is fixed in volume and does not accommodate any expansion of its contents. The cranial bones include the frontal bone, parietal bones, occipital bone, temporal bones, and the ethmoid and sphenoid bones. The base of the skull, composed of portions of the cranial bones, has openings for blood vessels, the spinal cord, and the auditory canals and exits for the cranial nerves. The cranial base has rough surfaces and is weakened from the openings. This makes it vulnerable to fracture, abrasion, laceration, and contusion. At the base is the foramen magnum, a large opening through which the spinal cord exits the cranium.

The meninges are three layers of tissue—the dura mater, the arachnoid, and the pia mater—that provide further protection for the brain. These are discussed in more detail in Chapter 11, Nervous System Trauma.

b. The structures that make up the face   **pp. 241–242**

The face, consisting of several bones covered with soft tissue, protects the special sense organs of sight, smell, hearing, balance, and taste and forms and protects the upper airway and the beginning of the alimentary canal. The brow ridge (a portion of the frontal bone), the nasal bones, and the cheek bone (zygoma) form the eye sockets and protect the eyes. The upper jaw (the maxilla) and the moveable lower jaw (mandible) provide the skeletal structures that form the opening of the mouth. The face is covered with thin, flexible skin, beneath which is a small layer of subcutaneous tissue and small muscles that control facial expression, the movements of the mouth, eyes, and eyelids. Cavities within this region (sinuses) help to provide shape to the face without increasing the weight of the head. The nasal bone and cartilage form the shape of the nose. Cartilage divides the nostrils into two openings, the nares. Inside, the nasal cavity provides an extended surface to warm, humidify, and cleanse incoming air. The lower border of the nasal cavity is formed by the hard palate. Posteriorly lies the soft palate, which closes off the nasal cavity during swallowing. The oral cavity houses the tongue and teeth and accommodates the early physical and chemical breakdown of food. Food exits the cavity through the pharynx, where it moves into the esophagus. Cranial nerves service the facial region and cavities providing for sensation, motor control, taste, and endocrine function.

c. The structures that make up the neck and spinal column   **pp. 244–250**

The neck is the conduit for many anatomical functions, including respiration, digestion, blood flow to the brain, lymph flow, and neural networks for sensation and muscle control. It contains two major endocrine glands, the thyroid and parathyroid glands, and houses the esophagus, multiple cranial nerves, lymphatic and thoracic ducts, and the brachial plexus. Major blood vessels traversing the neck include the carotid arteries and the jugular veins. Where the internal and external carotid arteries bifurcate are the carotid bodies and carotid sinuses, which monitor levels of carbon dioxide and oxygen in the blood and blood pressure, respectively. Airway structures begin with the larynx, which is formed by the thyroid and cricoid cartilages. The vocal cords surround the glottic opening into the trachea. They close to protect the trachea during swallowing and allow for speech production. Inferiorly, the trachea, comprised of C-shaped cartilaginous rings, extends to the sternum, where it bifurcates into the left and right bronchi.

The spinal column extends from the skull to the pelvis and consists of 33 bones called vertebrae. Nine of these fuse to form the sacrum and coccyx. Between most of the vertebrae are intervertebral discs, which cushion the vertebrae and absorb energy. The spinal column provides the main structural support for the body, while permitting significant motion and also protecting the spinal cord. The spinal cord runs through the spinal canal or vertebral foramen, which is formed by various vertebral structures. Ligaments hold the vertebral column in place. These ligaments help prevent hyperextension and hyperflexion and maintain the normal curvature of the spine. The spinal column can be divided into five anatomical regions: cervical spine, thoracic spine, lumbar spine, sacrum, and coccyx.

a. Cervical spine   **pp. 246–248**

The cervical spine is the vertebral column between the base of the skull and the thorax. It consists of seven irregular bones held firmly together by ligaments that both support the weight of the head and permit its motion while protecting the delicate spinal cord that runs through the central portion of these bones. The first two cervical vertebrae, C-1 (atlas) and C-2 (axis), have an usual structure and allow for rotation and nodding of the head. The last cervical vertebra (C-7) can be felt as the pronounced bony prominence along the spine just above the shoulders.

b. Thoracic spine   **pp. 248–249**

The thoracic vertebral column consists of 12 irregularly shaped bones, one corresponding to each rib pair. Their system of fixation to the ribs limits rib movement and increases the strength of the thoracic spine.

©2013 Pearson Education, Inc.
Paramedic Care: Principles & Practice, Vol. 5, 4th Ed.

    c. Lumbar spine **p. 249**

The lumbar spine consists of five lumbar vertebrae with massive vertebral bodies and thick intervertebral discs to support the weight of the head, neck, and thorax. They bear the forces of lifting and bending above the pelvis. Here the spinal cord ends at the juncture between L-1 and L-2 and nerve roots fill the spinal foramen from L-2 into the sacral spine.

    d. Sacrum **p. 250**

The sacrum consists of five vertebrae that are fused into a single plate forming the posterior portion of the pelvis. Together, the pelvis and sacrum protect the urinary and reproductive organs. The upper body balances on the sacrum, which articulates with the pelvis at the fixed sacroiliac joint. The sacrum serves as the point of attachment between the spinal column and lower extremities.

    e. Coccyx **p. 250**

The coccygeal region of the spine consists of three to five fused vertebrae that form the remnant of a tail. It serves no major function.

4. Anticipate specific types of injuries to the head, face, neck, and spinal column based on the mechanism of injury. **pp. 250–253**

Injuries to the head, face, neck, and spine occur secondary to blunt or penetrating mechanisms. The most common cause of serious blunt head trauma is the auto collision; other common mechanisms include falls, acts of violence, explosions, and sports-related activities. The head is especially vulnerable to blunt trauma because of its prominence. When struck, the borders of the scalp may tear, resulting in an avulsion. Blunt injury to the face is more likely to occur from intentional violence such as from a club or fist. Ears are subject to damage from the pressures associated with explosions or diving. The neck is well protected but it still may be impacted as the neck strikes the steering wheel or from a vehicle shoulder strap worn without a lap belt. Penetrating injury is not as common as blunt injury but can still endanger life. Typical mechanisms are gunshots and stabbings. High-energy gunshot wounds to the head devastate brain tissue and are frequently not survivable. Gunshot or stabbing wounds to the face and neck may also be life threatening because they may compromise the airway and distort facial and airway features. Explosions may propel objects into the head and facial regions. Penetrating injuries may also occur when a victim riding a recreational vehicle strikes a wire fence, is bitten by a dog, or is impaled by a fixed object.

    Spinal injuries may involve the vertebrae, spinal cord, nerve roots, tendons, ligaments, and muscles. Spinal column injury does not necessarily involve the spinal cord. Likewise, the cord may be injured in the absence of vertebral fracture or displacement. An injury to the spinal column, however, reduces its stability, posing a risk for cord damage if the patient is inappropriately moved. Spinal injury may result from numerous mechanisms, including extremes of normal anatomical movement, compression (axial loading), or traction (distraction). These injuries may occur as a direct result of penetrating or blunt trauma. Hyperextension or hyperflexion injuries most commonly affect the cervical or lumbar regions. Disk disruption, vertebral fracture, ligament stretching, or rupture and cord compression injury may result. Excessive rotation or lateral bending generally affect the cervical and lumbar regions. If a compression fracture occurs, bone fragments may be driven into the cord or the spinal column may become unstable from torn or stretched ligaments. Axial loading results from compression forces applied to the spinal axis. These injuries are seen when a person hits his head on a windshield, falls from a height landing on his heels, or when a diver strikes his head during a shallow dive. The impact is likely to compress, fracture, and crush the vertebrae or rupture disks. Common sites of axial loading injuries are T-12 and L-2 or the cervical region. Distraction injuries occur when the spinal column is stretched such as in a hanging. The upper cervical region is most commonly affected. Ligaments or the cord itself may be injured. Penetrating injuries may also damage the spine. Any type of spinal injury may have secondary consequences when swelling compresses the cord or interrupts blood flow.

5. Discuss the pathophysiology of: **pp. 253–260**

    a. Scalp and cranial injuries

Scalp injuries tend to bleed heavily and persistently because the blood vessels in the scalp do not constrict well. They also increase the risk for infection of the meninges. Scalp wounds may present as an outwardly projecting hematoma or be concealed when bleeding occurs under the skin into a depressed skull fracture. Because scalp tissue is loosely connected to the cranium, it may tear away (avulsion) exposing the skull.

Skull fractures require significant force to occur. Fractures may range from small cracks posing minimal danger to depressed skull fractures with significant intracranial damage. The temporal bone is the thinnest and most frequently fractured cranial bone. The base of the skull may also fracture, as it is weakened by the multiple foramina. Depending on the location, basilar skull fractures may present with "Battle's sign" when the lower lateral area of the skull is damaged or, "raccoon eyes" associated with orbital fractures. If the dura mater is torn, cerebrospinal fluid may leak from the ears or nose. A gunshot wound to the cranium may produce numerous cranial fractures and drive bone fragments into the brain or explode the skull outward. Impaled objects can cause extensive damage to delicate brain tissue. Cranial fractures alone do not threaten the brain; however, the force involved creates a high probability of interior brain injury.

b. **Facial and eye injuries**

Facial injuries involve the soft or skeletal structures of the face and may cause disfigurement. The facial area is extremely vascular and may bleed heavily, endangering the airway or causing vomiting. Soft tissue swelling occurs rapidly and can completely close or restrict the airway. Facial fractures may be open or closed and involve any of the skeletal structures of the area. They are generally associated with significant pain, swelling, deformity, or hemorrhage. The jaw may dislocate or break, with concomitant loss of teeth. Maxillary or facial bone fractures are classified according to Le Fort criteria. Leaking cerebral spinal fluid may endanger the nasal and oral cavities. These fractures are usually due to serious blunt trauma. Orbital blowout fractures involve the zygoma or maxilla. Pressure on the orbital region fractures the zygomatic arch and may interrupt muscle movement of the eye or jaw. Maxillary fractures cause swelling in the sinus region.

Although the eye is well protected from most blunt trauma by the surrounding skeletal structures, various eye injuries may occur. Depending on the injury, the victim may sustain permanent vision loss. Hyphema is a condition where blood fills the anterior chamber. Subconjunctival hemorrhage (a blood-red discoloration of the sclera) occurs when small blood vessels burst. If the orbital structures surrounding the eye are fractured, the eye may appear to protrude from the wound (eye avulsion). A depressed-appearing eye (enophthalmos) can result from compression or fracture of the orbital region. In retinal detachment, the retina separates from the posterior wall of the eye. Penetrating trauma may cause loss of the eye's fluids or entrap the small muscles that control it. Corneal abrasions or lacerations can occur if a foreign object is dragged across the eye's surface. If the eye or eyelid is lacerated, corneal lubrication or lacrimal duct function may be disrupted.

c. **Blunt and penetrating trauma to the neck**

Neck injury generally occurs from blunt or penetrating trauma to the anterior portion and can result in severe damage to the airway, spine, and blood vessels. Hematomas in the neck can rapidly expand, compressing the jugular veins. Laceration to the jugular veins or carotid arteries may cause significant brain hypoxia or exsanguination. Open neck wounds can draw air into them, forming an air embolism. If the larynx or trachea is fractured or crushed, destruction of the airway structures, swelling, and blood may seriously compromise respiration. Penetrating trauma involving the esophagus may allow gastric contents to enter the fascia, harming mediastinal structures or setting the stage for subsequent infection. If the vagus nerve is damaged, cardiovascular and gastrointestinal disruption occurs.

d. **Spinal column injuries**

The cervical spine is most commonly injured during spinal trauma, with C-1 and C-2 injuries most often associated with fatalities. Other spinal injuries often occur at the juncture between cervical spine regions where the differences in flexibility and rigidity of the transitioning regions make them more prone to damage. The spinal nerve roots extending beyond the L-1/L-2 region are more mobile and less prone to injury.

©2013 Pearson Education, Inc.
Paramedic Care: Principles & Practice, Vol. 5, 4th Ed.

6. **Demonstrate assessment of patients with head, face, neck, and spinal column injuries.**
pp. 260–267

Assessment of patients with head, face, neck, and spinal column injuries follows the standard assessment process using the techniques of observation, inspection, palpation, and auscultation. With these injuries, careful assessment of level of consciousness, airway, and breathing is critical. Begin with the scene size-up and analyze the mechanism of injury to develop an index of suspicion for possible injuries. Determine what forces were involved and how they were directed to the head, face, neck, and spine. Be aware that signs or symptoms may be masked by slow development, by the patient's use of alcohol or drugs, or other distracting injuries. If the mechanism of injury suggests, or the patient has any signs or symptoms of, spinal injury, the head and neck must be immediately manually immobilized and maintained until full mechanical immobilization is implemented. Form an initial impression of the patient's level of consciousness and orientation and recheck throughout care, as patients with these types of injuries are prone to deterioration. Also determine whether the patient experienced any loss of consciousness even if he was alert during your assessment. Evaluate the airway by examining the face and neck for any deformity, swelling, hemorrhage, or other injury that may threaten the airway. Anticipate vomiting, which can occur suddenly. Ensure that the mandible is stable and visualize the trachea for structural integrity and alignment. Determine the rate, volume, and adequacy of breathing. Look for bilateral chest excursion. Check pulse oximetry and apply oxygen if it is less than 96 percent. Monitor carbon dioxide levels with capnography. Check circulation by evaluating pulse rate and rhythm, and skin condition. Next assign a patient transport priority using the CUPS acronym.

Begin your secondary assessment with a rapid trauma assessment. Complete a full head-to-toe examination and manage any life-threatening injuries or conditions as you find them. Look at the head and sweep and gently palpate each region, checking for deformity and bleeding. Assume brain injury if a depressed or unstable skull fracture is identified. Examine the auditory canal with a penlight for evidence of leaking cerebrospinal fluid. Inspect the bones and soft tissues of the face for asymmetry, swelling, discoloration, deformity, instability, or crepitus. Observe the mouth for excessive secretions, blood, swelling, or dislodged teeth. Observe the eyes for pupil size, equality, and reactivity and check for proper movement. Ask the patient about any visual disturbances. Palpate the neck and note if frothy blood or subcutaneous emphysema is present. These indicate serious airway compromise. Examine the depth of any neck wounds to anticipate jugular or arterial damage. Assess the spine by observing the curvature. Look for swelling or discoloration and palpate for crepitus and deformity. Question the patient about pain, tenderness, weakness, or abnormal sensations. Note whether findings are unilateral or bilateral. Check the extremities for signs of decreased muscle tone, flaccid muscles, diminished sensation, or muscle strength.

Complete the secondary assessment by assigning the patient a baseline Glasgow Coma Scale score and obtaining vital signs. Note blood pressure, especially pulse pressure. Be alert for signs of Cushing's triad, which indicate increased intracranial pressure. During transport complete a detailed assessment after caring for all significant injuries. Injuries that were earlier masked may become apparent during this process. Frequently reassess the patient by repeating the primary assessment and reevaluating vital signs. Carefully monitor any changes in neurologic status for deterioration or improvement.

7. **Demonstrate proper techniques of manually stabilizing and immobilizing the spine.**
pp. 271–274

Immobilizing the spinal injury patient begins during the primary assessment with moving the patient to the neutral, in-line position, manually immobilizing the cervical spine, and applying a cervical collar after the neck is assessed. The primary objective of the entire process is maintaining the neutral, in-line position. The patient must first be moved from the position found into a supine, neutral, in-line position with the head facing directly forward and elevated 1 to 2 inches above the ground. If the patient is seated or standing, support the head by gently lifting it to reduce the head's weight on the spine. Align the nose, navel, and toes with the head facing forward and the shoulders and pelvis in a single plane with the body. If movement causes a significant increase in pain, meets with resistance, worsens neurologic signs, or you note a grossly deformed spine, immobilize the patient in the position found.

Manual in-line cervical immobilization is accomplished by approaching the patient from the front to prevent the patient from turning the head. A provider behind the patient should immobilize the head by placing the hands up along the patient's ears, using the little fingers to support the mandible and the heels of the hand to engage the mastoid region of the skull. If the patient is supine, support the head by placing the hands along the lateral and inferior surfaces of the head with the little fingers and heels of the hand lateral to the skull's occipital region. Lift the head 1 to 3 inches off the ground and elevate the shoulders of an infant or small child with a blanket or towel. Apply a cervical collar that has been appropriately sized snugly around the neck after the neck has been assessed. The cervical collar limits movement but does not completely prevent it, so manual stabilization must be maintained until the patient is mechanically immobilized.

If a patient with suspected spinal injury is walking around on scene, employ the procedures indicated above and use a standing takedown procedure to maintain spinal alignment. The provider at the head manually stabilizes the head while directing the process. If the patient is wearing a helmet, carefully assess whether the helmet should be removed. If the helmet interferes with airway or breathing, does not immobilize the head within, or cannot be secured to the spine board, it should be removed using proper technique to prevent movement of the head.

8. **Demonstrate proper techniques of handling, moving, and positioning patients with injuries to the head, face, neck, and spinal column.**   pp. 274–278

The primary goal of spinal immobilization is to ensure the patient remains in a neutral, in-line position. All movements should prevent any flexion/extension, rotation, or lateral bending. Movement to a long spine board should be carefully planned, well coordinated, and slowly executed. Several techniques are suitable for moving the spinal-injured patient, including the log roll, straddle slide, rope-sling slide, orthopedic stretcher lift, application of a vest-type device or short spine board, and rapid extrication. Regardless of technique, the provider at the head should always direct the move. A log roll is used to rotate a patient 90 degrees if found in a supine position or 180 degrees if in a prone position. After the patient has been manually immobilized and a C-collar applied, ideally, a four-person team performs the log roll. Extend the patient's arm above his head and roll the body toward the providers. Slide or pull a long spine board to the patient's side and gently roll the patient onto the board. If the patient is prone, the providers should reach across the board to grasp the patient and bring the patient to the board. The straddle slide is beneficial when there is not enough room to place a board along the patient lengthwise. One provider holds the head while two providers straddle the patient, grasping the shoulders and pelvis. They then lift the patient while a fourth provider slides the board underneath the patient from either the patient's head or feet.

A rope-sling slide is useful when there are only two providers available. The process utilizes a length of thick rope placed across the patient's chest and under the arms to pull axial traction and drag the patient onto the board. The first provider must hold cervical immobilization from the side or straddle the board and then ensure the head goes with the body as the patient is moved. Orthopedic or scoop stretchers separate into two halves for scooping the patient onto the device. Vest-type immobilization devices are often used to move a patient from a seated to a supine position on a long spine board, such as when moving a victim of an automobile crash. The device is placed behind the patient and secured. The patient is then rotated onto the buttocks and lowered to a supine position for further immobilization. Release the thigh straps after the patient is positioned on the board. A rapid extrication procedure is implemented when applying a vest-type device is too time consuming for a serious patient or because of scene safety considerations. The patient is extricated directly to a long board in a similar manner as with the vest-type device, ensuring that the spine, shoulders, pelvis, and legs are kept in line with the patient's nose, navel, and toes.

Once the patient is moved to the long spine board he should be properly centered and secured with the strappings. Straps should hold the shoulders and pelvis firmly to the board. The legs should be tied together and a rolled blanket placed under the knees to immobilize them in a flexed position. Last, the head should be immobilized to the board using a cervical immobilization device. Secure the head with forehead and chin straps without placing pressure on the neck or restricting jaw movement.

©2013 Pearson Education, Inc.
Paramedic Care: Principles & Practice, Vol. 5, 4th Ed.

Ideally the head should be elevated about 1 to 3 inches above the board's surface. Elevate the shoulders in a young child or infant. Padding may be used to fill the voids under the occiput and at the small of the back in adults. In the event of a diving injury, float a long spine board under the patient and secure him to the board before lifting and carrying him from the water.

9. **Describe the criteria that can be used as part of a spinal clearance protocol.**
                                                                                              pp. 261–262

If a patient presents with no serious signs or symptoms of injury and no significant mechanism of injury, you may consider whether to continue spinal precautions. In making this decision, remember that spinal cord injury can occur in the absence of column injury or neurological signs. Follow local spinal clearance protocol. Generally spinal precautions may be discontinued if three criteria are met: (1) the patient is alert and oriented; not under the influence of alcohol or drugs; and has a Glasgow Coma Scale (GCS) score of 15; (2) there are no distracting injuries or symptoms of abdominal pain or dyspnea; and (3) there are no signs or symptoms of spinal injury. Additionally, consider the age of the patient. Elderly and pediatric patients are not reliable reporters of spinal symptoms and some protocols call for spinal immobilization based on age parameters regardless of presenting signs and symptoms.

10. **Given a variety of scenarios, develop treatment plans for patients with injuries to the head, face, neck, and spinal column.**   pp. 263–265, 268–271, 278–279

Management priorities for patients with head, face, neck, and spinal column injury include spinal immobilization and airway management. Spinal precautions must begin immediately during the primary assessment. The patient should be moved to a supine, neutral, in-line position with the hips and knees somewhat flexed and the head elevated 1 to 2 inches above the ground. Next, immobilize the cervical spine to ensure no aggravation of any spinal injury. This manual immobilization is maintained and augmented by the application of a cervical collar, until the immobilization is continued by mechanical immobilization with an appropriate device. Airway management then takes precedence. Be prepared to suction aggressively in any patients with nasal, oral, or head trauma if blood or vomit is threatening the airway. Consider placement of an airway adjunct, but do not use a nasopharyngeal airway if basilar skull fracture is suspected. The decision to intubate should be made early in the care of an unresponsive patient or a patient with altered mental status. Remember, blood, vomit, and soft tissue trauma may cause swelling that can quickly progress from airway restriction to complete obstruction. Airway management techniques for head or spinal injury patients include use of extraglottic airways and orotracheal, retrograde, directed, and rapid sequence intubation. If the facial, neck, or airway structures are grossly distorted, percutaneous cricothyrotomy may be required. Ventilation should be guided by capnography. Maintain an end-tidal carbon dioxide (CO_2) reading of between 35 and 40 mmHg or slightly lower, 30 to 35 mmHg in patients with signs of herniation. If the patient is moving an adequate respiratory volume, administer high-concentration oxygen to maintain an oxygen saturation of at least 96 percent.

Manage circulation by controlling any serious hemorrhage and supporting blood pressure and cerebral perfusion. Although head and facial hemorrhage is usually easy to control, some injuries may bleed profusely, leading to hemorrhage and shock. Scalp injuries tend to bleed heavily. Control hemorrhage with direct pressure except when skull fracture is suspected. In that case, control bleeding with gentle pressure around the wound and place a loose dressing over it. Cover the ears and nose with gauze to ensure free outward movement of any cerebrospinal fluid. Glancing injuries may expose the skull and flap the scalp over on itself. Remove any gross contaminants by rinsing with normal saline. Then cover the exposed surfaces with a large, bulky, sterile dressing.

Facial injuries may involve fractures and/or soft tissue injury of the facial bones, eyes, ear, nose, throat, or mouth. Most eye wounds are best cared for by applying soft dressings to cover the closed, injured eye. If injury to one eye is severe, cover both eyes to prevent sympathetic motion. Use sterile dressings soaked in sterile saline to cover open eye wounds. Carefully remove embedded objects with a saline-moistened cotton swab. Irrigate gross contamination. If an eye is avulsed or has an impaled object, cover the eye and object with a protective device and dress and bandage both eyes.

Ear injury most commonly affects the pinna. External injury is cared for with dressing and bandaging; for internal injury, the ear is covered with gauze to permit the drainage of any fluids from the external auditory canal.

Nasal injury can involve the nasal cartilage and bones and cause fractures or dislocations. Hemorrhage in this area (epistaxis) can be very heavy. If possible, the patient's head should be brought forward to ensure that blood from the nasal cavity drains outward and not down the throat, which could irritate the stomach and increase the likelihood of vomiting.

Injuries to the oral cavity are related to fractures of the mandible, associated soft tissue destruction, or impaled objects. These injuries may result in serious hemorrhage and risk of soft tissue swelling and airway compromise. The airway should be maintained with suctioning, oral or nasal airway insertion, or intubation. Leave impaled objects in place unless they interfere with airway control. In this case, remove the object and control bleeding by direct pressure. Dislodged teeth should be wrapped in saline-soaked gauze and brought to the emergency department.

Neck injury may involve the structural integrity of the trachea or injury to major blood vessels. If the trachea is open to the environment, keep the area clear of blood and seal the wound. If frothy blood is noted, seal the wound on three sides with an occlusive dressing. Open neck wounds affecting the blood vessels present a risk for air embolism. Cover such wounds with occlusive dressings and secure them in place. Control bleeding with direct digital pressure. Position the patient's body head down on a backboard or stretcher if possible.

Case Study Review

Reread the case study on pages 238 and 239 in Paramedic Care: Trauma; *then, read the following discussion. This case highlights the precautions that must be taken whenever there is a possibility of spinal injury.*

Fred and Lisa respond to a blunt injury impact on the football field. They work with the team's athletic trainer and listen very carefully to his and the patient's description of the mechanism of injury as they begin their primary assessment. His torso was impacted from the side, probably displacing the chest laterally while the head and neck remained stationary. Either the impact caused the injury or injury was caused by the impact with the ground. As they begin their care for their patient, the paramedics don sterile gloves and form a general impression. He is an otherwise healthy young male who is able to speak in complete sentences and appears oriented to time, place, and persons. After a check of the player's distal pulse, Fred and Lisa quickly rule out any serious and immediate threats to his airway, breathing, and circulation.

As Fred and Lisa move to the focused trauma exam, they investigate the complaint of "tingling" and assess the spine from the base of the head to the sacrum and then determine which dermatomes are affected by the paraesthesia. They note tenderness around the 7th thoracic vertebra, a relatively common site for spine injury with lateral impact. The dermatomes affected are consistent with a lower cervical injury (most of the upper extremity is spared). With such conclusive evidence of a spinal column and cord injury, Fred and Lisa will be very careful in their helmet removal, movement of the patient to the long spine board, and spinal immobilization procedures. They will also carefully monitor for the signs and symptoms of neurogenic shock (warm lower limbs and cool upper limbs and the signs of hypovolemic compensation).

Fred and Lisa are presented with a dilemma regarding the helmet. It firmly immobilizes their patient's head within but because of its spherical nature it would be extremely difficult to affix to the flat surface of the long spine board. They choose to remove the helmet and secure his head directly to the spine board. They are also very attentive to the proper positioning of the player's head. Normally it would rest about 1 to 2 inches above the posterior body plane. However, because of his shoulder padding, to achieve proper positioning the head must be kept well above the playing field. They carefully remove the pads and lower the head, with the shoulders, to just slightly above the level of the field. They choose to use axial traction to move the player to the long spine board because it will help keep the spine in alignment during the move and requires fewer participants. As they move and secure him to the spine board, they ensure that the head rests the appropriate 1 to 1½ inches above the surface of the board.

During the entire procedure Lisa and Fred calm and reassure their patient that their actions are, for the most part, precautionary and explain each action before they perform it. This reduces the player's anxiety. Clearly the proper spinal precautions, as performed by this paramedic team, were responsible for limiting the seriousness of his injuries.

©2013 Pearson Education, Inc.
Paramedic Care: Principles & Practice, Vol. 5, 4th Ed.

Content Self-Evaluation

MULTIPLE CHOICE

_____ 1. The most common cause of trauma-related death is due to injury to the
- A. head.
- B. thorax.
- C. abdomen.
- D. pelvis.
- E. extremities.

_____ 2. What percentage of gunshot wounds to the cranium result in mortality?
- A. 30 to 40 percent
- B. 40 to 50 percent
- C. 65 to 70 percent
- D. 75 to 80 percent
- E. 90 to 95 percent

_____ 3. Which of the following is a layer of the scalp?
- A. The skin
- B. Connective tissue
- C. Galea aponeurotica
- D. Areolar tissue
- E. All of the above

_____ 4. Which of the following is NOT a bone of the cranium?
- A. Frontal
- B. Mandible
- C. Parietal
- D. Sphenoid
- E. Ethmoid

_____ 5. The largest opening in the cranium is the
- A. auditory canal.
- B. orbit of the eye.
- C. foramen magnum.
- D. tentorium.
- E. transverse foramen.

_____ 6. Which of the following is the lower and movable jaw bone?
- A. Maxilla
- B. Mandible
- C. Zygoma
- D. Stapes
- E. Pinna

_____ 7. Which of the following is the bone of the cheek?
- A. Maxilla
- B. Mandible
- C. Zygoma
- D. Stapes
- E. Pinna

_____ 8. The structure(s) responsible for our positional sense is (are) the
- A. ossicle.
- B. cochlea.
- C. semicircular canals.
- D. sinuses.
- E. vitreous humor.

_____ 9. Which of the following is the opening through which light travels to contact the light-sensing tissue in the eye?
- A. Retina
- B. Aqueous humor
- C. Vitreous humor
- D. Pupil
- E. Iris

_____ 10. Which of the following is the light-sensing tissue in the eye?
- A. Retina
- B. Aqueous humor
- C. Vitreous humor
- D. Pupil
- E. Iris

_____ 11. The white of the eye is the
- A. sclera.
- B. conjunctiva.
- C. cornea.
- D. aqueous humor.
- E. vitreous humor.

_____ 12. The delicate, clear tissue covering the pupil and iris is the
   A. sclera.
   B. conjunctiva.
   C. cornea.
   D. aqueous humor.
   E. vitreous humor.

_____ 13. The vertebral column is made up of how many vertebrae?
   A. 24
   B. 33
   C. 43
   D. 45
   E. 54

_____ 14. The functions of the ligaments supporting the spinal column include all of the following, EXCEPT
   A. preventing hyperextension.
   B. allowing straightening of the spine.
   C. connecting adjoining vertebrae.
   D. protecting the neck.
   E. securing the spinal cord.

_____ 15. The component of the vertebrae that protrudes posteriorly and can be felt in several regions of the spine is which of the following?
   A. Transverse process
   B. Spinous process
   C. Laminae
   D. Pedicles
   E. Foraminae

_____ 16. The region of the vertebral column that permits the greatest movement is the
   A. cervical.
   B. thoracic.
   C. lumbar.
   D. sacral.
   E. coccygeal.

_____ 17. The major weight-bearing component of the vertebral column is the
   A. spinous process.
   B. transverse process.
   C. vertebral body.
   D. spinal foramen.
   E. lamina.

_____ 18. The region of the vertebral column that has 12 vertebrae is the
   A. cervical.
   B. thoracic.
   C. lumbar.
   D. sacral.
   E. coccygeal.

_____ 19. The region of the vertebral column that has five separate vertebrae is the
   A. cervical.
   B. thoracic.
   C. lumbar.
   D. sacral.
   E. coccygeal.

_____ 20. Head trauma accounts for just over what percentage of motor vehicle–related deaths?
   A. 20 percent
   B. 40 percent
   C. 50 percent
   D. 80 percent
   E. 90 percent

_____ 21. Which of the following motions is likely to result from the rear-end auto impact?
   A. Hyperextension
   B. Hyperflexion
   C. Lateral bending
   D. Axial loading
   E. Distraction

_____ 22. Which of the following motions is likely to result from hanging?
   A. Hyperextension
   B. Hyperflexion
   C. Lateral bending
   D. Axial loading
   E. Distraction

_____ **23.** Spinal cord injury can occur without injury to the vertebral column or its associated ligaments.
- **A.** True
- **B.** False

_____ **24.** Serious scalp injury is unlikely to produce hypovolemia and shock because the arteries there frequently constrict and effectively limit blood loss.
- **A.** True
- **B.** False

_____ **25.** Which of the following statements is NOT true of scalp wounds?
- **A.** They pose a risk of meningeal infection.
- **B.** Wounds there tend to heal very well.
- **C.** Wounds there tend to bleed heavily.
- **D.** Contusions there swell outward noticeably.
- **E.** Avulsion of the scalp is not a likely injury.

_____ **26.** The most common type of skull fracture is
- **A.** depressed.
- **B.** basilar.
- **C.** linear.
- **D.** comminuted.
- **E.** spiral.

_____ **27.** The type of skull fracture most often associated with high-velocity bullet entry is
- **A.** depressed.
- **B.** basilar.
- **C.** linear.
- **D.** comminuted.
- **E.** spiral.

_____ **28.** It is common for the paramedic to observe either Battle's sign or bilateral periorbital ecchymosis in the patient who has just sustained a basilar skull fracture.
- **A.** True
- **B.** False

_____ **29.** The discoloration found around both eyes due to basilar skull fracture is
- **A.** retroauricular ecchymosis.
- **B.** bilateral periorbital ecchymosis.
- **C.** Cullen's sign.
- **D.** the halo sign.
- **E.** Gray's sign.

_____ **30.** Blood and CSF draining from the ear may display a
- **A.** speckled appearance.
- **B.** concentric light-yellow circle.
- **C.** congealed mass.
- **D.** greenish discoloration.
- **E.** light-red ring.

_____ **31.** A cranial fracture, by itself, is a skeletal injury that will heal with time; it is the injury underneath that is of most concern.
- **A.** True
- **B.** False

_____ **32.** With facial trauma, lower airway obstruction is more likely due to blood than other fluids or physical obstruction.
- **A.** True
- **B.** False

_____ **33.** According to the Le Fort criteria, a fracture involving just the maxilla and limited instability is classified as
- **A.** Le Fort I.
- **B.** Le Fort II.
- **C.** Le Fort III.
- **D.** Le Fort IV.
- **E.** Le Fort V.

_____ **34.** Which type of Le Fort fracture is likely to result in cerebrospinal fluid leakage?
- **A.** Le Fort I
- **B.** Le Fort II
- **C.** Le Fort II and III
- **D.** Le Fort I and II
- **E.** Le Fort I and III

35. Which of the following statements is TRUE regarding injuries to the pinna of the ear?
   A. They hemorrhage severely.
   B. Hemorrhage is difficult to control.
   C. Hemorrhage is limited.
   D. Wounds there do not heal very well.
   E. Both C and D.

36. Which of the following mechanisms is likely to injure the tympanum?
   A. Basilar skull fracture
   B. An explosion
   C. Diving injury
   D. An object forced into the ear
   E. All of the above

37. The collection of blood in front of a patient's pupil and iris due to blunt trauma is called a(n)
   A. hyphema.
   B. retinal detachment.
   C. aniscoria.
   D. anterior chamber hematoma.
   E. subconjunctival hemorrhage.

38. A sudden and painless loss of sight is most likely a(n)
   A. hyphema.
   B. retinal detachment.
   C. acute retinal artery occlusion.
   D. anterior chamber hematoma.
   E. subconjunctival hemorrhage.

39. Blood vessel injury in the neck region carries with it the hazards of all of the following, EXCEPT
   A. severe venous hemorrhage.
   B. severe arterial hemorrhage.
   C. development of subcutaneous emphysema.
   D. air aspiration.
   E. pulmonary emboli.

40. The region that accounts for more than half of spinal cord injuries is the
   A. cervical spine.
   B. thoracic spine.
   C. lumbar spine
   D. sacral spine.
   E. coccygeal spine.

41. Helmets reduce the incidence of both head and spine injury.
   A. True
   B. False

42. Manual immobilization should continue from the moment you arrive at the suspected spine-injured patient's side until a cervical collar is applied.
   A. True
   B. False

43. Which of the following is a criteria for discontinuing spinal precautions?
   A. The patient's only symptom is dyspnea.
   B. The patient is alert and partially oriented.
   C. The patient is free of significant distracting injuries.
   D. The patient is showing signs of sympathetic response.
   E. The patient is a very young child.

44. Which of the following is NOT a mechanism of injury likely to cause spinal injury?
   A. Fall from over three times the patient's height
   B. High-speed motor vehicle crash
   C. Serious blunt trauma above the shoulders
   D. Penetrating trauma directed to the lateral thorax
   E. Penetrating trauma directed to the spine

_____ 45. Oral intubation is generally more difficult in the patient who requires spinal precautions because the landmarks are more difficult to visualize.
  A. True
  B. False

_____ 46. During the initial assessment, you should be aware that exaggerated abdominal movement and limited chest excursions often suggest
  A. airway obstruction.
  B. the need to reposition the head and neck.
  C. diaphragmatic breathing.
  D. neurogenic shock.
  E. cardiac contusion.

_____ 47. Any significant open wound to the anterior or lateral neck should be covered with a(n)
  A. wet dressing.
  B. occlusive dressing.
  C. nonadherent dressing.
  D. adherent dressing.
  E. pressure dressing.

_____ 48. The major reason for allowing fluid to drain from the nose or ear is that
  A. it may speed the rise of intracranial pressure.
  B. its flow will prevent pathogens from entering the meninges.
  C. it is impossible to stop the flow anyway.
  D. regeneration of CSF is beneficial to the healing process.
  E. none of the above.

_____ 49. Conditions that may make it difficult to spinally immobilize a patient include all of the following, EXCEPT
  A. ankylosing spondylitis.
  B. kyphosis.
  C. scoliosis.
  D. herniated disk.
  E. bamboo spine.

_____ 50. Which of the following could be considered a component of Cushing's triad?
  A. Cheyne-Stokes respirations
  B. Decreasing pulse rate
  C. Increasing blood pressure
  D. Ataxic respirations
  E. All of the above

_____ 51. The head injury patient may vomit without warning, and the vomiting may be projectile in nature.
  A. True
  B. False

_____ 52. Which of the following airway techniques is NOT recommended for the patient with suspected basilar skull fracture?
  A. Nasopharyngeal airway insertion
  B. Directed intubation
  C. Digital intubation
  D. Orotracheal intubation
  E. Rapid-sequence intubation

_____ 53. Prolonged attempts at intubation can induce hypoxia and hypercarbia.
  A. True
  B. False

_____ 54. Which of the following is an acceptable method for confirming endotracheal tube placement in the head injury patient?
  A. Use of an end-tidal CO_2 monitor
  B. Use of a pulse oximeter
  C. Observing bilaterally equal chest rise
  D. Good and bilaterally equal breath sounds
  E. All of the above

55. For adequate ventilation through a needle cricothyrotomy, you must use a demand valve ventilator.
    A. True
    B. False

56. When locating the cricoid cartilage, either for Sellick's maneuver or the cricothyrotomy, it is the first hard rigid ring you feel as you move your fingers up the trachea from the suprasternal notch.
    A. True
    B. False

57. Proper immobilization of the patient with spinal injury should include placing a blanket roll under the knees.
    A. True
    B. False

58. Which of the following is a contraindication to continuing to move the head and spine toward the neutral, in-line position?
    A. You meet with significant resistance.
    B. Your patient complains of a significant increase in pain.
    C. You notice gross deformity along the spine.
    D. You notice an increase in the signs of neurologic injury.
    E. All of the above.

59. Some gentle axial traction on the head will make cervical immobilization more effective.
    A. True
    B. False

60. The ideal position for the small adult's or child's head during spinal immobilization is
    A. 1 to 3 inches above the spine board.
    B. level with the spine board.
    C. with padding under the shoulders and the head on the spine board.
    D. with the head slightly extended and level with the board.
    E. none of the above.

61. The standing takedown for the patient with spinal injuries requires a minimum of how many care providers?
    A. Two
    B. Three
    C. Four
    D. Five
    E. No less than six

62. Under which of the following circumstances should a helmet be removed from a patient?
    A. The head is not immobilized within the helmet.
    B. The helmet prevents airway maintenance.
    C. You cannot secure the helmet firmly to the long spine board.
    D. You anticipate breathing problems.
    E. All of the above.

63. A four-count cadence is preferable for moves because it better signals care providers when the move starts.
    A. True
    B. False

64. A log-roll is properly performed by
    A. crossing the patient's arms across the chest.
    B. placing a towel under the neck.
    C. placing a bulky blanket between the legs.
    D. securing the patient's hands together.
    E. rolling the patient 45 degrees onto the board.

©2013 Pearson Education, Inc.
Paramedic Care: Principles & Practice, Vol. 5, 4th Ed.

65. Newer orthopedic stretchers are rigid enough to be used for spinal immobilization by themselves.
    A. True
    B. False

66. The vest-type immobilization device is meant to permit rescuers to move the patient from a seated to a supine position in an auto crash by rotating the buttocks on the seat, then tilting the patient to the supine position.
    A. True
    B. False

67. Which of the following circumstances would NOT automatically merit employment of rapid extrication techniques?
    A. Toxic fumes
    B. An auto collision
    C. An immediate threat of fire
    D. Rising water
    E. None of the above

68. Once you immobilize the body to the long spine board, you can then secure the head to it.
    A. True
    B. False

69. The most ideal position for the adult head during spinal immobilization is
    A. 1 to 3 inches above the spine board.
    B. level with the spine board.
    C. with padding under the shoulders and the head on the spine board.
    D. with the head slightly extended and level with the board.
    E. none of the above.

70. The best technique for immobilizing a patient onto a long spine board who is in the water after sustaining a diving injury is
    A. log-rolling.
    B. straddle slide.
    C. rope-sling slide.
    D. applying a vest-type device.
    E. none of the above.

71. When treating an avulsed eye you should
    A. apply dry, sterile gauze.
    B. irrigate the eye.
    C. remove an embedded object.
    D. cover both eyes.
    E. invert the eyelid.

72. Dislodged teeth from a patient should be
    A. wrapped in gauze soaked in water.
    B. wrapped in gauze soaked in sterile saline.
    C. wrapped in dry gauze.
    D. kept dry but cool.
    E. replaced immediately.

Special Project

Recognizing Spinal Regions

Label the regions of the spine and the number of the vertebrae in each.

A. _____

B. _____

C. _____

D. _____

E. _____

Paramedic Care: Principles & Practice, Vol. 5, 4th Ed.

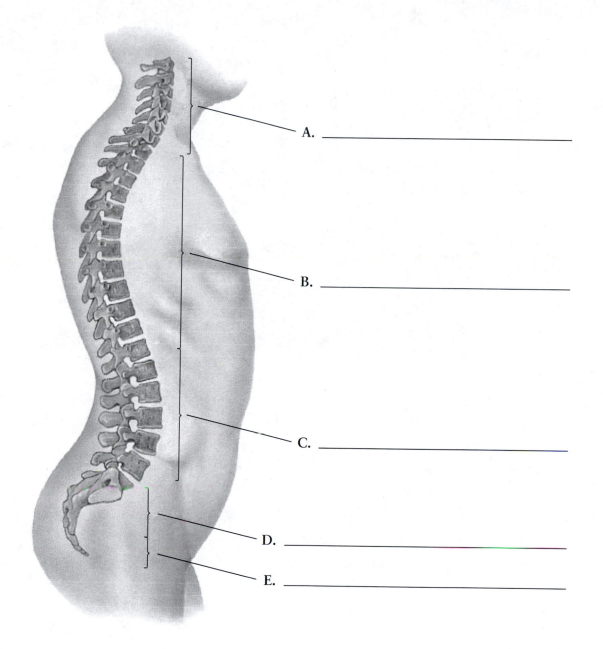

A. _____

B. _____

C. _____

D. _____

E. _____

11

Nervous System Trauma

Review of Chapter Objectives

After reading this chapter, you should be able to:

1. Define key terms introduced in this chapter.

Knowing and being able to apply the key terms in each chapter is critical to understanding chapter concepts. Write the list of key terms. Then write the definition of each one in your own words. Check your understanding by confirming the definitions in the text glossary. Correct any misunderstandings. Create a study aid by writing each key term on the front of an index card and the definition on the back. Use the cards to quiz yourself, or to have someone quiz you.

2. Describe the anatomy and physiology of the nervous system.   **pp. 284–293**

The nervous system is the central processing system of the body, enabling sensory and motor function as well as involuntary control of organs. The nervous system is comprised of two major components: the central nervous system (brain and spinal cord) and the peripheral nervous system (all other nerves of the body).

The brain and spinal cord are protected by skin and skeletal structures. Beneath these are connective tissues called the meninges. There are three layers of tissue—the dura mater, the arachnoid, and the pia mater—that surround the brain and spinal cord. The dura mater is a tough, fibrous layer that lines the interior of the skull and spinal foramen and is continuous with the inner periosteum of the cranium. The pia mater is a delicate membrane covering the convolutions of the brain and spinal cord. The arachnoid is a weblike structure between the dura mater and pia mater. Cerebrospinal fluid is a clear, colorless solution that surrounds the central nervous system. It fills the subarachnoid space and "floats" the brain and spinal cord to help absorb the energy of trauma. Cerebrospinal fluid is constantly regenerated. It also serves to bring nutrients to brain tissue and remove waste products.

The brain fills about 80 percent of the cranium and is comprised of the cerebrum, cerebellum, and brainstem. The cerebrum is the center of consciousness, personality, speech, motor control, and perception. The cerebrum occupies most of the cranial vault. It contains the frontal, parietal, and temporal lobes, which are further divided by the falx cerebri into right and left hemispheres controlling the activities of the opposite side of the body. The cerebellum lies behind and beneath the cerebrum. It is responsible for fine motor control, balance, and maintenance of muscle tone. The brainstem forms the communication relay area between the brain and spinal cord. It contains the midbrain, pons, and medulla oblongata. Structures within the brainstem are responsible for controlling the endocrine system, maintaining consciousness and regulating sleep, the vomiting reflex, temperature, and blood pressure. The lower portion of the brainstem performs critical regulatory functions for the cardiovascular and respiratory systems. Originating within the cranium and along the brainstem are the 12 cranial nerves, which innervate the facial area and also control other major body functions. The brain is perfused by a network of major arterial vessels. These all interconnect through the circle of Willis in the base of the brain, where additional arteries branch out to supply the brain's substance. The cranium maintains a slight pressure, called intracranial pressure (ICP), which is dynamic. Because the intracranial volume is fixed with respect to the rigid cranial vault, cerebrospinal fluid and blood must stay in balance to prevent a rise in ICP. A significant rise in ICP may displace the brain toward the opposite side of the cranium or herniate the cranial contents out through the foramen magnum.

The spine is the principal support system of the body. The vertebral column provides structural support for the head, thoracic cage, upper body, and pelvis. The spinal cord travels through the vertebral column, serving as the conduit for sensory input to the brain and outgoing motor impulses from the brain to the various muscles and organs. It also plays a role in the reflex system. The spinal cord is a long cylinder comprised of gray matter (neural cell bodies) and white matter (nerve fibers) surrounding the gray matter. Nerve cell pathways called axons are arranged in ascending and descending tracts, transmitting signals upward to the brain and downward through the cord, respectively. The ascending tracts carry sensory impulses of touch, pressure, vibration, positional sense, pain, and temperature. Descending tracts are responsible for voluntary muscle movement.

Contiguous with the brain are the spinal meninges, which similarly consist of the dura mater, arachnoid membrane, and pia mater. The meninges cover the entire spinal cord and the peripheral nerve roots as they exit the spinal column. Cerebrospinal fluid bathes the spinal cord, providing protection and serving as a medium for nutrient and waste product exchange. Branching out from the cord are 31 pairs of peripheral nerve roots, which exit through the intervertebral foramina. The nerve roots form clusters called a plexus, enabling the nerves to function as a group. The primary plexuses are the cervical, brachial, lumbar, and sacral. The sensory nerves innervate specific body surface areas called dermatomes. Myotomes are discrete tissues and muscles of the body innervated by the motor components of the spinal nerve roots. The spinal nerves are further subdivided into the parasympathetic and sympathetic components of the autonomic nervous system. The parasympathetic subdivision controls rest and regenerative functions, while the sympathetic nervous system controls metabolic activity and the "fight-or-flight" response.

3. **Explain the pathophysiology of direct (focal and diffuse) and indirect brain injuries.** pp. 293–296

Direct brain injury may be caused by deceleration or acceleration forces, penetrating injury, or jarring of the brain within the cranium. Coup injuries produce tissue damage at the point of impact. Contrecoup injuries cause damage away from the impact point as the brain rebounds and strikes the opposite side of the cranium. Direct injuries may be focal or diffuse.

Focal injuries include cerebral contusion and intracranial hemorrhage. Contusions are caused by blunt trauma, which results in capillary bleeding into the brain's substance at one or more sites in the brain. Dysfunction is localized to the injury site. Intracranial hemorrhage may occur above, below, or in any of the meninges or within the brain matter itself. Depending on severity these are often associated with progressive hemorrhage and ICP. An epidural hematoma involves bleeding between the dura mater and the skull's interior surface. It usually involves high-pressure arterial vessels, which causes rapidly increasing intracranial pressure. When bleeding occurs beneath the dura mater or within the subarachnoid space, it is called a subdural hematoma. Blood loss is usually due to small venous vessel rupture and progresses slowly. Neurologic signs and symptoms may be absent initially or subtle, manifesting hours or days after the incident. Intracerebral hemorrhage is the most damaging. Blood, usually from a ruptured artery, flows into the substance of the brain. Nervous tissue is irritated, causing tissue edema, which may progress rapidly, resulting in neurologic deficits and increased intracranial pressure.

Diffuse injuries involve mild to severe nerve tissue disruption. Axons are damaged when stretching, tearing, or shearing forces are applied to nerve fibers. If the injury is distributed throughout the brain it is considered a diffuse axonal injury (DAI). Acceleration, deceleration, or overpressure from an explosion are characteristic mechanisms. Concussions are a mild to moderate form of DAI. Structural damage may be minimal with a transient episode of nerve dysfunction. Moderate diffuse axonal injury involves limited brain tissue bruising from shearing, stretching, or tearing forces. The patient may be rendered unconscious or have sustained a basilar skull fracture. In severe DAI, major disruption of nerve tissue occurs in both cerebral hemispheres and possibly the brainstem. This serious injury may result in death or permanent neurologic impairment.

Indirect injury occurs after the initial injury and may have even more serious consequences. Two pathological processes are responsible. As intracranial pressure rises, intracranial perfusion decreases. This may be worsened by hypoxia, hypercarbia, and systemic hypotension. Initially, the body attempts to compensate for a rise in ICP. Venous blood vessels are compressed first by expansion of a mass in the brain. This triggers movement of cerebrospinal fluid out of the cranium into the spinal cord. However, this compensatory mechanism is limited and the continued rise of ICP causes arterial blood flow restriction, reducing perfusion to the brain. Blood pressure rises to offset this problem, but as blood pressure rises, so does ICP, leading to a potentially deadly cycle. Secondarily, the rising ICP begins to displace uninjured brain tissue, putting pressure on the brainstem. Ultimately, the process results in herniation, where brain tissue is pushed through openings in the upper or lower brainstem. Both pathologies worsen nervous tissue damage and reduce perfusion, leading to the progressive signs and symptoms associated with head injury.

4. Recognize the signs and symptoms of traumatic brain injury.   pp. 295–297

Signs and symptoms of traumatic brain injury occur both from the direct injury and as a result of the rise in intracranial pressure and brain tissue displacement. Signs and symptoms are related to the severity of injury. In mild to moderate diffuse axonal injury (concussion) the patient may experience an episode of unconsciousness followed by confusion, disorientation, and retrograde or anterograde amnesia. The victim may report headache, light sensitivity, and disturbances in smell or other senses. The patient may have focal neurologic deficits and experience anxiety or mood swings. With more severe injury, the patient may be unconscious for an extended period of time or initially present with an altered level of consciousness and orientation. Extensive cortical injury may cause the person to be unaware of what happened or lose recall of events both prior to and following the injury. The patient may become combative. Focal deficits, such as hemiplegia or hemiparesis, and seizures may result. The patient may display visual disturbances, speech problems, or undergo alterations in personality depending on the location of the injury. If the ascending reticular activating system in the brainstem, responsible for maintaining consciousness, is affected, the patient may become lethargic or comatose. Displacement of brain tissue as intracranial pressure rises can lead to vomiting, pupil dilation and fixation, or disturbances in breathing, blood pressure, and heart rate. Decerebrate or decorticate posturing may be apparent.

5. Relate patients' signs and symptoms to the progression of traumatic brain injury.   pp. 297–298

With significant cortical disruption, the patient undergoes a progression of signs and symptoms secondary to increased intracranial pressure and structural displacement. This pattern is known as the central syndrome. Upper brainstem compression results in Cushing's reflex. Blood pressure rises to maintain cerebral perfusion, while heart rate decreases in response to vagus nerve (parasympathetic) stimulation of the sinoatrial (SA) and atrioventricular (AV) nodes. A characteristic cyclic breathing pattern (Cheyne-Stokes respirations) of increasing, then decreasing respiratory volume followed by a period of apnea appears. Together, these classic signs are called Cushing's triad. If the hypothalamus is involved the patient may vomit. Pupils remain small and reactive. Decorticate posturing in response to painful stimuli may be obvious. As pressure continues to build the middle brainstem becomes involved. Pulse pressure widens and heart rate decreases. Respirations may be deep and rapid (central neurogenic hyperventilation). Pupils become bilaterally sluggish and nonreactive. Decerebrate posturing develops. Once the pressure reaches the lower brainstem, respirations become ataxic or cease. Pupils become fully dilated and unreactive. The pulse rate may be irregular and changeable. Electrocardiogram (ECG) disturbances are apparent. Hypotension ensues. The patient ceases to respond to painful stimuli and the skeletal muscles become flaccid. At this stage, patient survival is unlikely.

6. **Discuss differences between pediatric and adult head trauma pathophysiology and findings.** p. 298

Pediatric patients have softer skulls than adults. The skull contains more cartilaginous tissue, which results in greater direct damage to the brain tissue but permits more intracranial expansion from swelling. This slows the progression of increased intracranial pressure and its related pathologies. In infants, the swelling may be apparent from bulging fontanelles. Additionally, pediatric patients have proportionately larger heads and smaller total body fluid volume and reserves. While intracranial hemorrhage does not manifest early on as hypovolemia in adults, young patients may present with hypovolemia much sooner.

7. **Explain the pathophysiology of spinal cord injuries.** pp. 298–299

The spinal cord, like all central nervous system tissue, is extremely specialized and delicate and does not repair itself well, if at all. The spinal cord may be injured in much the same way as the brain by mechanisms including concussion, contusion, compression, laceration, hemorrhage, and transection. The concussion is a jarring that momentarily disrupts the cord function. Contusion results in some damage and bleeding into the cord but will likely repair itself. Compression may occur as a result of vertebral body displacement or as a result of cord edema; it deprives portions of the cord of blood, and ischemic damage may result. The degree of injury and its permanence is related to the amount of compression and the length of time the compression remains. Laceration occurs as bony fragments are driven into the cord and damage it. If the injury is severe, the injury is probably permanent. Hemorrhage into the cord results in compression and irritation of the cord tissue as blood crosses the blood–brain barrier. The injury may also restrict blood flow to a portion of the cord, extending the injury. Transection is a partial or complete severance of the cord with its function below the lesion, for the most part, lost.

8. **Recognize findings associated with spinal cord syndromes.** pp. 299–301

The signs and symptoms of spinal cord injury depend on the level of the injury and the degree of damage. Often they are classified as complete or incomplete. A complete cord injury completely severs the spinal cord, and the ability to send and receive nerve impulses below the site of the injury is lost. Results may include, depending on the site of injury, paraplegia, quadriplegia, incontinence, and partial or complete respiratory paralysis. With incomplete cord injury, the spinal cord is only partially severed. There is potential for some recovery of function. There are four primary types of incomplete injury.

Anterior cord syndrome Anterior cord syndrome is due to damage caused by bone fragments or pressure on the arteries that perfuse the anterior portion of the cord. The affected limbs are likely only to retain motion, vibration, and positional sensation, with motor and other sensory perceptions lost.

Central cord syndrome Central cord syndrome is related to hyperextension-type injuries and is often associated with a preexisting disease such as arthritis that narrows the spinal foramen. It usually results in motor weakness of the upper extremities and in some cases loss of bladder control. The prognosis for at least some recovery for the central cord syndrome is the best of all the cord syndromes.

Brown-Séquard syndrome Brown-Séquard syndrome is most often caused by a penetrating injury that affects one side of the cord (hemitransection). Sensory and motor loss is noted on the ipsilateral side, while pain and temperature sensation is lost on the contralateral side. The injury is rare but often associated with some recovery.

Cauda equina syndrome Cauda equina syndrome occurs when nerve roots at the lower end of the spinal cord are compressed. Sensory and motor control are disrupted, resulting in bladder and bowel incontinence, and weakness and altered sensation in the lower extremities.

Neurogenic shock occurs when the injury interferes with the brain's ability to control autonomic functions. The patient presents with low blood pressure; a slow heart rate; cool, moist, pale skin above the lesion; and warm, dry, flushed skin above the injury. Transient injury to the spine may result from injury that does not seriously or permanently damage the cord. With spinal shock, the patient may initially present with classic signs and symptoms of cord injury, including the inability to move the extremities, loss of sensation, incontinence, and priapism in males. Loss of body temperature control and hypotension may be present. A stinger is typically a contact-sport-related injury to the nerves in or near the neck or shoulder. The patient experiences painful electric sensations radiating through the neck or one of the arms. This does not result in permanent paralysis. Transient quadriplegia, while temporary, is a more serious injury. The cervical spinal cord is disrupted, causing numbness or pain, with or without weakness or paralysis in some or all extremities. The episode usually lasts less than 15 minutes but may take up to as long as 48 hours to resolve.

9. Discuss differences between pediatric and adult spinal injuries.   pp. 301–302

In general, pediatric spines are more mobile and elastic than in adults. This affords greater protection against spinal cord trauma. Pediatric patients present with different age-related spinal cord injury patterns. Infants have underdeveloped neck muscles, incompletely calcified vertebrae, and shallow, horizontally oriented facet joints. The head is large relative to the body. These developmental factors increase the likelihood of spine injury between the skull and first cervical vertebrae. Between ages 2 and 10 muscles and ligaments strengthen and calcified bone replaces cartilage. The size of the head becomes more proportionate to body size. These changes shift injury patterns to the lower cervical spine. Because of the more flexible spinal column, children, unlike adults, may sustain spinal cord injury without radiographic indication of vertebral column injury.

10. Demonstrate the assessment of patients suspected of having central nervous system injuries.   pp. 302–308

Head injury and sometimes spinal cord injuries may be present in the absence of obvious external evidence. Evaluating the mechanism of injury is critical to ensuring good patient outcomes. During your analysis, consider whether there may have been excessive flexion, extension, lateral, rotational, axial loading, or distraction of the head and neck. If there is any suspicion of spinal injury, immediately implement spinal precautions followed by full spinal immobilization as required. Begin your primary assessment by evaluating the patient's level of consciousness and orientation. Any confusion or amnesia suggests traumatic brain injury. Utilize the Simplified Motor Score (SMS) or the Glasgow Coma Scale (GCS) to quantify the condition of your patient's mental status. Remember that altered mental status may leave the patient unable to maintain the airway. Monitor the respiratory rate, depth, and rhythm. Check circulatory status and skin condition for evidence of hypovolemia or neurogenic shock.

The secondary assessment will include a rapid full body trauma assessment and vitals. Begin at the feet and move up the body to the head. Observe and palpate each body region. Note whether there is any line of demarcation in skin condition denoting a change from flush and warm to cool and clammy. Evaluate for changes in sensitivity to pain and light touch as well as noting any differences in muscle tone. Test for motor and sensory function in all extremities. If deficits are found, determine whether they are bilateral or unilateral. Ask the patient whether he has any abnormal feelings in the limb, such as paralysis, weakness, numbness, tingling, or pain. Any loss in the ability to move (paralysis) or muscular strength (paresis) is suggestive of spinal cord injury.

While performing the physical exam question the patient about other signs and symptoms. Ask the patient about his recall of the incident, including events preceding and following the injury to identify retrograde or anterograde amnesia. Obtain a SAMPLE history, paying close attention to pre-incident nervous system injury or illness and whether the patient is taking any anticoagulants. Remember that drug and/or alcohol intoxication may mask signs of central nervous system injury. Obtain vital signs and monitor blood pressure carefully. If the patient is hypotensive in the presence of traumatic brain injury, look for signs or symptoms suggesting internal hemorrhage. A widening pulse pressure (high systolic with normal diastolic) is a sign of increasing intracranial pressure.

Frequent reassessment is critical for head- or spine-injured patients. Reassess mental status, assigning a GCS score or SMS rating each time to monitor trends in condition. Reevaluate pupils for evidence of cerebral hypoxia or increasing intracranial pressure. Track changes in movement or sensory perception. Reassess vitals every 5 minutes. Watch pulse oximetry, capnography, and blood pressure readings to ensure that the patient becomes neither hypoxic or hypovolemic. If the patient's condition deteriorates, provide rapid transport to an appropriate trauma facility.

11. Relate assessment findings to the potential for particular central nervous system injuries.

pp. 302–308

Careful assessment of the trauma patient may reveal findings indicative of specific central nervous system injury. If the patient displays any alteration in mental status, including confusion or disorientation, suspect possible brain injury. Obtaining an early baseline against which to compare mental status throughout care can alert you to a deteriorating situation. Abnormal breathing patterns may be a significant indicator of increasing intracranial pressure. An increased respiratory rate and volume or erratic respirations suggest brainstem injury. Cerebral herniation should be suspected in a patient who presents with an irregular respiratory pattern coupled with increasing systolic blood pressure, and a slow, decreasing pulse (Cushing's triad). Skin that is warm and dry in the lower extremities while upper body regions show cool, clammy skin is indicative of spinal injury accompanied by neurogenic shock. Exam the pupils carefully, as eye reactivity reflects the brain's oxygenation status. Look for equality, reactivity, and size. Unilateral reactivity or gaze or eyes that move with the head suggest head injury. More specifically, the eyes can give indications of problems with cranial nerves, II, III, IV, and VI. Fixed and dilated pupils suggest increasing intracranial pressure on the oculomotor nerve (CN-III). The ipsilateral pupil will become sluggish, then dilated and fixed as the rising pressure interferes with parasympathetic nerve fibers.

During the physical exam, determine whether there is any loss of motor function or sensation. Note the level at which the patient first identifies sensation or pain. Assess muscle tone, looking for areas of muscle flaccidity. These neurologic signs indicate the level at which the spinal cord is disrupted. Identify how large of a region is involved. If multiple dermatomes are symptomatic, suspect spinal cord injury. If only a single dermatome is involved, suspect nerve root damage. Test for finger abduction/adduction in the upper extremities to ascertain injury at the level of T-1. Test finger or hand extension for injury at C-7. Assess grips for equality and firmness. Check for pain reception by (the spinothalamic tract) using a pointed object to induce slight point pain. Use a cotton swab or pad of a finger to assess light touch (several tracts). Responses to both pain and touch should be bilateral and equal. Evaluate the lower extremities for indications of neurological deficits. Evaluate the lower extremities for pain and touch sensation in a similar manner. Test plantar flexion (S-1 and S-2) by having the patient push the feet against your hands. Having the patient pull the toes and foot upward tests dorsiflexion (L-5). Perform a test for Babinsky's sign. Stroke the lateral aspect of the bottom of the foot. Fanning of the toes and lifting of the great toe is a positive sign suggesting injury along the pyramidal (descending spinal) tracts.

Monitor body temperature. Spinal injury patients are subject to fluctuations in body temperature, as they are unable to control the skin's heat regulating function. Look for priapism in the male patient. A patient with midcervical spine injury may present in the "hold-up" position. The patient's arms will rise above the shoulders and head. A head injury patient may complain of headache and light sensitivity. Be prepared for seizures and vomiting. These findings indicate head injury and may compromise airway and respirations while increasing intracranial pressure.

12. Describe the physiological goals for blood pressure, ventilation, end-tidal carbon dioxide, pulse oximetry, and blood glucose levels in patients with central nervous system trauma.

pp. 303–304, 306, 309, 311

Proper management of airway, breathing, and circulation are critical in the patient with central nervous system trauma. During the primary assessment, quickly determine the rate, depth, and rhythm of breathing. A patient who is breathing less than 10 times per minute or is moving less than 500 mL of air with each breath requires manual positive pressure ventilation. Ventilations should be guided by capnography. In the absence of signs of herniation, ventilate the patient to maintain an end-tidal carbon dioxide (CO_2) reading of between 35 and 40 mmHg. This is a ventilation rate of 10 breaths per minute for adults and 20 breaths per minute for children. For patients with suspected herniation, end-tidal CO_2 readings should range between 30 and 35 mmHg, using a ventilation rate about 10 breaths per minute greater than for patients without herniation. Closely monitor pulse oximetry in patients who are breathing adequately on their own. Apply oxygen by nonrebreather mask to maintain a saturation above 95 percent.

©2013 Pearson Education, Inc.
Paramedic Care: Principles & Practice, Vol. 5, 4th Ed.

Hypovolemia concurrent with brain injury can have significant negative outcomes. In the presence of increased intracranial pressure, the body attempts to maintain cerebral perfusion by increasing systolic blood pressure. If the patient is also hypovolemic, this compensatory mechanism may fail to adequately perfuse the brain. It is essential to maintain a systolic blood pressure of at least 90 mmHg with aggressive fluid resuscitation. Goals for systolic blood pressure are slightly lower and age-dependent in children.

Significant hypoglycemia or hyperglycemia are detrimental to patients with head injury. Any patient with significant hypoglycemia should receive glucose and thiamine. Check blood glucose levels on all unresponsive head injury patients, especially those with a history of diabetes or chronic alcoholism. Consult local protocols for dextrose administration guidelines.

13. Given a variety of scenarios, implement proper prehospital management of patients with central nervous system trauma. pp. 304–304, 308–309

Proper patient positioning is important when transporting patients with central nervous system injury. In the presence of suspected head injury with no indication of or mechanism for spinal damage, the patient should be transported in the recovery position or with the head and shoulders elevated 15 degrees. Patients with oral, nasal, or facial bleeding who are conscious and alert should be transported sitting up and leaning forward to facilitate drainage away from the posterior airway. Many head injury patients, however, require spinal precautions. Maintain manual C-spine stabilization until the patient is immobilized on a long backboard and the head is properly secured. If both head and spine injury are suspected, the patient should be immobilized and the head of the board elevated to about 30 degrees. Be prepared to turn the board and patient if the patient vomits. If the patient with spinal injury presents in the "hold-up" position, secure the patient's wrists to his belt to hold the limbs down for transport.

Proper management of airway and breathing is crucial. An extraglottic airway or endotracheal intubation is indicated in all unresponsive patients because they cannot protect the airway and are likely to vomit. A patient who meets the following criteria may require intubation using a rapid-sequence intubation (RSI) procedure: unable to protect the airway; has an altered level of consciousness but is not completely unresponsive; is experiencing clenched teeth; has serious facial trauma; or is at risk for rapid, progressive airway swelling. Use capnography to guide ventilations. Adjust ventilation rates to maintain an end-tidal CO_2 of between 35 and 40 mmHg for head injury patients without signs of herniation and between 30 and 35 mmHg if herniation is suspected. If the patient is breathing adequately, be sure to monitor pulse oximetry and maintain an oxygen saturation of 96 percent or above.

Adequate circulation is mandatory if head and spinal cord injury patients are to survive with positive outcomes, as hypotension and associated hypovolemia reduce oxygen transport to the brain. This is further compounded if there is any increase in intracranial pressure. Provide fluid resuscitation to the head injury patient to maintain a systolic blood pressure of 90 mmHg. Administer serial fluid boluses of 500 mL of an isotonic solution. In patients experiencing neurogenic shock, provide fluid boluses and keep the patient warm to protect against temperature fluctuations. Do not treat the hypertensive brain injury patient other than to elevate the head by 30 degrees.

In the event that the head-injured patient seizes, protect the patient from further injury and pay special attention to airway management. Consider the administration of diazepam. If the patient has a blood glucose reading of less than 60 mg/dL, administer D50 intravenously to maintain a glucose level between 60 and 100.

14. Describe indications, contraindications, advantages, disadvantages, precautions, and procedures for various pharmacological and non-pharmacological interventions for patients with central nervous system trauma. pp. 309–311

Patients who require RSI for airway control are premedicated with a sedative and paralytic. Because the patient generally has some level of consciousness, a sedative such as etomidate, diazepam, lorazepam, midazolam, fentanyl, or morphine is administered first. This is followed by a paralytic to paralyze skeletal muscle. Commonly used agents include succinylcholine, atracurium, and vecuronium. Atropine may be administered to limit muscle fasciculations.

Succinylcholine is a short-acting depolarizing skeletal muscle relaxant. It is used to achieve temporary paralysis in patients with muscle tone, spasms, or seizures. Succinylcholine induces complete paralysis in 30 to 60 seconds and persists for about 2 to 3 minutes. It may also be administered intramuscularly, although the onset is slow and effects may be erratic. Succinylcholine may transiently increase ICP, inducing vomiting. It should be used with caution in patients with head injury. It is contraindicated in patients with penetrating eye injuries, and should be used with caution in patients who are taking digitalis because of the risk of hypokalemia.

Atracurium and **Vecuronium** are nondepolarizing skeletal muscle relaxants. They do not cause muscle contractions and fasciculations. Both agents are used to paralyze patients with muscle tone, spasms, or seizures to permit endotracheal intubation. Both have a rapid onset of less than 1 minute and shorter duration (25 to 40 minutes) than other nondepolarizing agents. They also have fewer cardiovascular side effects than succinylcholine.

Diazepam is a benzodiazepine with both anti-anxiety and muscle relaxant qualities. Onset of action is almost immediate, with peak effectiveness occurring within 15 minutes. Its duration is 15 to 60 minutes.

Lorazepam is a very potent benzodiazepine with a shorter sedative half-life than diazepam. Administer 2 mg slowly IV, repeating with 1-mg IV as needed.

Midazolam is a benzodiazepine similar to diazepam but three to four times more potent. Onset of action occurs with 3 to 5 minutes. Midazolam may cause cardiorespiratory arrest and hypotension. The drug does not protect against ICP, which may result from administration of succinylcholine or pancuronium. It may also cause nausea and vomiting.

Etomidate is a rapid-acting, short-duration, nonbarbiturate hypnotic. Hypnosis occurs within 1 minute and lasts for 3 to 5 minutes. Etomidate lowers cerebral blood flow and oxygen consumption, so it is appropriate for head injury patients because it somewhat lowers ICP. It has minimal cardiovascular and respiratory effects.

Morphine is an opium alkaloid used as an analgesic, to sedate and reduce anxiety. Morphine may mildly increase ICP. It also may cause a decrease in blood pressure and so should be used cautiously in the hypovolemic patient. It may also cause respiratory depression and nausea and vomiting.

Fentanyl is an opiate narcotic used for pain control. It has a rapid onset and is more potent than morphine. It is an ideal agent for trauma, as it does not cause hypotension to the same degree as morphine.

Atropine is an anticholinergic agent used in RSI to reduce vagal stimulation, which may reduce heart rate during intubation. It is frequently used when intubating pediatric patients with RSI. Atropine use may also be considered in patients with upper spinal cord injury demonstrating signs and symptoms of neurogenic shock to counteract the unopposed vagal stimulation. Atropine may reduce oral and airway secretions associated with administration of succinylcholine.

A number of other pharmacological agents may be indicated for patients with central nervous system injury depending on protocol. These include diuretics, vasopressors, and medications for hypoglycemia and seizures. Sedatives may be indicated for combative or uncooperative patients who have sustained spinal cord or head injury to reduce anxiety and permit treatment.

Mannitol is an osmotic diuretic. It is administered to patients with severe head injury manifesting signs and symptoms of herniation, as it may reduce cerebral edema and ICP. It should not be used in patients with renal deficiency or in patients who are hypotensive (systolic blood pressure less than 90).

Dextrose is indicated in patients with hypoglycemia. It is not administered routinely to head injury patients unless indicated by a blood glucose level check.

Steroids are no longer routinely administered to spinal cord injury patients. Check local protocol.

©2013 Pearson Education, Inc.
Paramedic Care: Principles & Practice, Vol. 5, 4th Ed.

Case Study Review

Reread the case study on pages 283 and 284 in Paramedic Care: Trauma; *then, read the following discussion.*

This case study presentation addresses the considerations of CNS injury in the auto accident. It looks at the elements of scene size-up, patient assessment, care, and transport, all with regard to the patient with potential head and spine injury.

The paramedics of Unit 765 are dispatched to a typical auto collision with one patient. As Jan and Steve arrive at the scene, they note that the mechanism of injury is a frontal-impact auto crash with severe vehicle deformity. This suggests that the patient is a candidate for rapid transport to the trauma center (trauma triage criteria). They also know that the crumple zones for frontal impact are extensive and vehicle deformity may somewhat spare occupant injury. Their analysis of the mechanism of injury notes a single star-shaped break in the windshield, suggesting an unrestrained driver and a potential for serious head injury. The driver's door ajar might suggest ejection and an increase in the suspected patient injuries. Jan and Steve anticipate head, chest, and lower extremity fractures from their analysis of the mechanism of injury.

Before the medics approach the vehicle they are careful to rule out scene hazards. They look for downed power lines, leaking gas or other fluid, any source of ignition for fire, traffic, jagged metal, and broken glass. They will also don gloves and have goggles, masks, and disposable gowns ready, just in case the danger of body fluid contamination should merit their use. They also ensure that the fire department is on the scene to stabilize the auto and to be ready in case there is any suggestion of fire danger. The police officer's report of the patient's unconsciousness supports the probability of head injury and the need for rapid transport.

As the medics arrive at the distorted auto, Jan immediately immobilizes John's head in a neutral position, facing directly forward, while Steve explains this is just a precaution and that he and Jan are paramedics there to aid John. During the primary assessment Steve determines John's mental status and finds he is somewhat disoriented to time and event. He remains disoriented even though Steve explains what time it is and that John was in an auto collision. This, coupled with the history of unconsciousness, clearly establishes a neurologic problem, most likely associated with a head injury. They will move quickly to transport John to a neurocenter, if available, and will use the results of their initial neurologic assessment to trend any increase or decrease in John's orientation and level of consciousness. The airway appears fine because John is conscious, somewhat alert, and able to speak without encumbrance. Breathing is also adequate, but the patient's complaint of chest pain requires an investigation of the chest and reveals likely rib fractures, which may be limiting respiratory excursion and suggestive of pulmonary contusion underneath. Jan and Steve will frequently monitor breath sounds throughout their care to note any early development of pulmonary edema. They also attach electrocardiogram (ECG) electrodes to monitor the heart in case of any myocardial contusion. Circulation appears very adequate with a strong pulse, good capillary refill, and a high oximetry reading.

Monitoring of the vital signs and level of consciousness may give evidence of progressing intracranial hemorrhage. An increase in blood pressure, reduction in pulse rate, erratic respirations, or decrease in orientation or level of consciousness would support the diagnosis. These signs and any other neurologic deficits will be documented and relayed to medical direction to help identify the location of the injury and its progression.

Questioning by the paramedics during the primary assessment reveals a patient who cannot remember the events of the accident. This is a relatively common response, called retrograde amnesia. It is normal and by itself reflects a psychological response rather than a physiological injury. As time progresses, the patient may begin to remember the accident. The patient questioning also investigates any medical history (the AMPLE elements of the medical history) or other condition that could have been a cause of the collision.

As the assessment continues, John becomes less alert, then unconscious (responding with decerebrate posturing to painful stimuli), and his left pupil dilates. These findings suggest increasing intracranial pressure, a serious condition that can be corrected only at a neurocenter. As the patient continues to deteriorate, Jan and Steve employ rapid extrication techniques to move him to the long spine board.

He is secured quickly, and the crew begins transport to the neurocenter. Once John is unconscious and is no longer able to control his airway, Steve intubates him and ensures full breaths at 10 per minute. Capnography reveals a reading of 42 mmHg and will guide ventilations. Nevertheless, Jan and Steve will constantly monitor the patient's signs and symptoms for any indication of the early development of shock. While hyperventilation might increase oxygenation, it might also blow off excessive CO_2, constrict cerebral arteries, and further reduce blood flow to the brain. Steve places the endotracheal tube quickly to reduce the increase in intracranial pressure caused by vagal stimulation during intubation attempts. He may use a topical anesthetic spray such as lidocaine or benzocaine to reduce vagal stimulation or premedicate with atropine to prevent a vagal response and possible dysrhythmias.

Content Self-Evaluation

MULTIPLE CHOICE

_____ 1. Which of the following places the layers of the meninges in the correct order as they occur from the cerebrum to the skull?
   A. Dura mater, pia mater, arachnoid
   B. Dura mater, arachnoid, pia mater
   C. Arachnoid, pia mater, dura mater
   D. Arachnoid, dura mater, pia mater
   E. Pia mater, arachnoid, dura mater

_____ 2. The layer of the meninges that is strong and lines the interior of the cranium is the
   A. pia mater.
   B. falx cerebri.
   C. arachnoid.
   D. dura mater.
   E. tentorium.

_____ 3. The structure that divides the cerebrum into left and right halves is the
   A. pia mater.
   B. falx cerebri.
   C. arachnoid.
   D. dura mater.
   E. tentorium.

_____ 4. The cerebellum is the center of conscious thought and perception.
   A. True
   B. False

_____ 5. Which of the following is a function of the hypothalamus?
   A. Body temperature control
   B. Control of the ascending reticular activating system
   C. Control of respiration
   D. Responsibility for sleeping
   E. Maintaining balance

_____ 6. Which of the following is a function of the thalamus?
   A. Body temperature control
   B. Control of the ascending reticular activating system
   C. Control of respiration
   D. Responsibility for sleeping
   E. Maintaining balance

_____ 7. Which of the following is a function of the medulla oblongata?
   A. Body temperature control
   B. Control of the ascending reticular activating system
   C. Control of respiration
   D. Responsibility for sleeping
   E. Maintaining balance

©2013 Pearson Education, Inc.
Paramedic Care: Principles & Practice, Vol. 5, 4th Ed.

_____ 8. While the brain accounts for only 2 percent of the total body weight, it requires 15 percent of the cardiac output and 20 percent of the body's oxygen supply.
A. True
B. False

_____ 9. The capillaries serving the brain are thicker and less permeable than those in the rest of the body.
A. True
B. False

_____ 10. The normal intracranial pressure is
A. 120 mmHg.
B. 90 mmHg.
C. 50 mmHg.
D. 25 mmHg.
E. less than 10 mmHg.

_____ 11. Perfusion through the cerebrum is a factor of intracranial pressure and
A. systolic blood pressure.
B. diastolic blood pressure.
C. mean arterial pressure
D. cerebral perfusion pressure.
E. none of the above.

_____ 12. The reflex that increases the systemic blood pressure to maintain cerebral blood flow is called
A. the ascending reticular activating system.
B. the descending reticular activating system.
C. autoregulation.
D. Cushing's reflex.
E. mean arterial pressure.

_____ 13. Which of the following nerves is responsible for slowing the heart rate?
A. CN-I
B. CN-III
C. CN-VIII
D. CN-X
E. CN-XII

_____ 14. Which of the following nerves is responsible for voluntary movement of the tongue?
A. CN-I
B. CN-III
C. CN-VIII
D. CN-X
E. CN-XII

_____ 15. Which of the following nerves control eye movement?
A. CN-II
B. CN-III
C. CN-IV
D. CN-VI
E. all except A

_____ 16. The region of the vertebral column in which the spinal cord ends is the
A. cervical.
B. thoracic.
C. lumbar.
D. sacral.
E. coccygeal.

_____ 17. The nerve tissue(s) responsible for communicating sensory impulses to the brain is (are) the
A. white matter.
B. gray matter.
C. ascending tracts.
D. descending tracts.
E. myotomes.

_____ 18. The nerve tissue(s) consisting of nerve cell axons and making up the exterior portion of the spinal cord is (are) the
A. white matter.
B. gray matter.
C. ascending tracts.
D. descending tracts.
E. myotomes.

_____ 19. The structure of the meninges of the spinal column is similar to the structure of the meninges of the cranium.
   A. True
   B. False

_____ 20. The region of the spine with the closest tolerance between the spinal cord and the interior of the spinal foramen is the
   A. cervical spine.
   B. thoracic spine.
   C. lumbar spine.
   D. sacral spine.
   E. coccygeal spine.

_____ 21. The region of the spine that has one more pair of nerve roots than it does vertebrae is the
   A. cervical spine.
   B. thoracic spine.
   C. lumbar spine.
   D. sacral spine.
   E. coccygeal spine.

_____ 22. The S-1 nerve root controls the
   A. collar region.
   B. little finger.
   C. nipple line.
   D. umbilicus.
   E. small toe.

_____ 23. The T-10 nerve root controls the
   A. collar region.
   B. little finger.
   C. nipple line.
   D. umbilicus.
   E. small toe.

_____ 24. During your assessment of a patient, you find sensation is lost as you move from the lower extremities all the way up to the level of the collar. This is probably due to an injury at which spinal level?
   A. C-3
   B. T-1
   C. T-4
   D. T-10
   E. S-1

_____ 25. The type of injury that causes damage to the brain on the side opposite the impact is called
   A. coup.
   B. subdural hematoma.
   C. subluxation.
   D. contrecoup.
   E. concussion.

_____ 26. Which of the following is considered a focal injury?
   A. Cerebral contusion
   B. Epidural hematoma
   C. Subdural hematoma
   D. Intracerebral hemorrhage
   E. All of the above

_____ 27. Which of the following injuries is most likely to cause the patient to deteriorate rapidly?
   A. Cerebral contusion
   B. Epidural hematoma
   C. Subdural hematoma
   D. Intracerebral hemorrhage
   E. Concussion

_____ 28. Which of the following is an injury with venous bleeding into the arachnoid space?
   A. Cerebral contusion
   B. Epidural hematoma
   C. Subdural hematoma
   D. Intracerebral hemorrhage
   E. Concussion

_____ 29. Which of the following head injuries would you NOT expect to get worse with time?
   A. Intracerebral hemorrhage
   B. Subdural hematoma
   C. Concussion
   D. Epidural hematoma
   E. Intracranial hemorrhage

©2013 Pearson Education, Inc.
Paramedic Care: Principles & Practice, Vol. 5, 4th Ed.

30. The injury that classically presents with unconsciousness immediately after an accident followed by a lucid interval and then a decreasing level of consciousness is most likely a(n)
  A. concussion.
  B. epidural hematoma.
  C. subdural hematoma.
  D. cerebral hemorrhage.
  E. both A and B.

31. Indirect brain injury occurs as a result of, but after, initial injury.
  A. True
  B. False

32. All of the following result in indirect injury to the brain, EXCEPT
  A. diminishing circulation to brain tissue.
  B. hypoxia.
  C. displacement of brain tissue.
  D. hypertension.
  E. hypercarbia.

33. As intracranial hemorrhage begins, it first displaces which occupant of the cranium?
  A. Cerebrospinal fluid
  B. Venous blood
  C. Arterial blood
  D. Oxygen
  E. The pia matter

34. High levels of carbon dioxide in the blood will cause which of the following?
  A. Hyperventilation
  B. Cerebral artery constriction
  C. Cerebral artery dilation
  D. Hypertension
  E. None of the above

35. Vomiting, changes in the level of consciousness, and pupillary dilation result from herniation of the upper brainstem through the
  A. tentorium incisura.
  B. foramen magnum.
  C. falx cerebri.
  D. transverse sinus.
  E. tentorium cerebelli.

36. Cushing's triad includes which of the following?
  A. Erratic respirations
  B. Increasing blood pressure
  C. Slowing heart rate
  D. A and B
  E. A, B, and C

37. Which of the following respiratory patterns is NOT indicative of brain injury?
  A. Eupnea
  B. Ataxic respirations
  C. Central neurogenic hyperventilation
  D. Cheyne-Stokes respirations
  E. Agonal respirations

38. In the presence of increased intracranial pressure, the fontanelles of the infant will
  A. withdraw.
  B. become stiff.
  C. bulge.
  D. pulsate.
  E. atrophy.

39. A spinal cord concussion is likely to produce residual deficit.
  A. True
  B. False

40. A patient who presents with quadriplegia, incontinence, and respiratory paralysis has most likely sustained which type of spinal cord injury?
  A. Laceration
  B. Concussion
  C. Contusion
  D. Transection
  E. Compression

41. A spinal cord injury more commonly occurring in patients older than 50 years of age is
    A. autonomic hyperreflexia.
    B. central cord syndrome.
    C. anterior cord syndrome.
    D. Brown-Sequard syndrome.
    E. cauda equina syndrome.

42. A penetrating spinal cord injury affecting one side of the cord is known as
    A. Brown-Sequard syndrome.
    B. anterior cord syndrome.
    C. cauda equina syndrome.
    D. anterior cord syndrome.
    E. autonomic hyperreflexia.

43. Spinal shock is a temporary form of neurogenic shock.
    A. True
    B. False

44. Which of the following is a sign associated with neurogenic shock?
    A. Priapism
    B. Decreased heart rate
    C. Decreased peripheral vascular resistance
    D. Warm skin below the injury
    E. All of the above

45. Which of the following is associated with the resolution of shock due to cord injury and results in hypertension?
    A. Autonomic hyperreflexia syndrome
    B. Neurogenic shock
    C. Spinal shock
    D. Central cord syndrome
    E. Both B and D

46. An episode of transient quadriplegia usually lasts less than
    A. 30 minutes.
    B. 15 minutes.
    C. 45 minutes
    D. 10 minutes.
    E. 5 minutes.

47. Pediatric patients display different spinal injury patterns than adults for all of the following reasons, EXCEPT
    A. underdeveloped neck muscles.
    B. calcified, wedge-shaped vertebrae.
    C. shallow, horizontally oriented facet joints.
    D. proportionately larger head.
    E. increased spinal elasticity and mobility.

48. Capnography-guided ventilations for the patient without suspected cerebral herniation should keep the end-tidal CO_2 readings at
    A. 35 to 40 mmHg.
    B. 30 to 35 mmHg.
    C. 40 to 50 mmHg.
    D. 10 to 20 mmHg.
    E. 90 to 100 mmHg.

49. Endotracheal intubation is indicated in patients with a Simplified Motor Score of
    A. 15.
    B. 8.
    C. 3.
    D. 1.
    E. 0.

50. Oxygenation of the head injury patient, who is breathing adequately, should be guided by oximetry to maintain a saturation of at least
    A. 80 percent.
    B. 85 percent.
    C. 90 percent.
    D. 96 percent.
    E. 98 percent.

©2013 Pearson Education, Inc.
Paramedic Care: Principles & Practice, Vol. 5, 4th Ed.

51. The approximate rate of ventilation for the infant head injury patient is
   A. 10 breaths per minute.
   B. 20 breaths per minute.
   C. 25 breaths per minute.
   D. 12 breaths per minute.
   E. 30 breaths per minute.

52. Which of the following signs is indicative of cerebral herniation?
   A. Increasing blood pressure
   B. Decreasing heart rate
   C. Dilated and fixed pupil
   D. Erratic respirations
   E. All of the above

53. Which of the following is a probable sign of increasing intracranial pressure?
   A. Decreasing pulse strength
   B. Weakening pulse strength
   C. Slowing pulse rate
   D. Increasing pulse strength
   E. Both C and D

54. When light intensity changes in one eye and both respond, this response is called
   A. diplopia.
   B. aniscoria.
   C. consensual reactivity.
   D. synergism.
   E. photophobia.

55. When assessing limb sensation in the spine-injured patient, you should check for
   A. paralysis.
   B. paraparesis.
   C. anesthesia.
   D. paresthesia.
   E. all of the above.

56. A wide pulse pressure is a sign of cardiovascular compensation and decreasing intracranial pressure.
   A. True
   B. False

57. The Glasgow Coma Scale measures a patient's level of consciousness by assessing
   A. verbal response, motor response, and sensation.
   B. eye opening, verbal response, and pain.
   C. eye opening, verbal response, and motor response.
   D. sensation, pain response, and motor response.
   E. eye opening, sensation, and motor response.

58. During your assessment you determine that the patient exhibits confused speech, follows simple commands, and opens his eyes on his own. What Glasgow Coma Scale value would you assign?
   A. 15
   B. 14
   C. 12
   D. 10
   E. 7

59. The highest Glasgow Coma Scale score is
   A. 20.
   B. 15.
   C. 12.
   D. D+.
   E. a score that varies with each patient.

60. A patient who responds only to pain by withdrawing, mutters incomprehensible words when shouted at loudly, and opens his eyes only to pain is given what Glasgow Coma Scale score?
   A. 14
   B. 12
   C. 10
   D. 8
   E. 6

61. Priapism secondary to spinal injury is the result of
    A. unopposed parasympathetic stimulation.
    B. increased sympathetic stimulation.
    C. loss of motor function.
    D. loss of sensory pathways.
    E. increased blood pressure.

62. When a patient reports sensitivity to light, this is an example of
    A. diplopia.
    B. aniscoria.
    C. consensual reactivity.
    D. synergism.
    E. photophobia.

63. If the head injury patient is found without any other suspected injuries, what positioning would be best for him?
    A. Recovery position with the head of the stretcher raised 30 degrees
    B. With the head of the spine board elevated 30 degrees
    C. The Trendelenburg position
    D. Immobilized completely and rolled to his side
    E. None of the above

64. If the patient has sustained an open neck injury with danger of air embolism, what positioning would be best for him?
    A. The Trendelenburg position
    B. With the head of the spine board elevated 30 degrees
    C. Left lateral recumbent position
    D. Immobilized completely and rolled to his side
    E. None of the above

65. All of the following are indications for rapid-sequence intubation EXCEPT for a patient who
    A. is experiencing trismus.
    B. is completely unresponsive.
    C. has serious oral trauma.
    D. is at risk of rapid airway swelling.
    E. none of the above.

66. Care for the patient with increasing intracranial pressure must NOT include aggressive fluid resuscitation, even if the patient's blood pressure drops below 80 mmHg.
    A. True
    B. False

67. The minimum blood pressure necessary to maintain cerebral perfusion in the adult patient with serious head injury is
    A. 90 mmHg.
    B. 80 mmHg.
    C. 75 mmHg.
    D. 65 mmHg.
    E. 50 mmHg.

68. Which of the following paralytics increases intracranial pressure and should be used with caution, if at all, in head injury patients?
    A. Diazepam
    B. Mannitol
    C. Vecuronium
    D. Succinylcholine
    E. Midazolam

69. Diazepam is used to premedicate patients prior to inserting a supraglottic airway.
    A. True
    B. False

70. Which of the following drugs will reverse the effects of diazepam and midazolam?
    A. Naloxone
    B. Flumazenil
    C. Atropine
    D. Thiamine
    E. None of the above

71. Which of the following actions of atropine make it a desirable adjunct to rapid-sequence intubation?
  A. It reduces vagal stimulation.
  B. It reduces airway secretions.
  C. It reduces fasciculations.
  D. It helps maintain heart rate during intubation.
  E. All of the above.

72. Which of the following is used in the prehospital setting for the treatment of spine injuries?
  A. Mannitol
  B. Methylprednisolone
  C. Dexamethasone
  D. Furosemide
  E. None of the above

73. To address bradycardia in the suspected spinally injured patient, which drug would you consider?
  A. Methylprednisolone
  B. Atropine
  C. Furosemide
  D. Dopamine
  E. Diazepam

74. Dextrose is administered to the head injury patient
  A. routinely.
  B. for hyperglycemia only.
  C. for hypoglycemia only.
  D. for suspected diabetes or alcoholism.
  E. with hetastarch.

75. If a suspected spinally injured patient does not respond to fluid resuscitation, which drug would you consider?
  A. Methylprednisolone
  B. Atropine
  C. Furosemide
  D. Dopamine
  E. Diazepam

Special Project

Composing a Radio Message and Run Report

Preparing both the radio message to the receiving hospital and the written run report are two of the most important tasks you will perform as a paramedic. Reread the case study on pages 283 and 284 of Paramedic Care: Trauma; *then, read the additional information about the call provided below. From this information compose a radio message and complete the run report for this call.*

The Call

Dispatch to the call comes from the 911 center at 2:15 A.M. It directs Unit 765 to an auto crash at the junction of Highway 127 and Country Trunk H in Wilbur Township. They arrive at the scene at 2:32 to find one 31-year-old male occupant of the vehicle.

The initial care of the patient includes spinal immobilization (2:33), cervical collar (2:34), vitals (2:36), and oxygen at 15 L via nonrebreather mask (2:36). A second set of vitals is taken just after the patient becomes unconscious. They reveal a pulse of 52, respirations of 22 that are deep and labored, blood pressure of 136/8, and a pulse oximeter reading of 98 percent. The patient is responsive to painful stimuli only (2:41). The patient is immobilized to a long spine board (2:41), loaded on the stretcher, and moved to the ambulance at 2:42 with transport begun immediately.

En route, an initial IV is started in the left forearm with a 16-gauge angiocatheter to run normal saline (1,000 mL) at a "to-keep-open" rate. You are headed to the Community Hospital, the closest facility and the base of your medical direction.

Medical direction is contacted and you call in the following:

_____

_____

_____

_____

The medical direction physician instructs you to bring your patient to the medical center and orders that an endotracheal tube be placed if possible. An 8.0-mm tube is positioned orally via digital technique with good bilateral breath sounds auscultated (2:51). The vitals are repeated (pulse, 62; blood pressure, 142/92; respirations, 20 ventilations per minute; pulse oximeter, 97; $ETCO_2$ –38 percent).

You contact medical direction and provide the following update:

_____

_____

_____

_____

Your ETA to the medical center is now 15 minutes. The second set of vital signs taken en route show the following: blood pressure, 140/90; pulse, 50 and bounding; respirations, 20 (assisted by BVM $ETCO_2$ –38 percent), and pulse oximetry of 97 percent (3:01). The patient is delivered to the medical center at 3:15, and you report for service at 3:55.

Complete the prehospital care report on the next page using the information contained in the narrative of this call. Now, compare the radio message and the run report form that you prepared against the examples in the Answer Key of this workbook. As you make this comparison, keep in mind that there are many "correct" ways to communicate this body of information. Ensure that you have recorded the major points of your assessment and care and enough other material to describe the patient and his condition to the receiving physician and anyone who might review the form. Remember that this document may be the only record of your assessment and care for this patient. When you are done, it should be a complete accounting of your actions.

©2013 Pearson Education, Inc.
Paramedic Care: Principles & Practice, Vol. 5, 4th Ed.

Date		Emergency Medical Services Run Report		Run # 913

Patient Information

Service Information

Times

Name:			

Address:			

City:	St:	Zip:	

Age:	Birth: / /	Sex: [M][F]	

Nature of Call:

Chief Complaint:

Agency:	Rcvd	:
Location:	Enrt	:
Call Origin:	Scne	:
Type: Emrg[ ] Non[ ] Trnsfr[ ]	LvSn	:
	ArHsp	:
	InSv	:

Description of Current Problem:

Medical Problems

Past		Present
[ ]	Cardiac	[ ]
[ ]	Stroke	[ ]
[ ]	Acute Abdomen	[ ]
[ ]	Diabetes	[ ]
[ ]	Psychiatric	[ ]
[ ]	Epilepsy	[ ]
[ ]	Drug/Alcohol	[ ]
[ ]	Poisoning	[ ]
[ ]	Allergy/Asthma	[ ]
[ ]	Syncope	[ ]
[ ]	Obstetrical	[ ]
[ ]	GYN	[ ]

Other:

Trauma Scr: Glasgow:

On-Scene Care:	First Aid:
	By Whom?

O_2 @ L : Via	C-Collar :	S-Immob. :	Stretcher :

Allergies/Meds:

Past Med Hx:

Time	Pulse	Resp.	BP S/D	LOC	ECG
:	R: [r][i]	R: [s][l]	/	[a][v][p][u]	
Care/Comments:					
:	R: [r][i]	R: [s][l]	/	[a][v][p][u]	
Care/Comments:					
:	R: [r][i]	R: [s][l]	/	[a][v][p][u]	
Care/Comments:					
:	R: [r][i]	R: [s][l]	/	[a][v][p][u]	
Care/Comments:					

Destination:	Personnel:	Certification
Reason:[ ]pt [ ]Closest [ ]M.D. [ ]Other	1.	[P][E][O]
Contacted: [ ]Radio [ ]Tele [ ]Direct	2.	[P][E][O]
Ar Status: [ ]Better [ ]UnC [ ]Worse	3.	[P][E][O]

Recognizing Dermatomes

In the spaces provided below, write in the areas of the body affected by each of the dermatomes indicated.

C–3 _____

T–1 _____

T–4 _____

T–10 _____

S–1 _____

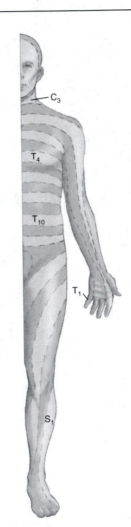

Drugs Used for Nervous System Injuries

Emergency management for head injury utilizes many of the pharmacological agents that are available to the paramedic. Please review and memorize the various names/class, descriptions, indications, contraindications, precautions, and dosages/routes for the following, with special attention to those used in your system. The drug flash cards found at the back of the Workbook for Volume 1 will be helpful for this activity.

Mannitol	Midazolam	Dopamine	Dextrose
Succinylcholine	Morphine	Etomidate	Thiamine
Atracurium	Fentanyl	Diazepam	
Vecuronium	Atropine		

©2013 Pearson Education, Inc.
Paramedic Care: Principles & Practice, Vol. 5, 4th Ed.

12

Environmental Trauma

Review of Chapter Objectives

After reading this chapter, you should be able to:

1. **Define key terms introduced in this chapter.**

   Knowing and being able to apply the key terms in each chapter is critical to understanding chapter concepts. Write the list of key terms. Then write the definition of each one in your own words. Check your understanding by confirming the definitions in the text glossary. Correct any misunderstandings. Create a study aid by writing each key term on the front of an index card and the definition on the back. Use the cards to quiz yourself, or to have someone quiz you.

2. **Identify factors that place patients at particular risk for environmental emergencies.**
   p. 317

   General risk factors that place an individual at greater risk for an environmental emergency include age (very young and very old), poor general health, fatigue, predisposing medical conditions, and certain medications, either prescription or over-the-counter. Drugs and alcohol raise the risk factor, as do environmental considerations. Geographic regions where climate conditions change rapidly, atmospheric (high altitude) or hydrostatic (underwater) pressure, local weather patterns, and types of terrain all affect risk for environmental emergencies.

3. **Describe the homeostasis of body temperature, including discussion of the following:**
   pp. 317–320

   Homeostasis is the body's ability to maintain a steady and normal internal environment despite changing external conditions.

   a. Mechanisms of heat loss and heat production
   The body gains and loses heat through internal mechanisms and the external environment. Heat loss or gain from the environment depends on the thermal gradient. The body loses heat to a cooler environment and gains heat when the ambient air is warmer than the body. The body also generates heat through a process called thermogenesis. There are three types of thermogenesis. The most basic and vital type is thermoregulatory thermogenesis, in which the nervous system and endocrine system work together to control the rate of cellular metabolism, which in turn increases heat production. In work-induced thermogenesis, heat is produced through the work of skeletal muscles during exercise. In a cool or cold environment, muscles will produce some additional heat through shivering. The last type of heat generation is diet-induced thermogenesis, and it reflects the heat generated by cells as they process food and nutrients and eventually metabolize the breakdown products.

The loss of heat is called thermolysis. The body loses heat to the environment by conduction, convection, radiation, evaporation, and respiration. Evaporation and respiration account for significant amounts of heat loss through the skin and lungs.

b. **Physiology of thermoregulation**

The body's thermal regulation is achieved through coordination of the nervous and endocrine systems. The hypothalamus, a structure at the base of the brain, acts as a thermostat. The hypothalamus depends on a negative feedback system to control temperature. Based on the temperature of core body blood and temperature sensors located in other parts of the body, neurosecretions shut on or off mechanisms that stimulate heat production and loss. Additional sensor cells for core temperature are located in the spinal cord, abdomen, and around the great veins in the chest. Peripheral sensors are in the skin and subcutaneous tissue. Additionally, the body adjusts the metabolic rate to maintain core temperature. Heat is produced when more nutrients are metabolized. The cardiovascular system plays a role in body temperature maintenance by dilating and constricting vessels to direct blood flow to the periphery for heat dissipation or by shunting warm blood away from the skin back to the core. Shivering also increases metabolism and generates heat.

c. **Factors that can interfere with thermoregulation**

Thermoregulation is a critical function that can become overwhelmed and fail in certain circumstances. Hyperthermia, a state of extremely high body temperature, results from excessive heat transfer from the environment, excessive generation of heat within the body, or as a result of certain medications. Age, health, certain chronic illnesses, medications, level of acclimation, length and intensity of exposure, and environmental factors all affect the thermoregulatory balance.

4. **Describe the pathophysiology of heat-related illnesses.**   pp. 320–324

As the body overheats, it attempts to eliminate the heat through sweating and vasodilation. As hyperthermia continues, the thermoregulatory mechanisms can no longer adequately compensate. The patient will display altered mentation or altered level of consciousness. Hyperthermia is progressive if left untreated.

Heat cramps are caused by overexertion and dehydration in a hot environment. When temperature- and exercise-induced sweating depletes the body of water and electrolytes, primarily sodium, skeletal muscle cramps occur.

Heat exhaustion, which is considered a mild heat illness, is an acute reaction to heat exposure, and it is the most common heat-related illness seen by EMS providers. The loss of water and electrolytes (notably sodium) from working in a hot environment, combined with general vasodilation as a heat-dissipating mechanism, leads to decreased circulating blood volume, venous pooling, and reduced cardiac output. The presenting symptoms are due to dehydration and sodium loss secondary to sweating. Because the symptoms are not unique to heat exhaustion, diagnosis requires a history of heat exposure. Left untreated, heat exhaustion can progress to heatstroke.

Heatstroke is a true life-threatening emergency in which the body's hypothalamic temperature regulation is lost. The ensuing uncompensated hyperthermia results in cell death and damage to the brain, liver, and kidneys. Generally, heatstroke is characterized by body temperature above 105°F (40.6°C), central nervous system (CNS) disturbances, and (usually) cessation of perspiration. It is thought that sweating stops either because of destruction of sweat glands or because of sensory overload resulting in their temporary dysfunction. There are two classifications of heatstroke. Classic heatstroke presents in patients with chronic illnesses affecting thermoregulatory function. Exertional heatstroke affects those who are usually in general good health and have been exposed to overwhelming heat stress.

Fever is a reaction to pathogens causing infection. The infection stimulates the production of pyrogens, which reset the hypothalamic thermostat to a higher level. Increased metabolism then causes temperature elevation. Increases body temperature helps to fight infection by making the host environment less hospitable to the invading organisms.

5. **Given a variety of scenarios, assess and manage patients with heat-related illnesses.**   pp. 320–325

Heat cramps are caused by overexertion and dehydration. Signs and symptoms include cramping in the fingers, arms, legs, or abdominal muscles. Patients are generally mentally alert with a feeling of

©2013 Pearson Education, Inc.
Paramedic Care: Principles & Practice, Vol. 5, 4th Ed.

weakness, but they may be dizzy or faint. Vital signs are stable, although temperature may be normal or slightly elevated. Skin is likely to be moist and warm. Note that heat cramps may be painful but they are NOT considered to be an actual heat illness. Treatment for heat cramps is usually easily accomplished. First, remove the patient from the hot environment to a cooler one such as a shady area or an air-conditioned ambulance. Administer water or a sports electrolyte drink. Do not use salt tablets. If the patient cannot take liquids readily, an IV of normal saline may be needed. Palliative care may include muscle massage or moist towels over the patient's head and the cramping muscles.

Dehydration and electrolyte loss from sweating account for the signs and symptoms of heat exhaustion. These include increased body temperature (over 100°F, 37.8°C); cool, clammy skin with heavy perspiration; rapid, shallow breathing; and a weak pulse. The patient may have vision disturbances, diarrhea, nausea/vomiting, and abdominal and muscle cramps. The patient will feel weak and may lose consciousness. There also may be CNS symptoms such as headache, anxiety, paresthesia, and impaired judgment or even psychosis. Assess for orthostatic hypotension. Treatment focuses on immediate cooling and fluid replacement. Remove the patient from the hot environment and place in the supine position. Administer water or a sports drink. Do NOT use salt tablets. Consider anti-emetic medications to assist the patient with oral intake. Consider normal saline IV if the patient cannot take liquids readily. Remove some clothing and fan the patient to increase heat dissipation. Be careful not to cool the patient to the point of chilling him. Stop fanning if shivering develops, and consider covering the patient lightly. If shock is suspected, treat accordingly. If symptoms do not resolve, consider the possibility of increased core body temperature and evolution of heatstroke.

Heatstroke is a life-threatening condition. It is generally characterized by a body temperature of at least 105°F, CNS disturbances, and usually cessation of sweating. Signs and symptoms include hot skin that is either moist or dry (depending on whether sweat has dried), very high core temperatures, deep respirations that become shallow and rapid respirations that may later slow, a rapid and full pulse that may slow later, hypotension with low or absent diastolic reading, confusion or disorientation or unconsciousness, and possible seizures. Field management centers on immediate cooling of the patient's body and replacement of fluids. First, remove the patient from the environment. Initiate rapid active body cooling to a target temperature of 102°F (39°C). Remove the patient's clothing and cover with sheets soaked in tepid water. If necessary, either fanning or misting may be used. Avoid overcooling because this can trigger reflex hypothermia. Do not use ice packs or cold water immersion. Administer high-flow oxygen and assist respirations if they are shallow. Use pulse oximetry if available. Administer fluid therapy orally (if possible) along with antiemetics. In many cases, sports drinks will suffice. If IVs are needed, initiate one or two and run fluid wide open. Be sure to monitor the electrocardiogram (ECG) because dysrhythmias can develop at any time. Avoid vasopressors and anticholinergic drugs. Last, monitor body temperature for trends.

Although fever typically presents in a setting of infectious disease, it may be difficult to distinguish from heatstroke. In some cases patients with heatstroke do not have a history of exposure to high temperatures. If you are unsure of diagnosis, treat for heatstroke. Treatment for fever should be undertaken when the patient is uncomfortable or when a child has a history of febrile seizures. Remove extra layers of clothing or bedclothes to allow passive cooling. Consider use of an antipyretic agent such as acetaminophen or ibuprofen. Note that sponge baths and cool water immersion should not be used because they can cause a rapid drop in temperature with reflex shivering and subsequent increase in body temperature.

6. **Describe the pathophysiology of cold-related disorders.**   pp. 325–327, 331

Hypothermia is defined as a state of low core body temperature, which can be due to inadequate heat generation, excessive cold stress, or a combination of both. Compensatory mechanisms including pilo-erection, shivering, increased muscle tone, peripheral vasoconstriction, and increased cardiac output attempt to conserve and generate heat. Body temperature falls when these compensatory mechanisms are overwhelmed. Hypothermia presents as a continuum and can be mild (core temperature greater than 90°F or 32°C), moderate (core temperature between 82° and 90° F), or severe (core temperature less than 90°F). In both forms, signs and symptoms of hypothermia are present. Onset of symptoms can be acute (falling through ice into a lake), subacute (hikers trapped on a mountain during a winter snow-storm), or chronic (homeless individuals living outdoors during the winter). In other cases, an individual with impaired capacity for compensation due to a medical condition is exposed to normal or cool conditions and develops hypothermia when a healthy individual would not.

Frostbite is an environmentally induced freezing of body tissues. As tissues freeze due to the excessive cold, ice crystals form within cells and water is drawn from cells into the extracellular space. As the ice crystals expand, cells are destroyed. Damage to blood vessels from ice-crystal formation causes loss of vascular integrity, which results in further tissue swelling and loss of distal blood flow. Peripheral tissues are more exposed to cold and thus more likely to be involved in frostbite. Thus, frostbite is largely seen in the extremities and in areas of the head and face. Patients with poor peripheral circulation make the extremities more vulnerable to frostbite. Two types of frostbite are defined based on the extent of tissue freezing: superficial and deep frostbite. Superficial frostbite (also called frostnip) involves some freezing of epidermal tissue, resulting in initial redness followed by blanching and diminished sensation. Deep frostbite involves both the epidermal and subcutaneous layers; there is a white, hardened appearance. Sensation is lost. Subfreezing temperatures are necessary for frostbite but are not necessary for hypothermia. You will find that many patients with frostbite also have hypothermia.

7. **Given a variety of scenarios, assess and manage patients with cold-related disorders.**   pp. 328, 331

Your assessment of an individual with mild hypothermia will likely reveal lethargy; mild confusion; shivering; poor coordination; pale, cold, dry skin; and an early rise in blood pressure, heart rate, and respiratory rates. In severe hypothermia, you may find disorientation; no shivering; loss of coordination; stiff, rigid muscles; hypotension; and an unpredictable pulse and respiration. On the ECG, you may find dysrhythmias, with the most common being atrial fibrillation. With progressive cooling of the body core, a variety of dysrhythmias may appear, with eventual bradycardia. As the body's core temperature falls below 86°F, ventricular fibrillation is probable. Management includes: (1) removal of wet garments; (2) protection against further heat loss and wind chill (calling for passive external warming with blankets, moisture barriers, and so on); (3) maintenance of patient in horizontal position; (4) avoidance of rough handling, which can trigger dysrhythmias; (5) monitoring of core temperature; and (6) monitoring of cardiac rhythm.

Persons with mild hypothermia may be rewarmed with active external techniques such as warmed blankets or heat packs applied to the base of the neck, the axilla, and the groin. In contrast, active rewarming of the severely hypothermic patient is best carried out in the hospital because of the possibility of complications such as ventricular fibrillation. If transport to the hospital will require more than 15 minutes, you may need to begin active rewarming in the field. Beware of rewarming shock, which can cause a return of cool blood and acids to the core, resulting in a further drop in temperature. and hypotension. Additionally, cold diuresis may occur when the kidneys remove excess fluid secondary to core vasoconstriction. Use of warmed crystalloid IV fluids can offset these problems. If the patient is conscious and can maintain his airway, he may be given warmed, sweetened fluids. Because of myocardial irritability, patients should be transported gently. Keep the patient level or slightly inclined with the head down.

You will also find that there is tremendous variation in presentation of frostbite. Some patients will feel little pain at the outset, whereas others will complain of bitter pain. Physical exam is a better indicator of the extent of frostbite. In superficial frostbite, there will be some degree of compliance felt beneath the frozen layer upon palpation; in deep frostbite, the frozen part will be hard and noncompliant. Treatment involves the following steps. First, do not thaw the affected area if there is any possibility of refreezing and do not massage the frozen area or rub with snow. Both may result in more extensive damage. Do administer analgesia before thawing, and do transport to the hospital for rewarming by immersion. If transport will be delayed, thaw the frozen part in a 102 to 104°F water bath. Water will need to be changed frequently as it cools. Cover the thawed part with loosely applied, dry, sterile dressings and elevate and immobilize the thawed part. Do not puncture or drain blisters, and do not rewarm frozen feet if they are required for walking out of a hazardous situation.

8. **Discuss measures to prevent heat-related and cold-related disorders.**   pp. 320, 325

Preventive measures for heat disorders include three major elements. First, maintenance of adequate fluid intake is vital, and remember that thirst alone is an inadequate indicator for dehydration. Second, you should allow yourself time for acclimatization to the hot environment, which results in more

©2013 Pearson Education, Inc.
Paramedic Care: Principles & Practice, Vol. 5, 4th Ed.

perspiration with lower salt concentration, thus conserving body-fluid volume. Last, it is important to limit exposure to hot environments.

Preventive measures can decrease the morbidity of cold-related injury. These include dressing warmly; being rested, which maximizes the ability of the heat-generating mechanisms to replenish energy reserves; eating appropriately at regular intervals to support metabolism; and limiting exposure to cold environments.

Remember that certain medications can predispose the individual to hyper- or hypothermia in less extreme climates.

9. Describe the pathophysiology of drowning. pp. 332–333

Drowning is defined as submersion or immersion in a liquid that results in a primary respiratory impairment. Following submersion, a conscious person will have complete apnea for up to 3 minutes as an involuntary reflex as he struggles to keep his head above water, and during this period blood is shunted to the heart and brain. During apnea, $PaCO_2$ will rise to greater than 50 mmHg, while PaO_2 falls to less than 50 mmHg. The hypoxic stimulus eventually overrides the sedative effects of the hypercarbia, resulting in CNS stimulation. While conscious, the panicky victim typically swallows a lot of water, stimulating severe laryngospasm and bronchospasm. This effect prevents significant influx of water into the lungs (and is thus termed a dry drowning). Another effect of laryngospasm is worsening hypoxia, which causes a deepening coma. Reflex swallowing continues, resulting in gastric distention and increased risk of vomiting and aspiration. The presence of water washes away surfactant, causing alveolar collapse. Deoxygenated blood is now shunted from the damaged alveoli back to the bloodstream. If untreated, hypotension, bradycardia, and death result. Water in the lungs of a drowning survivor may cause lower-airway disease.

Morbidity or delayed mortality in drowning is primarily due to brain injury from airway obstruction, laryngospasm, or aspirated water. Survival may be affected by water temperature. In general, the colder the water, the greater the chance for survival. Usually, you expect brain death after 4 to 6 minutes without oxygen. However, some patients in cold water (below 68°F) may be resuscitated after 30 minutes or more in cardiac arrest. A possible physiological factor in this phenomenon is the mammalian diving reflex. When a person dives into cold water, the submersion of the face inhibits breathing, drops heart rate, and causes vasoconstriction in tissues relatively resistant to asphyxia even as blood flow to the heart and brain continues. The colder the water, the greater the shunting of blood to the brain and heart. This is the origin of the saying "the cold-water drowning victim is not dead until he is warm and dead."

10. Given a variety of scenarios, assess and manage patients who have drowned. pp. 333–334

Field treatment for drownings in either saltwater or freshwater is similar. The first goal is to correct the profound hypoxia. Treatment includes the following steps. Remove the patient from the water. If possible, initiate ventilation while the victim is still in the water. Note that both steps require a trained, equipped rescue swimmer. Suspect head and neck injury if there was a fall or a dive involved; rapidly place the patient on a long backboard and use C-spine precautions. Then, protect from heat loss by removing wet clothing, laying the patient on a warm surface, and covering the body to the extent possible. The remaining steps are familiar to all resuscitations: Examine for airway patency, breathing, and pulse. If needed, begin cardiopulmonary resuscitation (CPR) and defibrillation. Manage the airway as needed with suctioning and airway adjuncts. Administer 100 percent oxygen. Use respiratory rewarming, if available, and if transport time will exceed 15 minutes. Establish an IV of lactated Ringer's solution or normal saline for venous access and run at 75 mL/hr. Follow ACLS protocols if the patient is normothermic. If hypothermic, the patient should be treated for hypothermia as discussed in the text.

Note: Resuscitation is NOT indicated if immersion is known to have been extremely prolonged (unless hypothermia IS present) or if there is evidence of decomposition. All drowning victims should be admitted for observation for possible late complications, including acute respiratory distress syndrome (ARDS).

11. **Describe the pathophysiology of diving emergencies, including the application of gas laws.**   p. 335

Three laws pertaining to the behavior of gases under different physical conditions relate to environmental emergencies.

- *Boyle's law* states that a volume of gas is inversely proportional to its pressure when temperature remains constant. As you increase pressure (as happens during a dive), gas is compressed into increasingly smaller volumes.
- *Dalton's law* states that the total pressure of a mixture of gases (such as air) is equal to the sum of the partial pressures of each individual gas. Air is roughly 78 percent nitrogen, 21 percent oxygen, and 1 percent carbon dioxide and other trace gases. As altitude changes (upward or downward), those proportions remain the same. The fraction of oxygen in air does not change.
- *Henry's law* states that the amount of a gas dissolved in a given volume of fluid is proportional to the pressure of the gas above it. This law is most relevant to diving.

The underlying physiology of diving emergencies is based on dissolution of gases in water, specifically, oxygen, carbon dioxide nitrogen, and other gases. As a diver descends to greater depths, oxygen is increasingly used up in cellular metabolism, whereas nitrogen, which is inert, does not change in quantity. Instead, it dissolves in blood plasma and body tissues. The volume of the gas is smaller because of increased pressure. During ascent, decreasing pressure allows gases to come out of solution, and they are eliminated gradually through respiration. If ascent is too rapid, however, dissolved gases, primarily nitrogen, come out of solution and expand in volume quickly, forming bubbles in the blood, brain, spinal cord, inner ear, muscles, and joints. There they can cause occlusion of small blood vessels known as decompression illness. SCUBA diving injuries are due to barotrauma (changes in pressure), pulmonary overpressure, arterial gas embolism, decompression illness, cold, panic, or a combination of these.

12. **Given a variety of scenarios, assess and manage patients with diving injuries including the following:**   pp. 336–339

Accidents generally occur at one of four phases of the dive: on the surface, during descent, at the bottom, or during ascent.

   a. **Surface injuries**
   Surface injuries generally involve risk factors at the surface. Lines or kelp can entangle the diver. Cold water might induce shivering or even blackout. Boats or other large objects in the area are potential sources of injury.

   b. **Descent injuries**
   Barotrauma during descent is commonly caused "the squeeze." If the diver cannot equilibrate the pressure between the nasopharynx and middle ear, he can experience severe pain, ringing in the ears, dizziness, and hearing loss, any of which can cause disorientation or panic. A similar problem of disequilibration can occur in the sinuses, producing frontal headache or pain below the eyes.

   c. **Bottom injuries**
   Emergencies at the bottom often involve nitrogen narcosis, a state of stupor commonly called "rapture of the deep." It results from the affects of nitrogen on brain function. Divers may take unnecessary risks. Other emergencies occur when a diver begins to run out of oxygen and panics.

   d. **Ascent injuries**
   Injury during ascent can involve barotrauma or decompression illness, "the bends." Decompression illness, or the bends, is due to nitrogen bubbles coming out of solution in the blood and tissues, causing increased pressure on various body structures and occluding circulation in small blood vessels. This occurs in joints, tendons, the spinal cord, skin, brain, and inner ear. The trigger is a rapid ascent after exposure to a depth of 33 feet or more for a time sufficient to allow body tissues to become saturated with nitrogen. The most serious form of barotrauma is pulmonary overpressure, a condition in which air trapped in the lungs expands, causing rupture of the alveoli. Air may leak through the visceral pleura, causing a pneumothorax. Air may also enter the circulatory system, causing an arterial gas embolism. From there, the embolism can lodge in various parts of the body,

where it obstructs blood flow, causing ischemia and possible infarct. Pneumomediastinum occurs when air leaks into the mediastinum and pericardial sac.

In a diving emergency, do not try to distinguish the exact problem. Obtain a diving history. Specific questions center on the timing and nature of the phases of the dive, including the depth, number, and duration of dives. Inquire about the diver's experience and state of equipment. Obtain a history of previous diving problems, medications, and use of alcohol.

13. Describe the pathophysiology of high-altitude illnesses.   p. 340

High-altitude illnesses are due to decreased ambient pressure creating a low-oxygen environment. As barometric pressure decreases at higher altitudes, lower oxygen availability can both trigger related disorders and aggravate existing medical conditions such as angina, congestive heart failure, chronic obstructive pulmonary disease (COPD), and hypertension. Even in very healthy individuals, rapid ascent to high altitudes without time for acclimatization can cause illness. It is difficult to predict who will be affected by altitude illness. High-altitude illness begins to be manifest at approximately 8,000 ft (2,400 m) above sea level. The range considered high altitude is 4,900 to 11,500 ft. Here, the hypoxic environment causes decreased exercise tolerance, although without major disruption of normal oxygen transport in the blood. The range for very high altitude is 11,500 to 18,000 ft, and this causes extreme hypoxia during exercise or sleep. Extreme altitude (greater than 18,000 ft) will cause severe illness in virtually everyone.

14. Discuss ways to prevent high-altitude illnesses.   pp. 340–341

The most important prevention consideration is acclimatization through gradual ascent. This allows the body to adjust to the induced hypoxia. Acclimatization occurs through ventilatory, cardiovascular, and blood changes. Over time the body will reset the normal ventilation rate and operating level of carbon dioxide (CO_2). The heart rate will increase to deliver more oxygen. Peripheral veins constrict to increase central blood volume. Because pulmonary circulation also constricts, however, this can cause or exacerbate preexisting conditions or predispose persons to pulmonary edema. Additionally, the body will make more red blood cells to increase the oxygen-carrying capacity of the blood. Other prevention strategies include limiting exertion at high altitude and sleeping at lower altitudes. Eating a diet high in carbohydrates will provide quick energy. Acetazolamide and Nifedipine are medications that may assist in acclimatization. Acetazolamide acts as a diuretic, forcing bicarbonate out of the body and allowing the hypoxic ventilatory response to reach a new set point more quickly. Nifedipine causes vasodilation, which can help reduce the risk of pulmonary edema.

15. Given a variety of scenarios, assess and manage patients with high-altitude illnesses.   pp. 341–342

When a person ascends rapidly to high altitude, signs and symptoms may range from fatigue and decreased exercise tolerance to headache, sleep disturbance, and respiratory distress. Specific disorders include acute mountain sickness, high-altitude pulmonary edema, and high-altitude cerebral edema.

Acute mountain sickness (AMS) usually manifests in an unacclimatized person who ascends rapidly to an altitude of 2,000 m (6,600 ft) or higher. Signs and symptoms include lightheadedness, breathlessness, weakness, headache, and nausea and vomiting. More serious signs can develop, especially if the person continues to ascend: severe weakness, severe vomiting, decreased urine output, shortness of breath, and altered level of consciousness. Mild AMS is self-limiting and often improves in one or two days if no further ascent occurs. Treatment for AMS consists of halting ascent or possibly lowering altitude, and use of acetazolamide and antinauseants as needed. Supplemental oxygen will relieve symptoms but is typically used only in severe cases. Definitive treatment for all high-altitude illnesses is descent.

High-altitude pulmonary edema (HAPE) results from increased pulmonary pressure and hypertension caused by changed blood flow in higher altitude. Initial symptoms include dry cough, mild shortness of breath on exertion, and slight crackles in the lungs progressing to severe dyspnea and cyanosis, coughing productive of frothy sputum, and weakness that may progress to coma and death. In its early stages, HAPE is completely reversed by descent and/or use of oxygen. An alternative is a portable hyperbaric bag. Acetazolamide may decrease symptoms. Other medications such as morphine, nifedipine, and furosemide may be useful but carry risk for complications such as hypotension and dehydration.

High-altitude cerebral edema (HACE) usually manifests with deteriorating neurological status in a patient with AMS or HAPE. It reflects increased intracranial pressure due to increased fluid in the brain. Symptoms include altered mental status, poor coordination, decreased level of consciousness, and coma. If descent isn't possible, oxygen, sildenafil, steroids, and a hyperbaric bag may help. If coma develops, it may persist for days after descent to sea level. Although it usually resolves, residual disability may result.

Case Study Review

Reread the case study on page 316 in Paramedic Care: Trauma; *then, read the following discussion.*

This case study demonstrates how paramedics react to a relatively common wintertime emergency: a patient with apparent hypothermia. The case study demonstrates how assessment findings reveal diagnosis, and, as presentation changes, how diagnosis and treatment change as well. The case study also demonstrates how contraindications to certain management steps appear at different stages of hypothermia.

The EMS team is en route to work on a winter day described as "bitterly cold" when they hear a priority call for an unconscious man found lying in snow. As they respond, they do not know any particulars regarding age, possible medical conditions, or even how long the man has been exposed to the snow and cold air.

They find a young man who is huddled and shivering on ice-covered ground. Breathing is shallow and irregular; the approximate number of respirations per minute is not given. The man is conscious, and, although confused, gives a brief, plausible history. He had been out celebrating and passed out. (The case study does not state whether the man admitted to use of alcohol or other drugs during the celebration, substances that may increase vulnerability to hypothermia.) The patient adds he may have been exposed to the elements for a "couple of hours." Important assessment findings include bradycardia, mild hypotension, and a core temperature of 86°F.

At this point, the assessment contains a few elements suggesting mild hypothermia and others pointing to severe hypothermia. Findings consistent with mild hypothermia include the presence of shivering, detectable although irregular respirations, and a level of consciousness sufficient to give a brief history. In contrast, there are also more ominous signs of severe hypothermia: bradycardia and hypotension. The core temperature of 86°F defines the case as severe hypothermia (core temperature less than 90°F).

The team knows that the man has severe hypothermia, and they know they must act quickly, as they can expect his condition to continue to deteriorate, perhaps precipitously, as long as he is in the cold environment. Indeed, before they can intervene, the patient's presentation does decline: shivering stops and speech becomes unintelligible.

The partners quickly move the man into the warm ambulance, remove his wet clothing, apply cardiac and core temperature monitors, and then begin active external rewarming with water bottles at the head, neck, chest, and groin. (The study does not note if the patient was covered with blankets or other insulating material, but you can assume that he was because the other initial actions taken by the team comply with management guidelines.) During this period core temperature does continue to drop, to 85°F.

Findings from the cardiac monitor are not given but presumably are stable, as no action is taken against dysrhythmia.

The temperature drop below 86°F signals a new level of urgency. At this temperature, active internal rewarming is mandated with measures such as warm IV fluid and warm humid oxygen, as well as the possible steps of peritoneal lavage, extracorporeal rewarming, and esophageal rewarming tubes. In the prehospital setting, the measures most likely to be available are the warm IV fluid and warm humid oxygen. The team also knows that they have reached a critical temperature in terms of cardiac instability. Dysrhythmias or asystole are now very real possibilities, and, indeed, the rough handling associated with road construction triggers ventricular fibrillation. A single defibrillation is unsuccessful (an expected finding as hearts are generally considered to be incapable of response to defibrillation at temperatures below 86°F).

The providers respond with traditional support for the ABCs: intubation, ventilation with warmed oxygen, and chest compressions. The team makes another correct decision for treatment at this low temperature: They refrain from giving medications via the IV because they know drug metabolism is significantly

©2013 Pearson Education, Inc.
Paramedic Care: Principles & Practice, Vol. 5, 4th Ed.

decreased at this low core body temperature. The drugs may not be useful in the short term and may accumulate to a toxic level once the body core is rewarmed.

At the emergency department, more resources are available to rewarm the patient, and, after core temperature rises over 86°F, the usual ACLS protocols are used to stabilize the patient, who eventually recovers fully.

Content Self-Evaluation

MULTIPLE CHOICE

_____ 1. General risk factors that predispose a person to developing an environmental illness include all of the following, EXCEPT
    A. predisposing medical conditions such as diabetes.
    B. fatigue.
    C. high levels of fluid intake.
    D. use of certain over-the-counter or prescription medications.
    E. age: either very young or very old persons.

_____ 2. Homeostasis is the body's ability to maintain a steady, normal internal environment in the face of changing external conditions.
    A. True
    B. False

_____ 3. Which process is NOT one that results in body heat loss into the environment?
    A. Evaporation   D. Radiation
    B. Convection   E. Diffusion
    C. Respiration

_____ 4. Which group of medications does NOT predispose a person to hyperthermia?
    A. Psychotropics   D. Beta blockers
    B. Antiepileptics   E. Antihistamines
    C. Diuretics

_____ 5. Thirst is an adequate indicator of dehydration.
    A. True
    B. False

_____ 6. Dehydration is often intimately associated with heat disorders because it inhibits peripheral vasodilation and limits sweating.
    A. True
    B. False

_____ 7. In situations where it is unclear whether the diagnosis is fever or heatstroke, always treat for both conditions.
    A. True
    B. False

_____ 8. Medical conditions that may predispose to hypothermia include all of the following, EXCEPT
    A. hypothyroidism.   D. thin body build.
    B. malnutrition.   E. hypoglycemia.
    C. Parkinson's disease.

_____ 9. Most patients who die during rewarming die from ventricular fibrillation.
    A. True
    B. False

10. Which is NOT appropriate as a rewarming measure for mild to moderate hypothermia?
    A. Warmed blankets
    B. Warmed IV fluids
    C. Peritoneal lavage
    D. Heat packs
    E. Heat lamp

11. Which of the following management guidelines for frostbite is NOT correct?
    A. Do not thaw affected area if possibility of refreezing exists.
    B. Do not massage the frozen area or rub with snow.
    C. Do not puncture or drain any blisters.
    D. Do not warm frozen feet if patient will need to walk out of hostile environment.
    E. Do not give analgesia before thawing.

12. The physiology of freshwater and saltwater drownings differs, and these differences contribute to differences in prognosis and field management.
    A. True
    B. False

13. Resuscitation of a drowning victim is not indicated when
    A. respirations have ceased.
    B. cardiac asystole exists.
    C. the patient has been pulled from freezing water and is very cold.
    D. immersion is known to have been extremely long.
    E. head or neck injury due to trauma is evident.

14. Which of the following might be administered via IV to a drowning patient?
    A. Plasmanate
    B. Dextran
    C. Lactated Ringer's
    D. D_5W
    E. Hetastarch

15. One of the most severe complications of drowning is
    A. "the squeeze."
    B. ARDS.
    C. DAN.
    D. barotrauma.
    E. pneumomediastinum.

16. Which gas law is most applicable to decompression illness?
    A. Boyle's law
    B. Dalton's law
    C. Henry's law
    D. Ohm's law
    E. Venturi's law

17. The condition whose chief signs and symptoms include altered levels of consciousness and impaired judgment is
    A. AGE.
    B. "the squeeze."
    C. "the bends."
    D. pneumomediastinum.
    E. nitrogen narcosis.

18. The most common symptom of decompression sickness is
    A. vomiting.
    B. rash.
    C. hyperactivity.
    D. joint pain.
    E. chest pain.

19. The condition whose signs and symptoms include substernal chest pain, irregular pulse, abnormal heart sounds, reduced blood pressure and narrow pulse pressure, and a change in voice is
    A. AGE.
    B. "the squeeze."
    C. "the bends."
    D. pneumomediastinum.
    E. nitrogen narcosis.

20. Acclimatization occurs through all of the following, EXCEPT
    A. peripheral venous dilation.
    B. hypoxic ventilatory response.
    C. increased central blood volume.
    D. erythropoiesis.
    E. increased heart rate.

©2013 Pearson Education, Inc.
Paramedic Care: Principles & Practice, Vol. 5, 4th Ed.

_____ **21.** High-altitude pulmonary edema develops as a result of
  A. tachycardia.
  B. hypertension.
  C. vasodilation.
  D. hyperventilation.
  E. none of the above.

_____ **22.** The condition whose signs and symptoms include altered mental status, ataxia, decreased level of consciousness, and coma is
  A. AGE.
  B. DAN.
  C. HACE.
  D. HAPE.
  E. AMS.

MATCHING

Write the letter of the term in the space provided next to the definition that describes it.

  A. basal metabolic rate

  B. core temperature

  C. acclimatization

  D. thermolysis

  E. thermoregulation

  F. hypothalamus

  G. negative feedback

  H. heat disorder

_____ **23.** The temperature of deep body tissues

_____ **24.** Maintenance of a particular body temperature

_____ **25.** Control mechanism through which a substance turns off its further production

_____ **26.** Regulatory structure that serves as part of the neurological and endocrine systems

_____ **27.** Increased core body temperature due to inadequate heat dissipation

_____ **28.** Metabolism required simply to maintain body stability

_____ **29.** Loss of body heat to external environment

_____ **30.** Reversible changes in the body that compensate for environmental change

Write the letter of the approximate core body temperature range in the space provided next to the physiological or pathophysiological state with which it occurs.

  A. 90° to 95°F

  B. 100° to 105°F

  C. 82° to 90°F

  D. 97° to 100°F

  E. Less than 82°F

  F. 105° to 110°F

_____ **31.** Moderate hypothermia

_____ **32.** Heat exhaustion

_____ **33.** Severe hypothermia with poor prognosis for cardiac stability/resuscitation

_____ **34.** Heatstroke

_____ **35.** Mild hypothermia

_____ **36.** Normal range

Write the letter of the disorder in the space provided next to the appropriate clinical characteristics.

A. heat exhaustion

B. deep frostbite

C. high-altitude cerebral edema

D. severe hypothermia

E. acute mountain sickness (early phase)

F. heatstroke

G. pulmonary overpressure

H. nitrogen narcosis

I. mild hypothermia

J. decompression illness

K. high-altitude pulmonary edema

_____ **37.** Moderately decreased core temperature, shivering, lethargy, early rise in heart and respiratory rates

_____ **38.** Dry cough and dyspnea progressing to cough productive of frothy sputum and severe dyspnea

_____ **39.** Severe pain and CNS disturbances that develop during a rapid ascent from a dive to depth below 40 feet

_____ **40.** Environmentally induced freezing of skin and subcutaneous tissues with hardness on palpation, no sensation

_____ **41.** Altered mental status and decreasing level of consciousness, ataxia

_____ **42.** Substernal chest pain that develops during ascent, often from shallow depths, associated with respiratory distress and diminished breath sounds

_____ **43.** Light-headedness, shortness of breath, nausea after rapid ascent to altitude of 6,600 feet or more

_____ **44.** State of stupor that develops during deep dives rather than during descent or ascent

_____ **45.** Severely increased core temperature, loss of sweating, hypotension, possible seizures

_____ **46.** Somewhat increased core temperature, rapid and shallow respirations, weak pulses

_____ **47.** Severely decreased core temperature, no shivering, hypotension, dysrhythmias, undetectable pulse and respirations

Write the letter of the disorder in the space provided next to the key prevention measures to which it applies.

A. heat disorders (heat cramps, heat exhaustion, heatstroke)

B. high-altitude illness

C. cold disorders (hypothermia)

_____ **48.** Maintain adequate fluid intake, limit exposure to hostile environment, and allow acclimatization

_____ **49.** Dress appropriately, get plenty of rest, eat appropriately, and limit exposure to hostile environment

_____ **50.** Limit exertion, eat properly, consider prophylactic medications, and allow acclimatization

©2013 Pearson Education, Inc.
Paramedic Care: Principles & Practice, Vol. 5, 4th Ed.

LISTING

51. List the three forms of thermogenesis.

_____

_____

_____

52. List the two major mechanisms for heat dissipation.

_____

_____

_____

53. List the two major mechanisms for heat conservation.

_____

_____

_____

13

Special Considerations in Trauma

Review of Chapter Objectives

After reading this chapter, you should be able to:

1. **Define key terms introduced in this chapter.**

   Knowing and being able to apply the key terms in each chapter is critical to understanding chapter concepts. Write the list of key terms. Then write the definition of each one in your own words. Check your understanding by confirming the definitions in the text glossary. Correct any misunderstandings. Create a study aid by writing each key term on the front of an index card and the definition on the back. Use the cards to quiz yourself, or to have someone quiz you.

2. **Describe the importance of an organized system of trauma care to reducing trauma morbidity and mortality.**

   pp. 347–348

   In the mid-1960s, health care leaders recognized that no organized system of care existed for treatment of trauma victims. This prompted the initial development of today's emergency medical system. EMS is now a highly sophisticated system integrated into a large continuum of trauma care. Even so, 177,000 persons die each year from trauma. Efforts must focus on evidence-based research and practice to ensure that EMS skills and actions actually result in better patient outcomes. Reducing and preventing trauma should take precedence to prevent morbidity and mortality. EMS should engage in prevention programs and function as an integrated part of the health care system within their communities.

3. **Describe the potential impact of full engagement of EMS in injury prevention initiatives.**

   p. 348

   To maintain a leadership role in prehospital emergency care, EMS must emphasize injury prevention by encouraging and conducting prevention programs within the community. Prevention shows the greatest promise for reducing the death toll from many types of trauma. EMS can look to the fire service as a role model in this initiative. Some progressive emergency service systems have begun programs for the public that make people aware of the steps they can take to make their homes safer, to reduce childhood accidents, and to promote the use of helmets and other protective equipment for sports and motorcycling safety. The high rate of injury among males between 13 and 35 years of age is an area of opportunity for education to encourage behavioral change. These programs can make the EMS system a more prominent presence in the community, fostering a good public image.

4. **Describe the key actions and decisions in each phase of trauma assessment.**   pp. 348–363

The assessment of the trauma patient follows the standard format for assessment, including the special components that relate to trauma. The assessment progresses through the scene size-up, primary assessment, secondary assessment including a rapid trauma assessment (for the serious or critical patient) or the focused assessment and history, detailed physical exam (in rare cases), and, finally, ongoing reassessments.

During the scene size-up, you evaluate the scene to investigate and determine the mechanism of injury and, from that, identify an index of suspicion for specific injuries. You also analyze the potential hazards of the scene, including the need for Standard Precautions. You should search out and identify all patients. And, finally, you identify and summon all resources needed to manage the patients and scene.

In the primary assessment, you quickly apply spinal precautions and form a general patient impression and then determine the patient's mental status. Then evaluate the patient's airway and breathing and perform any needed interventions (oxygen, oral or nasal airway or endotracheal intubation, and ventilation). Evaluate circulation by checking pulse and skin condition. Make a visual sweep for bleeding and control external obvious hemorrhage. If hypovolemia and shock are suspected, initiate at least one large-bore IV. At the conclusion of the primary assessment, the patient is categorized as needing the rapid trauma assessment (critical patients) or the focused trauma exam. Make a preliminary assignment of the patient to a priority category for care and transport.

During the rapid trauma assessment, you examine areas where significant injury is expected either from the mechanism of injury analysis or the primary assessment. Use techniques of questioning, inspection, palpation, auscultation, and percussion during your assessment. Ask about the patient's chief and minor complaints, as time and priority permit. In general, during this assessment you should look in detail at the head, neck, chest, abdomen, and pelvis, because these are the areas likely to produce life-threatening injury. Take a quick set of vital signs and an abbreviated patient history. At the end of the rapid trauma assessment, decide the priority of the patient for transport. That decision is made by comparing the assessment findings against the trauma triage criteria used in your system.

The focused trauma assessment is used for the patient with limited mechanism of injury and expected, isolated, and moderate to minor injuries. During the focused assessment, you direct consideration to the likely injuries and the specific patient complaints. It usually concludes with slow transport to a nearby emergency department or, in some cases, treatment and release.

The detailed physical exam is a comprehensive head-to-toe assessment of the patient while you search for signs and symptoms of injury. This procedure is useful for the unconscious patient for whom all other known or suspected life threats have been attended to, and it is then provided only during transport. However, portions of the techniques and process of the detailed assessment are used for elements of the primary and secondary assessments.

During the reassessment, you re-check mental status; reevaluate airway, breathing, and circulation; retake vital signs; reevaluate chief or serious patient complaints and significant signs of injury; and recheck any interventions you have performed. Reassess seriously injured patients every 5 minutes, every 15 minutes for stable patients. Also perform the reassessment after every major intervention or any sign that the patient's condition has changed or is changing. Compare results of each reassessment to baseline findings and those from previous reassessments to identify deterioration or improvement in patient status.

5. **Given a variety of trauma patient scenarios, identify signs and symptoms of injury.**   pp. 353–359

The signs and symptoms of injury in multiple-trauma patients are discovered by applying the systematic assessment process. Begin this process with the scene size-up, where you determine the mechanism of injury and develop an index of suspicion for possible injury. As you begin your assessment, remember to treat any life threats as soon as they are identified. If the patient's mental status is altered or the patient is unresponsive, think head injury, serious internal damage, or shock. Early signs of shock may also include increasing anxiety, restlessness, or combativeness. When evaluating airway and breathing, broken or irregular speech, unusual airway sounds, very rapid or slow respirations, or inadequate volume suggest inadequate brain perfusion and/or traumatic injury. Stridor, snoring, gurgling sounds, or wheezing indicate partial airway obstruction. Soft tissue trauma should alert you to the potential for

©2013 Pearson Education, Inc.
Paramedic Care: Principles & Practice, Vol. 5, 4th Ed.

swelling and airway occlusion. Drainage of fluid from the mouth or nose may be cerebrospinal fluid suggestive of skull fracture. Other signs of basilar skull fracture include bilateral periorbital ecchymosis (racoon eyes) and retroauricular ecchymosis (Battle's sign). Abnormal pupillary responses may suggest cranial nerve injury or orbital fracture and muscle entrapment. Poor chest excursion, paradoxical motion, and unilateral diminished or absent breath sounds suggest flail chest or pneumothorax. If the area is dull to percussion, a hemothorax may be present. Crackles on auscultation may represent pulmonary edema, usually due to pulmonary contusion. Inspect for open wounds. Grating sensations or complaints of pain on palpation of the chest may indicate rib fracture. Crackling sensations are indicative of subcutaneous emphysema.

Evaluating circulation and vital signs will provide clues to development of shock. Rapid, weak, and thready pulses and narrowing pulse pressure along with cool, clammy, pale skin suggest shock compensation. Ashen, cyanotic, or pale skin suggests possible hypovolemia, hypoventilation, or hypothermia. Hypotension indicates hypovolemia and late signs of shock. Muffled or distant heart sounds and hypotension suggest pericardial tamponade. Extreme jugular venous distension (JVD) implicates tension pneumothorax, pericardial tamponade, or traumatic asphyxia. Abdominal injury may present with muscle spasm, tenderness, or unusual masses. Suspect fracture and serious internal injury if crepitus or instability is noted during examination of the pelvis. Extremity discoloration suggests circulation problems.

Deformity of the extremities may present as enlargement or angulation. Suspect contusion if fluid accumulation is noted or fracture if a limb is abnormally positioned. Check for muscle tone, distal pulses, motor response, sensory response, and limb strength. Abnormal findings suggest damage to the nervous or circulatory system, including possible spinal injury. Slight deformities, minor reddening, or subtle pain and tenderness in the back further indicate spinal column damage. External wounds are more obvious. Abrasions, lacerations, openings in the skin, discoloration, or blistering indicate blunt or penetrating trauma or burns. Reddening in the absence of an open wound may indicate soft tissue damage or underlying organ injury.

6. **Given a variety of trauma patient scenarios, demonstrate assessment-based decision making, including treatment and transport decisions.**
pp. 354–356, 360, 365, 374–375

The components of shock trauma resuscitation include protecting the spine, ensuring airway patency, providing adequate ventilation, and supporting the circulatory system to maintain adequate perfusion.

The spine is protected from the moment that injury is suspected with manual immobilization of the head until the patient reliably reports the absence of spinal injury symptoms or the patient is immobilized on a long spine board. The airway must be maintained mechanically for any patient who is not capable of maintaining his own airway. Airway adjuncts, supraglottic airway devices, and/or endotracheal intubation will be required. Early intubation should be considered when physiological conditions (airway burns or airway soft tissue or structural damage) will become progressively worse, making later intubation more difficult or impossible or if vomiting and aspiration is a risk. If intubation cannot be accomplished, cricothyrotomy may be necessary.

Ventilation is employed for the patient who is not maintaining adequate air exchange on his own. If the patient has some respirations, overdrive ventilation is required and should be coordinated with the patient's attempts at respiration, if possible. Overdrive ventilation is of great value for the patient with flail chest or rib fractures. Apply with caution for patients with internal chest injury because it may convert a pneumothorax into a tension pneumothorax. High-concentration oxygen should be administered to maintain saturation at no less than 96 percent. Ventilations should be guided by capnography.

External hemorrhage must be controlled with direct pressure, elevation, pressure points, and, if absolutely necessary, a tourniquet. Large-bore IVs should be introduced using nonrestrictive administration sets and either normal saline or lactated Ringer's solution for serious hemorrhage and signs and symptoms of shock. Titrate fluid volume to patient needs, keeping in mind that prehospital fluid administration is usually limited to 3,000 mL.

Transport decisions are made throughout care. At the conclusion of the primary assessment, a preliminary priority should be assigned. If the patient meets any of the trauma triage criteria, either a mechanism of injury recognized during the scene size-up, a recognized anatomic injury, or a physical condition including vital signs identified during the primary assessment, consider the patient a priority for rapid transport. If the patient is in cardiac arrest, follow local protocol for discontinuing or not initiating resuscitation. Reprioritize the patient for immediate transport to a trauma center anytime during the assessment at the first signs of hypovolemic compensation. The final decision as to where to transport a patient and the priority for that transport is made at the end of the rapid or focused trauma assessment. This decision is based on the Centers for Disease Control trauma triage criteria. Transportation should begin once on-scene care has stabilized injuries and the patient is packaged appropriately to limit further injury. Make every effort to limit on-scene time to no more than 10 minutes. Consider using air medical service if it will substantially reduce transport time to definitive care. As a general rule, if transport by ground will exceed 45 minutes, request a helicopter. For serious trauma calls, consider placing the helicopter on standby early. Initiate the response or cancel the flight once you are on scene and have made an initial assessment of the situation and patient condition.

7. **Recognize the need for immediate life-saving interventions, including airway management, ensuring adequate oxygenation and ventilation, controlling external hemorrhage, providing appropriate fluid resuscitation, and performing pleural decompression.** pp. 363–364

Shock trauma resuscitation refers to care for multiple-system trauma to support the seriously injured patient. Trauma often induces hypovolemia, hypotension, and hypoperfusion. Recognizing these life-threatening conditions and immediately treating them take priority. Manage airway and breathing by providing oxygen to maintain an oxygen saturation of at least 96 percent. Consider overdrive ventilation if the respiratory rate is either less than 10 or greater than 29. Secure the airway if needed by using a supraglottic airway or performing endotracheal intubation. Replace volume loss by initiating a large-bore IVs and administering fluid rapidly to maintain a systolic blood pressure of 80 mmHg or 90 mmHg in the case of head injury. Be alert for signs and symptoms of a developing tension pneumothorax and decompress the affected side of the chest. Control significant hemorrhage with direct pressure and consider a tourniquet if bleeding is uncontrollable.

8. **Describe the importance of recognizing, preventing, and treating hypothermia in trauma patients.** pp. 364–365

Patients with serious trauma and shock are more prone to hypothermia and are at risk for suffering negative consequences as a result. Sympathetic stimulation causes the body to direct blood to critical organs and not temperature-regulation activities. Energy and heat production decrease as the patient is stabilized. Often fluid resuscitation is accomplished with cool fluids. Patients may be exposed for assessment and not adequately covered back up. Shivering in response to cold depletes the body's energy reserves, making the impact of injury worse. Additionally, a drop in core body temperature prolongs clotting time and negatively affects enzymes, which can disrupt oxygen utilization, decrease metabolism, and worsen acidosis. Treatment should include fluids at or near body temperature, blankets to keep the patient warm, and an ambulance temperature of 85 degrees.

9. **Describe the differences in anatomy, physiology, pathophysiology, assessment, and management of pediatric trauma patients.** pp. 366–369

Pediatric patients are anatomically smaller than adults and present with several anatomical and physiological considerations that affect their response to trauma. Their smaller size means that they have a larger ratio of body surface area to total body mass and volume. They are more prone to rapid heat loss or gain and suffer proportionally greater fluid loss with extensive body surface injuries such as burns or abrasions. Blood and fluid losses are consequential because these patients have smaller reserves to restore such losses. Their smaller size also affects the location and severity of injury. Traumatic injury often occurs higher on the anatomy, while shorter arms and legs are less able to protect the trunk and head from trauma. Internal organs are closer together and less protected by subcutaneous fat and muscle, making multisystem trauma more likely. The proportionately larger head subjects children to a greater incidence of neck and head injury. Airway structures are also different. The larger tongue is more likely to obstruct the airway, while the shorter, more delicate trachea can kink or be damaged during intubation. Softer, more cartilaginous bones allow flexibility but provide less protection for the brain and intrathoracic organs. Because bones are developing, future growth may be disrupted if an

©2013 Pearson Education, Inc.
Paramedic Care: Principles & Practice, Vol. 5, 4th Ed.

injury occurs to the growth plates. Seriously injured children will generally compensate for blood loss well, hiding the severity of internal injuries, then deteriorate rapidly when compensatory mechanisms fail. Pediatric patients also have less respiratory reserve, causing them to tire more quickly. Vital signs are also different from those of adults, and providers need to be familiar with normal ranges for different age groups.

Trauma assessment and care must be tailored to the anatomical needs of children. For infants, maintain neutral position by padding under the shoulders of an infant to avoid blockage of the airway. Oral airways should be inserted with a tongue blade. Use uncuffed endotracheal tubes and frequently recheck patency, as they are more prone to dislodge. Fluids and medications should be administered via intravenous (IV) or intraosseus (IO) route. Fluid boluses for volume replacement should be administered early at a rate of 20 mL/kg boluses.

10. **Describe the differences in anatomy, physiology, pathophysiology, assessment, and management of pregnant trauma patients.** pp. 369–371

Traumatic injury in pregnancy affects both the fetus and the mother. Several physiological changes during pregnancy alter the mother's response to injury and blood loss. Blood volume is greater, heart rate increases, and blood pressure will be lower in the second trimester, returning to normal near term. As the uterus grows it displaces abdominal contents upward. During the first two trimesters the fetus is generally well protected. However, in the third trimester the uterus is thinner and the fetus is larger and more exposed. The fetus is at greater risk for direct injury from blunt trauma, which may also cause the placenta to separate from the uterine wall, abruptio placentae. Conversely, the abdominal contents of the mother may be better protected. Although seat belts reduce the risk of injury, a lap belt worn alone may lead to uterine rupture or abruptio placentae during a collision. With serious trauma, hypovolemia, shock, or hypoxia affects the fetus before it endangers the mother. Be watchful for signs of shock and treat early, ensuring adequate airway, ventilation, and circulation. If blood loss is suspected, provide aggressive fluid resuscitation. The pregnant mother can lose a significant amount of blood and endanger the fetus while displaying limited signs and symptoms of hypovolemia. Transport pregnant patients in the left lateral recumbent position to avoid supine hypotensive syndrome. If the patient is spinally immobilized, tilt the board on its side 15 degrees.

11. **Describe the differences in anatomy, physiology, pathophysiology, assessment, and management of bariatric trauma patients.** p. 371

Obesity is a growing problem. Assessment, care, and transport can be challenging for EMS providers. Obese patients usually have increased blood volume and cardiac output due to increased oxygen demand. This may lead to cardiac problems and hypertension, making the patient less able to accommodate the stress of traumatic injury and shock. Respiratory effort is also increased due to intra-abdominal pressure and greater chest wall resistance. Oxygen should be initiated early. Obese patients are more subject to multiple organ involvement, more serious pulmonary complications, and have higher mortality. They are more likely to suffer pulmonary contusions and pelvic, rib, and extremity fractures. Therefore, pay closer attention to the thorax and pelvic ring during assessment. Vital signs will be more difficult to obtain, requiring greater attention. Equipment modifications may be required for proper care. Providers should also ensure the availability of adequate resources during lifting and moving to avoid injury.

12. **Describe the differences in anatomy, physiology, pathophysiology, assessment, and management of geriatric trauma patients.** p. 372

Geriatric patients pose some challenges to assessment and care. These patients are subject to both the effects of aging and to the accumulating effects of chronic disease. Diminished reflexes, hearing, and sight make them more prone to trauma. Brittle bones fracture more easily and heal poorly. Decreased brain mass makes brain injuries more common as the organ moves about in the cranium. They have smaller cardiac reserves and less resilient vascular structures, which limits the ability to increase heart rate and stroke volume in response to hypovolemia. Geriatric patients have reduced fluid reserves, which negatively affects their response to fluid loss while, alternatively, large fluid infusions can overwhelm the body, causing pulmonary edema. Respiratory systems are less compliant with smaller reserves. Poor heat regulation predisposes them to hypothermia. Preexisting disease may further reduce cardiac and respiratory reserves. These conditions may also affect their ability to compensate for hypovolemia and the stresses of shock. Assessment of geriatric patients can be complicated by reduced mental acuity and diminished ability to perceive pain.

Shock care for geriatric patients must be initiated early. Provide fluids but closely monitor lung sounds for pulmonary edema. Use smaller catheters appropriate for thin skin, and small, delicate veins. Use electrocardiogram (ECG) monitoring, especially for patients with preexisting cardiac disease. Administer oxygen early but be careful when ventilating with a bag-valve mask (BVM) to avoid creating a pneumothorax. Prevent hypothermia by covering the patient with warm blankets.

Case Study Review

Reread the case study on page 346 and 347 in Paramedic Care: Trauma; *then, read the following discussion.*

The patient presented in this case study has the typical signs and symptoms of shock and is cared for with the aggressiveness required if shock resuscitation is to be successful.

Alex responds to a call of an auto collision where two vehicles have had serious frontal impact with air-bag deployment. Once on scene he finds the area has already been secured and the driver of one of the vehicles seems to be responsive and unharmed. Alex then approaches the other vehicle with an unresponsive 20-something female. He directs the EMT to help in initiating spinal precautions, where the snoring airway sounds clear once they bring her head and neck from flexion to the neutral position. Alex then moves on to check her radial pulse, capillary refill, and breaths. By looking at the condition of the car, Alex can see that the female patient is trapped against the seat. Given these factors the patient is categorized as unstable.

A rapid trauma assessment is performed as the equipment is prepared to remove the patient. Alex notes that the patient's skin is slightly pale, and her left pupil is slowly reactive to his penlight, but given the patient's positioning he cannot access her right pupil. Her neck appears to be symmetrical and has flat jugular veins. Alex palpates the upper chest and finds a "crackling life" feeling, and auscultation shows quiet breath sounds on the right side and somewhat louder sounds on the left. The patient's respiratory rate is increasing and is now about 26 breaths per minute. The position of the patient prevents Alex from performing the remainder of the rapid trauma assessment.

Once the patient is removed from the vehicle and placed on a stretcher with a cervical collar, they notice that she is pregnant and is likely in the late second or early third trimester. Her lower extremities appear distorted and Alex suspects bilateral femur fractures along with a possible pelvic facture. As Alex assesses the patient he notices a grating feeling when he compresses the ribs inward and notices reduced breath sounds over the entire left thorax. The EMT reports that the blood pressure is 66, the pulse is greater than 140, and pulse oximetry reads 84 percent. High-concentration oxygen is given to the patient as Alex prepares for a needle decompression of the chest. Alex decides that this patient is a candidate for rapid transport and starts and IV en route.

In the ambulance Alex tilts the spineboard to elevate the right side, and provides a 500-mL bolus of normal saline through an IV and then re-checks the vitals. Blood pressure is now 72/46, pulse is 148, and oxygen saturation is 92; however, the women does not respond to painful stimuli. During reassessment, Alex does notice that breath sounds on the left and right are now equal. Given the situation, Alex inspects for vaginal bleeding and finds a small amount of hemorrhage. On arrival at the emergency department, Alex reports this information as the trauma team inserts a chest tube and arranges for a CT scan of the head, neck, chest, and abdomen, and an ultrasound of the uterus and fetus.

Once arriving back at the station, Alex learns from the trauma center that the women had a placental abruption and miscarried after her arrival. She had an apparent concussion and has since regained consciousness; although she is in serious condition, she is expected to recover.

©2013 Pearson Education, Inc.
Paramedic Care: Principles & Practice, Vol. 5, 4th Ed.

Content Self-Evaluation

MULTIPLE CHOICE

_____ 1. The number of lives lost each year to trauma is
- A. 77,000.
- B. 177,000.
- C. 257,000.
- D. 300,000.
- E. 375,000.

_____ 2. Injury prevention steps for EMS include which of the following?
- A. Supporting preexisting programs that support prevention
- B. Acquainting the population with EMS
- C. Alerting society to hazards
- D. Performing home inspections
- E. All of the above

_____ 3. An EMS home inspection might examine for
- A. hot water temperature.
- B. pool fencing.
- C. smoke detector battery levels.
- D. crib slat spacing.
- E. all of the above.

_____ 4. Which of the following is a group especially at risk for trauma?
- A. Young women
- B. Young men
- C. Middle-aged females
- D. Middle-aged males
- E. Elderly women

_____ 5. The dispatch information is likely to provide you with which of the following?
- A. Location of the incident
- B. Any suspected scene hazards
- C. Any suspected danger of violence
- D. Other units responding
- E. All of the above

_____ 6. When approaching a scene of suspected violence, you should
- A. enter the scene immediately.
- B. enter the scene if it seems calm.
- C. enter the scene if the police are there.
- D. enter the scene if you are told it is safe by the police.
- E. none of the above.

_____ 7. What level of Standard Precautions will you employ at all trauma scenes?
- A. Gloves
- B. Goggles
- C. Gloves and goggles
- D. Gown
- E. Gloves and gown

_____ 8. The analysis of the mechanism of injury provides you with which item of patient information that is used during the primary and rapid trauma assessments?
- A. Number of patients
- B. Type of impact
- C. Resources needed
- D. Index of suspicion
- E. Hazards at the scene

_____ 9. Once you identify the type and nature of a hazardous material, attempt to enter the scene and remove the patient if there is any danger present.
- A. True
- B. False

_____ 10. The risk of contamination and resultant disease from contact with body substances is greater for you than for your patient.
- A. True
- B. False

11. In the case where you are assessing several patients, some with hemorrhage, you should
    A. use one glove set per patient.
    B. use one glove set per patient contact.
    C. use one set of gloves for all patient contacts.
    D. wash your hands (with gloves on) between contacts.
    E. none of the above.

12. If you arrive at a scene where a patient is covered with blood and has it spurting from an open facial wound, appropriate Standard Precautions include
    A. gloves.
    B. gloves and goggles.
    C. gloves and gown.
    D. gloves and mask.
    E. gloves, goggles, mask, and gown.

13. Air medical service should be summoned for any serious trauma scene if transport time will exceed
    A. 15 minutes.
    B. 15 to 20 minutes.
    C. 20 to 30 minutes.
    D. 45 minutes.
    E. 1 hour.

14. The reason for calling in additional resources before arriving at the patient's side is to ensure the needed resources arrive in a timely manner.
    A. True
    B. False

15. Which of the following is an element of the primary assessment?
    A. Spinal precautions
    B. General patient impression
    C. Mental status evaluation
    D. Airway maintenance
    E. All of the above

16. Which of the following injury mechanisms would suggest the need for spinal precautions?
    A. Severe flexion/extension
    B. Severe lateral bending
    C. Severe distraction
    D. Severe axial loading
    E. All of the above

17. The general impression of the patient is a difficult impression to make accurately early in a paramedic's career.
    A. True
    B. False

18. If your impression of a patient conflicts with the seriousness of potential injuries suggested by the mechanism of injury analysis, you should
    A. act according to your general impression.
    B. reanalyze the mechanism of injury analysis.
    C. determine vital signs and then determine patient priority.
    D. suspect the worst of the indicators is correct and act accordingly.
    E. not worry, as the patient's true condition will become more evident with time.

19. The "A" of the AVPU mnemonic stands for
    A. altered mental status.
    B. alert.
    C. adjusted to time.
    D. accurate.
    E. attitude.

20. Which is the order in which levels of orientation are lost?
    A. Time, persons, place
    B. Time, place, persons
    C. Persons, place, time
    D. Persons, time, place
    E. Place, persons, time

©2013 Pearson Education, Inc.
Paramedic Care: Principles & Practice, Vol. 5, 4th Ed.

_____ 21. The movement by the patient away from a painful stimulus is termed
A. purposeful.
B. purposeless.
C. decorticate posturing.
D. decerebrate posturing.
E. painful.

_____ 22. The movement by the patient to a position of muscular extension with the elbows flexing is termed
A. purposeful.
B. purposeless.
C. decorticate posturing.
D. decerebrate posturing.
E. painful.

_____ 23. It is easy to determine that the airway of a conscious and alert patient is patent when he can speak clearly in normal sentences.
A. True
B. False

_____ 24. If the patient does not have a protective airway reflex, when should you intubate him?
A. At the end of the assessment
B. Once there are signs of emesis
C. Immediately
D. Delay intubation but insert an oral airway
E. None of the above

_____ 25. If you find it necessary to ventilate a patient, you should do so at a rate of
A. 10 to 12 times per minute.
B. 12 to 20 times per minute.
C. 12 to 24 times per minute.
D. 16 to 30 times per minute.
E. 30 to 40 times per minute.

_____ 26. Capillary refill is no longer of value in the assessment of the pediatric patient.
A. True
B. False

_____ 27. Which of the following will affect the rate of capillary refill in the adult patient?
A. Smoking
B. Low ambient temperatures
C. Preexisting disease
D. Use of certain medications
E. All of the above

_____ 28. A weak, thready pulse suggests shock compensation.
A. True
B. False

_____ 29. In people with pigmented skin, examine for discoloration of the
A. lips.
B. sclera.
C. palms.
D. soles of the feet.
E. all of the above.

_____ 30. Hyperresonance on percussion of the chest suggests
A. blood accumulation.
B. fluid accumulation.
C. air.
D. air under pressure.
E. both C and D.

_____ 31. The detailed physical exam is used rarely in prehospital trauma care.
A. True
B. False

_____ 32. When one eye is shaded, the opposite pupil should
A. remain as it is.
B. dilate briskly.
C. dilate slowly.
D. constrict briskly.
E. constrict slowly.

33. You notice flat jugular veins in the supine patient. This suggests
   A. tension pneumothorax.
   B. pericardial tamponade.
   C. a normotensive patient.
   D. a hypovolemic patient.
   E. infection.

34. Allergies to which of the following drugs may be important in the treatment of the trauma patient?
   A. "Caine" drugs
   B. Antibiotics
   C. Tetanus toxoid
   D. Analgesics
   E. All of the above

35. Which of the following is NOT indicative of shock compensation?
   A. Falling blood pressure
   B. Increasing pulse rate
   C. Decreasing level of consciousness
   D. Decreasing pulse strength
   E. Cool and clammy skin

36. A trauma patient is breathing at 12 times per minute, has normal respiratory expansion, a blood pressure of 96 systolic, delayed capillary refill of 4 seconds, and a Glasgow Coma Scale score of 10. What should you report as the trauma score to medical direction?
   A. 7
   B. 9
   C. 10
   D. 11
   E. 15

37. Transport decisions for serious trauma patients are determined by the use of
   A. trauma score.
   B. Glasgow Coma Scale score.
   C. trauma triage criteria.
   D. vital signs.
   E. helicopter availability.

38. Reassessment should be performed every 15 minutes on the seriously injured trauma patient.
   A. True
   B. False

39. Which of the following terms refers to the reduction of fluid volume within the cardiovascular system?
   A. Hypovolemia
   B. Hypoperfusion
   C. Hypotension
   D. Anemia
   E. Mimesis

40. Which of the following terms refers to a low blood pressure?
   A. Hypovolemia
   B. Hypoperfusion
   C. Hypotension
   D. Anemia
   E. None of the above

41. Normally, the prehospital infusion of crystalloids in the resuscitation of a shock patient should be limited to
   A. 500 mL.
   B. 1,000 mL.
   C. 2,000 mL.
   D. 3,000 mL.
   E. 5,000 mL.

42. Hypothermia is a serious complication of shock that compromises the patient's clotting mechanisms.
   A. True
   B. False

©2013 Pearson Education, Inc.
Paramedic Care: Principles & Practice, Vol. 5, 4th Ed.

_____ 43. What percentage of trauma responses are for noncritical cases?
- A. 30 percent
- B. 50 percent
- C. 65 percent
- D. 80 percent
- E. 95 percent

_____ 44. Which of the following statements is NOT true regarding the pediatric patient as compared to the adult patient?
- A. The child's surface-area-to-volume ratio is greater.
- B. The child's organs are closer together.
- C. The child's airway is smaller.
- D. The child compensates for blood loss poorly.
- E. The child's skeletal components are more flexible.

_____ 45. The healthy pediatric patient may compensate for blood loss up to what percentage before signs appear?
- A. 25 percent
- B. 35 percent
- C. 45 percent
- D. 50 percent
- E. 60 percent

_____ 46. Which of the following is NOT true regarding pediatric vital signs as the child ages?
- A. The temperature rises.
- B. The pulse rate decreases.
- C. The tidal volume increases.
- D. The blood pressure increases.
- E. The respirations slow.

_____ 47. For the pediatric patient, the oral airway should be inserted by rotating it 180 degrees during insertion.
- A. True
- B. False

_____ 48. An alternative pediatric IV access site for administering medications and IV fluids is the:
- A. subclavian vein.
- B. intraosseous site.
- C. antecubital fossa.
- D. popliteal vein.
- E. scalp vein.

_____ 49. The recommended size of the initial fluid bolus for a pediatric trauma patient is
- A. 100 mL.
- B. 250 mL.
- C. 20 mL/kg.
- D. 60 mL/kg.
- E. 80 mL/kg.

_____ 50. Because a pregnant trauma patient has greater blood volume, the fetus is at less risk from maternal hypovolemia.
- A. True
- B. False

_____ 51. Which of the following is NOT true of pregnant patients?
- A. Cardiac rate decreases.
- B. Oxygen demands decrease.
- C. Abdominal contents displace upward.
- D. Blood pressure decreases.
- E. Tidal volume increases.

_____ 52. Blunt trauma to the gravid uterus may result in
- A. placenta previa.
- B. uterine rupture.
- C. abruptio placenta.
- D. A, B, and C.
- E. B and C.

_____ 53. Obese patients are likely to have
     A. decreased blood volume.
     B. lower minute volume.
     C. increased chest wall resistance.
     D. greater incidence of head injury.
     E. decreased cardiac output.

_____ 54. Most EMS equipment is designed to accommodate obese patients safely.
     A. True
     B. False

_____ 55. Which is the fastest-growing group of EMS patients?
     A. The elderly   D. Young females
     B. Pediatric patients   E. Middle-aged patients
     C. Young males

_____ 56. Which of the following statements is NOT true regarding elderly patients?
     A. They have a lower pain tolerance.
     B. Renal function is decreased.
     C. Brain mass and volume are decreased.
     D. Lung function is decreased.
     E. Cardiac stroke volume is decreased.

_____ 57. Because of chronic and preexisting diseases, geriatric patients move into which of these conditions more quickly than healthy adults?
     A. Shock compensation   D. Death
     B. Decompensated shock   E. All of the above
     C. Irreversible shock

_____ 58. Assessment of the geriatric patient is often difficult because the underlying problem that leads the patient to call EMS is often masked or confused by signs and symptoms of preexisting disease.
     A. True
     B. False

_____ 59. Key elements of the oral patient care report include all of the following, EXCEPT
     A. mechanism of injury.   D. interventions.
     B. response times.   E. results of interventions.
     C. results of assessment.

_____ 60. Which of the following is NOT an advantage to air medical transport of the trauma patient?
     A. The helicopter travels at very high speeds.
     B. The helicopter provides a superior working environment.
     C. The helicopter can bypass traffic congestion.
     D. The helicopter can travel in a straight line.
     E. None of the above.

_____ 61. As a general rule, you should request a helicopter if ground transport will exceed:
     A. 15 minutes.
     B. 20 minutes.
     C. 30 minutes.
     D. 45 minutes.
     E. 60 minutes.

_____ 62. Putting helicopters on standby delays response time.
     A. True
     B. False

©2013 Pearson Education, Inc.
Paramedic Care: Principles & Practice, Vol. 5, 4th Ed.

_____ **63.** Helicopters are capable of all of the following, EXCEPT:
- **A.** searching rough terrain.
- **B.** landing in icy conditions.
- **C.** illuminating scenes.
- **D.** transporting from remote areas.
- **E.** vertical lifts.

_____ **64.** Fluid resuscitation in the trauma patient is critical for:
- **A.** maintaining clotting factors.
- **B.** preserving red blood cells.
- **C.** preventing embolisms.
- **D.** preserving brain perfusion in head trauma.
- **E.** limiting internal hemorrhage.

TRAUMA
Content Review
Content Self-Evaluation

Chapter 1: Trauma and Trauma Systems

_____ 1. Trauma accounts for about what death toll each year?
   A. 77,000 deaths
   B. 177,000 deaths
   C. 257,000 deaths
   D. 300,000 deaths
   E. 375,000 deaths

_____ 2. Serious life-threatening injury occurs in about 30 percent of all trauma.
   A. True
   B. False

_____ 3. Surgical intervention rates for serious trauma are greatest in
   A. intentional trauma.
   B. penetrating trauma.
   C. accidental trauma.
   D. physical trauma.
   E. blunt trauma.

_____ 4. A Level III trauma center is a(n)
   A. community hospital.
   B. teaching hospital.
   C. emergency department with 24-hour service.
   D. nonemergency health care facility.
   E. regional center.

_____ 5. The guidelines that help determine the need of a trauma patient for the services of the trauma center are called the
   A. mechanism of injury.
   B. index of suspicion.
   C. trauma triage criteria.
   D. surgical guidelines.
   E. Golden Period.

_____ 6. The result of the analysis of the mechanism of injury is the
   A. Golden Period concept.
   B. kinetic analysis of the trauma.
   C. scene size-up.
   D. index of suspicion.
   E. expected injury algorithm.

_____ 7. The major advantage to helicopter transport of the trauma patient is that helicopters travel much faster than ground units and in a straight line.
   A. True
   B. False

_____ 8. Because paramedics are usually at the side of seriously injured patients so quickly, the signs and symptoms of serious injury and shock will be apparent.
   A. True
   B. False

_____ 9. One of the most effective methods of reducing trauma morbidity and mortality is through injury prevention programs.
   A. True
   B. False

_____ 10. Which of the following indicates a trauma patient's need for immediate transport to a trauma center?
   A. Systolic blood pressure less than 90 mmHg
   B. Flail chest
   C. Ejection from a vehicle
   D. Fall from greater than three times the victim's height
   E. All of the above

Chapter 2: Blunt Trauma

_____ 11. The capacity to do work is termed
   A. kinetics.
   B. velocity.
   C. energy.
   D. inertia.
   E. momentum.

_____ 12. Blunt trauma does not cause injury beneath the skin.
   A. True
   B. False

_____ 13. Auto collisions account for about what number of deaths each year?
   A. 23,500
   B. 28,500
   C. 34,500
   D. 50,500
   E. 70,500

_____ 14. Which of the following places the events of an auto collision in the order in which they occur?
   A. Body collision, vehicle collision, organ collision, secondary collisions
   B. Organ collision, vehicle collision, body collision, secondary collisions
   C. Vehicle collision, secondary collisions, body collision, organ collision
   D. Vehicle collision, body collision, organ collision, secondary collisions
   E. Body collision, vehicle collision, secondary collisions, organ collision

_____ 15. Which of the following have played a substantial role in reducing highway-collision-related deaths?
   A. Shoulder belts
   B. Passenger air bags
   C. Driver air bags
   D. Child seats
   E. All of the above

_____ 16. The seat belt is very effective at reducing injuries related to intrusion into the auto passenger compartment.
   A. True
   B. False

_____ 17. Which of the following are injuries that air-bag inflation may cause?
   A. Hand injuries
   B. Finger injuries
   C. Facial injuries
   D. Nasal fractures
   E. All of the above

_____ 18. The up-and-over pathway is most commonly associated with which auto collision type?
   A. Lateral
   B. Rotational
   C. Frontal
   D. Rear-end
   E. Rollover

©2013 Pearson Education, Inc.
Paramedic Care: Principles & Practice, Vol. 5, 4th Ed.

_____ 19. When analyzing the frontal-impact injury mechanism, the paramedic should assign a higher index of suspicion for serious life-threatening injury than with other types of impacts.
   A. True
   B. False

_____ 20. The type of injury most commonly associated with the rear-end impact is
   A. head injury.
   B. pelvic injury.
   C. neck injury.
   D. foot fracture.
   E. abdominal injury.

_____ 21. When you encounter the intoxicated patient, the mechanism of injury analysis becomes even more important.
   A. True
   B. False

_____ 22. The helmet reduces the incidence of head injury by about what percent?
   A. 25
   B. 35
   C. 50
   D. 65
   E. 80

_____ 23. In the auto/adult pedestrian collision, you would expect the victim to turn away from the impact.
   A. True
   B. False

_____ 24. In the terms of physics, a fall is nothing more than the release of stored gravitational energy.
   A. True
   B. False

_____ 25. A victim standing and facing the epicenter of a blast is more likely to sustain serious injury than a victim lying on the ground with his feet toward the blast epicenter.
   A. True
   B. False

_____ 26. Shrapnel is small, arrow-like objects within a bomb casing that extend its injury potential and range.
   A. True
   B. False

_____ 27. Which of the following are primary blast injuries?
   A. Heat injuries
   B. Pressure injuries
   C. Projectile injuries
   D. Injuries caused by structural collapse
   E. Both A and B

_____ 28. The closer a victim was to the blast epicenter, the higher should be the paramedic's index of suspicion for more serious injuries.
   A. True
   B. False

_____ 29. Ear injuries associated with an explosion, even those affecting as much as one-third of the eardrum with a tear, may improve with time.
   A. True
   B. False

_____ 30. Sports injuries are frequently associated with the mechanism(s) of
   A. compression.
   B. extension/flexion.
   C. compression/distraction.
   D. rotation.
   E. all of the above.

Chapter 3: Penetrating Trauma

_____ 31. An object that weighs twice as much as another object traveling at the same speed has
   A. twice the kinetic energy.
   B. three times the kinetic energy.
   C. four times the kinetic energy.
   D. five times the kinetic energy.
   E. six times the kinetic energy.

_____ 32. Wounds from a handgun are two to four times more lethal than those from a rifle.
   A. True
   B. False

_____ 33. The diameter of a projectile is its
   A. caliber.
   B. profile.
   C. drag.
   D. yaw.
   E. expansion factor.

_____ 34. Which of the following is a characteristic of a handgun bullet in contrast to a rifle bullet?
   A. It is a heavier projectile.
   B. It travels at a greater velocity.
   C. It has a blunter shape.
   D. It is more likely to fragment.
   E. All of the above.

_____ 35. With low-velocity penetrating objects, damage is usually more extensive than just the direct contact points between the object and human tissue.
   A. True
   B. False

_____ 36. Which element of the projectile injury process describes the region filled with air and tissue debris after the bullet has passed?
   A. Direct injury
   B. Pressure wave
   C. Temporary cavity
   D. Permanent cavity
   E. Zone of injury

_____ 37. The tissue structures that are very dense and usually sustain significant damage (often breaking apart) with the passage of a projectile are the
   A. solid organs.
   B. hollow organs.
   C. connective tissues.
   D. bones.
   E. lungs.

_____ 38. The tissue structures that are very resilient and usually sustain the smallest amount of damage associated with the passage of a projectile are the
   A. solid organs.
   B. hollow organs.
   C. connective tissues.
   D. bones.
   E. lungs.

_____ 39. The abdominal organ rather tolerant to the passage of a projectile is the
   A. bowel.
   B. liver.
   C. spleen.
   D. kidneys.
   E. pancreas.

_____ 40. The impact of a bullet with the ribs may induce an explosive energy exchange that injures the surrounding tissue with numerous bony fragments.
   A. True
   B. False

©2013 Pearson Education, Inc.
Paramedic Care: Principles & Practice, Vol. 5, 4th Ed.

_____ 41. A penetrating wound to the area of the rib margin should be suspected of involving the
   A. spleen or liver.
   B. kidneys.
   C. abdominal and thoracic organs.
   D. left, right, or both lung fields.
   E. all of the above.

_____ 42. Generally, powder burns and subcutaneous emphysema around the entrance wound suggest use of a
   A. gun at close range.
   B. high-powered rifle.
   C. handgun.
   D. black powder weapon.
   E. shotgun.

_____ 43. Which of the following is frequently associated with an exit wound?
   A. Tattooing
   B. A small ridge of discoloration around the wound
   C. A blown-out appearance
   D. Subcutaneous emphysema
   E. Propellant residue on the surrounding tissue

_____ 44. The exit wound is usually more likely to reflect the actual damaging potential of the projectile.
   A. True
   B. False

_____ 45. A relatively small bullet wound to the chest is all that is necessary to produce an open pneumothorax.
   A. True
   B. False

Chapter 4: Hemorrhage and Shock

_____ 46. Which of the following affects the cardiac output of the heart?
   A. Preload
   B. Afterload
   C. Cardiac contractility
   D. Heart rate
   E. All of the above

_____ 47. Approximately what volume of the body's blood is contained within the capillaries?
   A. 7 percent
   B. 13 percent
   C. 64 percent
   D. 23 percent
   E. 45 percent

_____ 48. The red blood cells account for what percentage of the total blood volume?
   A. 45 percent
   B. 78 percent
   C. 86 percent
   D. 92 percent
   E. 99 percent

_____ 49. Which of the following types of hemorrhage is characterized by slow-oozing bright red blood?
   A. Capillary bleeding
   B. Venous bleeding
   C. Arterial bleeding
   D. Both A and C
   E. None of the above

_____ 50. Which of the following is the phase of clotting in which smooth muscle contracts?
   A. Intrinsic phase
   B. Vascular phase
   C. Platelet phase
   D. Coagulation phase
   E. Aggregation phase

_____ **51.** Blood vessels that are lacerated longitudinally generally do not bleed very severely or for very long.
  A. True
  B. False

_____ **52.** Which of the following is likely to adversely affect the clotting process?
  A. Aggressive fluid resuscitation
  B. Hypothermia
  C. Movement at the site of injury
  D. Drugs such as aspirin
  E. All of the above

_____ **53.** Fractures of the tibia or humerus can account for a blood loss of
  A. less than 500 mL.
  B. from 500 to 750 mL.
  C. up to 1,500 mL.
  D. from 1,500 to 2,000 mL.
  E. in excess of 2,000 mL.

_____ **54.** In which stage of hemorrhage does the patient first display ineffective respiration?
  A. Class I
  B. Class II
  C. Class III
  D. Class IV
  E. Class V

_____ **55.** The female in late pregnancy is likely to have a blood volume that is
  A. much less than normal.
  B. slightly less than normal.
  C. slightly greater than normal.
  D. much greater than normal.
  E. normal.

_____ **56.** Which of the following is a result of sympathetic nervous system stimulation?
  A. Increased heart rate
  B. Increased peripheral vascular resistance
  C. Increased cardiac contractility
  D. Skeletal muscle vasodilation
  E. All of the above

_____ **57.** Which of the following is a catecholamine?
  A. Glucagon
  B. Insulin
  C. Norepinephrine
  D. Adrenocorticotropic hormone
  E. Erythropoietin

_____ **58.** Which of the following is a potent system vasoconstrictor?
  A. Antidiuretic hormone
  B. Angiotensin II
  C. Aldosterone
  D. Epinephrine
  E. Erythropoietin

_____ **59.** The opening of postcapillary sphincters and the resulting release of potassium, acids, and hypoxic blood is called
  A. ischemia.
  B. rouleaux.
  C. washout.
  D. hydrostatic release.
  E. none of the above.

_____ **60.** During which stage of shock is it difficult to determine if the patient is suffering from the effects of hypovolemia?
  A. Compensated
  B. Decompensated
  C. Irreversible
  D. Hypovolemic
  E. Cardiogenic

_____ 61. Which of the following does NOT first occur during the decompensated stage of shock?
   A. Pulses become unpalpable.
   B. Respirations slow or cease.
   C. Blood pressure decreases precipitously.
   D. The skin becomes cool and clammy.
   E. The patient becomes unconscious.

_____ 62. Under which of the following shock types would septic shock fall?
   A. Hypovolemic
   B. Distributive
   C. Obstructive
   D. Cardiogenic
   E. Respiratory

_____ 63. Under which of the following shock types would pericardial tamponade fall?
   A. Hypovolemic
   B. Distributive
   C. Cardiogenic
   D. Obstructive
   E. Respiratory

_____ 64. The color, temperature, and general appearance of the skin can indicate shock before there are changes in the blood pressure.
   A. True
   B. False

_____ 65. A fast and weak pulse may be the first indication of developing shock in the trauma patient.
   A. True
   B. False

_____ 66. In the normovolemic patient the jugular veins should be full when the patient is supine.
   A. True
   B. False

_____ 67. Large hematomas can account for a blood loss of
   A. up to 500 mL.
   B. from 500 to 750 mL.
   C. up to 1,500 mL.
   D. from 1,500 to 2,000 mL.
   E. in excess of 2,000 mL.

_____ 68. Frank blood in the stool is called
   A. hemoptysis.
   B. melena.
   C. hematuria.
   D. hematochezia.
   E. hematemesis.

_____ 69. For the patient in compensated shock, you should perform a reassessment
   A. every 5 minutes.
   B. every 15 minutes.
   C. after every major intervention.
   D. after noting any change in signs or symptoms.
   E. all except B.

_____ 70. Which of the following will permit the least fluid flow through a catheter?
   A. Short length, small lumen
   B. Short length, large lumen
   C. Long length, small lumen
   D. Long length, large lumen
   E. Large lumen and either long or short length

_____ 71. The preferred solution for the patient who is losing blood is
   A. normal saline.
   B. dextrose 5 percent in water.
   C. lactated Ringer's solution.
   D. hypertonic saline.
   E. whole blood.

Chapter 5: Soft-Tissue Trauma

_____ 72. Which of the following glands secrete a waxy substance?
   A. Sudoriferous glands
   B. Sebaceous glands
   C. Subcutaneous glands
   D. Adrenal glands
   E. Pituitary glands

_____ 73. The layer of skin that is made up of mostly dead cells and provides the waterproof envelope that contains the body is the
   A. dermis.
   B. subcutaneous layer.
   C. epidermis.
   D. sebum.
   E. corium.

_____ 74. Identify the layers of the arteries and veins in order from exterior to interior.
   A. Intima, media, adventitia
   B. Media, intima, adventitia
   C. Adventitia, intima, media
   D. Adventitia, media, intima
   E. Intima, adventitia, media

_____ 75. The blood vessels that have a wall only one cell thick are the
   A. arteries.
   B. arterioles.
   C. capillaries.
   D. venules.
   E. veins.

_____ 76. In the limbs, fascia define compartments with relatively fixed volumes.
   A. True
   B. False

_____ 77. Lacerations perpendicular to skin tension lines will cause the wound to gape.
   A. True
   B. False

_____ 78. The wound type characterized by a collection of blood under the skin is the
   A. abrasion.
   B. contusion.
   C. laceration.
   D. hematoma.
   E. avulsion.

_____ 79. The wound type characterized by a deep wound whose opening closes after injury is the
   A. abrasion.
   B. contusion.
   C. laceration.
   D. hematoma.
   E. puncture.

_____ 80. Prolonged crush injury (crush syndrome) permits the accumulation of
   A. myoglobin.
   B. potassium.
   C. lactic acid.
   D. uric acid.
   E. all of the above.

_____ 81. A likely cause of an avulsion is a(n)
   A. animal bite.
   B. severe glancing blow to the scalp.
   C. machinery accident.
   D. degloving injury.
   E. all of the above.

_____ 82. The natural ability of the body to halt blood loss is
   A. anemia.
   B. homeostasis.
   C. hemostasis.
   D. coagulation.
   E. metabolism.

_____ 83. Most blood vessels, when cut cleanly, will withdraw and constrict, limiting the rate of hemorrhage.
A. True
B. False

_____ 84. The cells that attack invading pathogens directly or through an antibody response are
A. macrophages.
B. lymphocytes.
C. chemotactic factors.
D. granulocytes.
E. both A and D.

_____ 85. The stage of the healing process in which skin cells regenerate to restore a uniform layer of skin cells along the wound border is
A. inflammation.
B. epithelialization.
C. neovascularization.
D. collagen synthesis.
E. none of the above.

_____ 86. The stage of the healing process in which capillaries grow to perfuse the healing tissue is
A. inflammation.
B. epithelialization.
C. neovascularization.
D. collagen synthesis.
E. none of the above.

_____ 87. Which of the following is a soft tissue wound infection risk factor?
A. HIV
B. Smoking
C. Avulsion
D. COPD
E. All of the above

_____ 88. The booster for tetanus is effective for
A. 1 year.
B. 2 to 4 years.
C. 5 years.
D. 10 years.
E. 25 years.

_____ 89. Which of the following can interfere with normal clotting?
A. Aspirin
B. Heparin
C. tPA
D. Clopidogrel
E. All of the above

_____ 90. The excessive growth of scar tissue beyond the boundaries of the wound is
A. hypertrophic scar formation.
B. keloid scar formation.
C. anatropic scar formation.
D. residual scar formation.
E. reactive scar formation.

_____ 91. The patient is not likely to experience pressure injury, even when immobilized for a lengthy period on a long spine board, PASG, or rigid splint.
A. True
B. False

_____ 92. The process of actual tissue death is
A. necrosis.
B. ischemia.
C. rhabdomyolysis.
D. gangrene.
E. mitosis.

_____ 93. Most dressings used in prehospital emergency care are sterile, nonocclusive, nonadherent, absorbent dressings.
A. True
B. False

_____ 94. The type of dressing that promotes clot development is
    A. adherent.
    B. nonadherent.
    C. absorbent.
    D. occlusive.
    E. nonocclusive.

_____ 95. The type of bandage that has limited stretch and conforms well to the body contours is the
    A. elastic bandage.
    B. self-adherent roller bandage.
    C. gauze bandage.
    D. adhesive bandage.
    E. none of the above.

_____ 96. If bleeding from a wound is difficult to control you should
    A. apply direct pressure around the wound.
    B. apply direct pressure over the entire wound.
    C. remove the dressing and bandage.
    D. reapply a dressing and bandage.
    E. apply direct digital pressure to the wound.

_____ 97. The dangers of a tourniquet include
    A. increased hemorrhage if pressure is not sufficient.
    B. possible loss of limb.
    C. accumulation of toxins in the limb.
    D. tissue damage beneath the tourniquet.
    E. all of the above.

_____ 98. The restoration of circulation once a tourniquet is released may cause all of the following, EXCEPT
    A. emboli.
    B. shock.
    C. lethal dysrhythmias.
    D. massive vasoconstriction.
    E. renal failure.

_____ 99. You should remove gross contamination from a wound if you can do so quickly and without further injury.
    A. True
    B. False

_____ 100. Scalp hemorrhage is rarely severe or difficult to control.
    A. True
    B. False

_____ 101. The ideal position for splinting a limb is halfway between extension and flexion and is called the
    A. anatomical position.
    B. physiological position.
    C. neutral position.
    D. position of function.
    E. recovery position.

_____ 102. The recommended procedure for packaging an amputated part for transport includes
    A. packing it in ice.
    B. keeping it at body temperature.
    C. keeping it moist and cool.
    D. keeping it wet and cool.
    E. freezing it immediately.

_____ 103. Most patients of crush syndrome can be identified before extrication is complete.
    A. True
    B. False

_____ 104. Recognition of compartment syndrome is usually straightforward.
    A. True
    B. False

©2013 Pearson Education, Inc.
Paramedic Care: Principles & Practice, Vol. 5, 4th Ed.

_____**105.** With compartment syndrome, motor and sensory function are frequently normal.
    A. True
    B. False

_____**106.** A wound involving which of the following requires transport?
    A. Nerves
    B. Blood vessels
    C. Tendons
    D. Ligaments
    E. All of the above

Chapter 6: Burn Trauma

_____**107.** The incidence of burn injury has been on the increase over the past decade.
    A. True
    B. False

_____**108.** The layer of skin with capillary beds and sensory nerve endings is the
    A. dermis.
    B. subcutaneous layer.
    C. epidermis.
    D. sebum.
    E. corium.

_____**109.** Which of the following is NOT a function of the skin?
    A. Protecting the body from bacterial infection
    B. Aiding in temperature regulation
    C. Permitting joint movement
    D. Encouraging fluid loss in cold weather
    E. Accommodating body movement

_____**110.** Place the following phases of the body's burn response in the order in which they would be expected to occur.
    A. Emergent, fluid shift, hypermetabolic, resolution
    B. Fluid shift, hypermetabolic, resolution, emergent
    C. Fluid shift, resolution, emergent, hypermetabolic
    D. Hypermetabolic, fluid shift, emergent, resolution
    E. Emergent, resolution, hypermetabolic, fluid shift

_____**111.** The area of a burn that is characterized by reduced blood flow is generally the zone of
    A. hyperemia.
    B. denaturing.
    C. stasis.
    D. coagulation.
    E. most resistance.

_____**112.** Which of the following skin types has the least resistance to the passage of electrical current?
    A. Mucous membranes
    B. Wet skin
    C. Calluses
    D. The skin on the inside of the arm
    E. The skin on the inside of the thigh

_____**113.** Electrical arc or flash burns may be hot enough to vaporize body tissue.
    A. True
    B. False

_____**114.** Burns due to strong acids are likely to be less deep than burns due to strong alkalis because acids produce liquefaction necrosis.
    A. True
    B. False

115. Which of the following radiation types is least powerful?
  A. Neutron
  B. Alpha
  C. Gamma
  D. Beta
  E. Delta

116. As radiation exposure increases, the signs of exposure become more evident and occur sooner.
  A. True
  B. False

117. Carbon monoxide has an affinity for hemoglobin that is how many times greater than the affinity of oxygen for hemoglobin?
  A. 10
  B. 100
  C. 200
  D. 250
  E. 325

118. Thermal airway burns occur more frequently than toxic inhalation injuries.
  A. True
  B. False

119. The burn characterized by erythema and pain only is the
  A. superficial burn.
  B. partial-thickness burn.
  C. full-thickness burn.
  D. electrical burn.
  E. chemical burn.

120. The burn characterized by discoloration and lack of pain is the
  A. superficial burn.
  B. partial-thickness burn.
  C. full-thickness burn.
  D. electrical burn.
  E. chemical burn.

121. A child patient has received burns to the entire anterior chest and to the entire left upper extremity circumferentially. Based on the rule of nines, what is the percentage of body surface area (BSA) involved?
  A. 9 percent
  B. 18 percent
  C. 27 percent
  D. 36 percent
  E. 48 percent

122. An adult patient receives burns to his entire head and neck and upper back. Based on the rule of nines, what is the percentage of BSA involved?
  A. 9 percent
  B. 10 percent
  C. 18 percent
  D. 19 percent
  E. 27 percent

123. Which of the following is a systemic complication that you should suspect with all serious burns?
  A. Hypothermia
  B. Hypovolemia
  C. Infection
  D. Eschar formation
  E. All of the above

124. Once the suspected inhalation injury patient displays any signs of airway restriction, intubation should not be attempted because it will traumatize the airway tissue, increase swelling, and further restrict the airway.
  A. True
  B. False

125. High-concentration oxygen (100 percent) will reduce the half-life of carbon monoxide in the blood by up to two-thirds.
  A. True
  B. False

©2013 Pearson Education, Inc.
Paramedic Care: Principles & Practice, Vol. 5, 4th Ed.

_____ 126. The patient you are attending has her entire left lower extremity seriously burned. The leg and foot are very painful and reddened, while the thigh is relatively painless and a dark red color. What percentage of the BSA and burn depth would you assign this patient?
  A. 18 percent full-thickness burn
  B. 18 percent partial-thickness burn
  C. 9 percent full-thickness burn
  D. 9 percent partial-thickness burn
  E. 9 percent partial-thickness and 9 percent full-thickness burn

_____ 127. Your assessment reveals a burn patient with partial-thickness burns to 27 percent of the body. What classification of burn severity would you assign her?
  A. Minor   D. Critical
  B. Moderate   E. None of the above
  C. Serious

_____ 128. Your assessment reveals a burn patient with superficial burns to more than half of the body. What classification of burn severity would you assign her?
  A. Minor   D. Critical
  B. Moderate   E. None of the above
  C. Serious

_____ 129. Your assessment reveals a burn patient with partial-thickness burns to the face, though you have ruled out inhalation injury. What classification of burn severity would you assign her?
  A. Minor   D. Critical
  B. Moderate   E. None of the above
  C. Serious

_____ 130. Which of the following burns would NOT be considered a critical burn?
  A. Circumferential third-degree burn to the chest
  B. Superficial facial burns with sooty residue
  C. 10 percent superficial and partial-thickness burns
  D. Full-thickness burns to the elbow and hand
  E. 25 percent partial-thickness burns in the geriatric patient

_____ 131. Local and minor burns (superficial and partial-thickness) may be cared for with
  A. direct pressure.
  B. immediate cool water immersion.
  C. prolonged application of ice.
  D. warm water immersion.
  E. A and D.

_____ 132. In general, moderate to severe burns should be cared for with
  A. moist occlusive dressings.
  B. dry sterile dressings.
  C. cool water immersion.
  D. plastic wrap covered by a soft dressing.
  E. warm water immersion.

_____ 133. Nonadherent padding should be placed between full-thickness burns of the fingers and toes to prevent adhesion and damage when they are separated.
  A. True
  B. False

134. Even though there are no other intravenous sites available on a patient, you should not introduce an intravenous catheter through a region that has partial-thickness burns.
   A. True
   B. False

135. What special facility/service might benefit the patient with carbon monoxide poisoning?
   A. Burn center
   B. Trauma center
   C. Hospital with thoracic surgery available
   D. Hyperbaric chamber
   E. None of the above

136. The cyanide antidote kit contains which of the following?
   A. Amyl nitrate
   B. Sodium nitrate
   C. Sodium thiosulfate
   D. All of the above
   E. None of the above

137. The paramedic can presume that a high-tension electrical line is not energized when it no longer sparks or gives off a blue glow.
   A. True
   B. False

138. Lightning strikes account for approximately how many deaths per year?
   A. 5
   B. 25
   C. 50
   D. 75
   E. 100

139. Which chemical burn should be covered with the oil used to hold the agent that caused it?
   A. Phenol
   B. Dry lime
   C. Sodium
   D. Riot control agents
   E. Organophosphate

140. When chemicals are splashed into the eyes of the patient with contacts, the contacts should be left in place because they will protect the underlying corneas.
   A. True
   B. False

141. If it is necessary to enter a radiation zone to remove a patient, which provider is the best candidate to perform the maneuver?
   A. A young female care provider
   B. A young male care provider
   C. The oldest care provider
   D. The fastest care provider
   E. The heaviest care provider

Chapter 7: Orthopedic Trauma

142. What percentage of multisystem trauma patients has significant musculoskeletal injuries?
   A. 20 percent
   B. 40 percent
   C. 50 percent
   D. 60 percent
   E. 80 percent

143. The bone cell responsible for laying down new bone tissue is the
   A. osteoblast.
   B. osteoclast.
   C. osteocyte.
   D. osteocrit.
   E. osteophage.

©2013 Pearson Education, Inc.
Paramedic Care: Principles & Practice, Vol. 5, 4th Ed.

_____144. The widened end of a long bone is called the
A. diaphysis.
B. epiphysis.
C. metaphysis.
D. cancellous bone.
E. compact bone.

_____145. The bone tissue making up the central portion of the long bone is called the
A. diaphysis.
B. epiphysis.
C. metaphysis.
D. cancellous bone.
E. compact bone.

_____146. The penetration through the compact bone that permits blood vessels to enter and exit the shaft of the long bones is the
A. periosteum.
B. peritoneum.
C. perforating canal.
D. osteocyte.
E. epiphysis.

_____147. The body joints that permit free movement are termed
A. synovial joints.
B. synarthroses.
C. amphiarthroses.
D. diarthroses.
E. A or D.

_____148. The shoulder and hip are examples of which type of joint?
A. Monaxial
B. Biaxial
C. Triaxial
D. Synarthrosis
E. Amphiarthrosis

_____149. Which of the following is a bone of the forearm?
A. Humerus
B. Radius
C. Olecranon
D. Phalange
E. Carpal

_____150. Which of the following is the bump of the elbow?
A. Humerus
B. Radius
C. Olecranon
D. Phalange
E. Carpal

_____151. Which of the following is the major bone of the lower leg?
A. Tarsal
B. Tibia
C. Fibula
D. Femur
E. Phalange

_____152. At what age does the degeneration of bone tissue generally begin?
A. 10
B. 20
C. 40
D. 50
E. 62

_____153. Which of the following is NOT a classification of muscle tissue?
A. Cardiac
B. Smooth
C. Voluntary
D. Involuntary
E. Contractile

_____154. The strong bands of connective tissue securing muscle to bone are the
A. bursae.
B. tendons.
C. ligaments.
D. cartilages.
E. meninges.

_____155. The muscle attachment to the bone that does NOT move when the muscle mass contracts is the
A. flexor.
B. extensor.
C. origin.
D. insertion.
E. articulation.

_____ 156. The condition that is caused by overstretching of some muscle fibers and that produces pain in the affected muscle group is called
A. cramp.
B. fatigue.
C. strain.
D. sprain.
E. spasm.

_____ 157. The partial displacement of a bone end from its location within a joint capsule is a
A. strain.
B. sprain.
C. cramp.
D. spasm.
E. subluxation.

_____ 158. Which of the following fractures is caused by a rotational injury mechanism?
A. Hairline
B. Oblique
C. Transverse
D. Comminuted
E. Spiral

_____ 159. The greenstick fracture is an incomplete fracture that occasionally must be completely broken to permit proper healing.
A. True
B. False

_____ 160. A common and serious type of fracture occurring in the pediatric patient that may prevent normal bone growth is the
A. hairline.
B. oblique.
C. epiphyseal.
D. comminuted.
E. spiral.

_____ 161. A chronic, systemic, and progressive deterioration of the connective tissue in the peripheral joints describes
A. gout.
B. rheumatoid arthritis.
C. osteoarthritis.
D. bursitis.
E. tendinitis.

_____ 162. A degenerative disease related to the normal wear and tear of the joint tissue describes:
A. gout.
B. rheumatoid arthritis.
C. osteoarthritis.
D. bursitis.
E. tendinitis.

_____ 163. If a fracture of the pelvis or bilateral femurs is suspected and patient vital signs are stable, the PASG should be
A. inflated to pop-off pressure.
B. inflated until immobilization is achieved.
C. applied but not inflated until vital signs begin to fall.
D. withheld and the long spine board and traction splint used instead.
E. none of the above.

_____ 164. Which of the following signs is reflective of a fracture?
A. Distal pulse loss
B. Crepitus
C. False motion
D. Deformity
E. All of the above

_____ 165. An elderly patient who has suffered a fracture due to bone degeneration is expected to experience what level of pain when compared to the traumatic fracture pain experienced by a younger adult patient?
A. About the same
B. More pain
C. Less pain
D. No pain at all
E. Extreme pain

_____166. Musculoskeletal injuries associated with sports are generally less severe than trauma-induced injuries and should merit a quick return to competition if possible.
   A. True
   B. False

_____167. Only attempt manipulation of a dislocation if a neurovascular deficit is noted.
   A. True
   B. False

_____168. In general, most fractures should be left in the position found because the splints of today are very effective in immobilizing a limb in that position.
   A. True
   B. False

_____169. Descending in altitude in a helicopter will cause the pressure in the air splint to
   A. increase.
   B. decrease.
   C. remain the same.
   D. become less uniform.
   E. become more uniform.

_____170. The traction splint is designed to splint which musculoskeletal injury?
   A. Knee dislocation
   B. Hip dislocation
   C. Pelvic fracture
   D. Femur fracture
   E. All of the above

_____171. Align an angulated long-bone fracture unless
   A. pulses are absent distal to the injury.
   B. there is a significant increase in pain.
   C. both sensation and pulses are intact.
   D. sensation is absent distal to the injury.
   E. motor function is absent distal to the injury.

_____172. If after moving a limb to alignment you notice distal sensation is absent, you should
   A. splint the limb, as is.
   B. gently move the limb to restore the pulse.
   C. return the limb to the original positioning.
   D. elevate the limb and then splint it.
   E. none of the above.

_____173. Signs that a reduction of a dislocation has been effective include which of the following?
   A. Feeling a "pop"
   B. Patient reports less pain
   C. Joint becomes more mobile
   D. Joint deformity lessens
   E. All of the above

_____174. If the reduction is successful and pulses and sensation are intact, splint the limb in the position of function and transport.
   A. True
   B. False

_____175. The splinting device recommended for a pelvic fracture is the
   A. traction splint.
   B. pelvic sling.
   C. spine board and padding.
   D. long padded board splint.
   E. air splint.

_____176. The traction splint is recommended for treatment of the following
   A. femur fracture with pelvic injury.
   B. midshaft femur fracture.
   C. proximal femur fracture.
   D. femur fracture with knee injury.
   E. all of the above.

_____ 177. The splinting device recommended for an isolated fracture of the clavicle is the
A. traction splint.
B. PASG.
C. spine board and padding.
D. air splint.
E. sling and swathe.

_____ 178. A posterior hip dislocation normally presents with the
A. foot turned outward.
B. foot turned inward.
C. knee flexed.
D. knee turned inward.
E. all except A.

_____ 179. The ankle is deformed with the foot pointing downward. Which type of ankle dislocation do you suspect?
A. Anterior
B. Posterior
C. Lateral
D. Medial
E. Inferior

_____ 180. The patient's arm is internally rotated and the elbow and forearm are held away from the chest. What type of dislocation of the shoulder should you suspect?
A. Anterior
B. Inferior
C. Superior
D. Posterior
E. Lateral

_____ 181. The arm is held locked above the head. What type of dislocation of the shoulder do you suspect?
A. Anterior
B. Inferior
C. Superior
D. Posterior
E. Lateral

_____ 182. The elbow dislocation should NOT be reduced in the field.
A. True
B. False

_____ 183. Which of the following injuries can be adequately splinted using the full-arm air splint and placing the hand in the position of function?
A. Radial fracture
B. Ulnar fracture
C. Wrist fracture
D. Finger fracture
E. All of the above

_____ 184. The normal initial dose of fentanyl for pain is
A. 2 mg.
B. 10 mg.
C. 2 to 10 mcg.
D. 25 to 50 mcg.
E. 100 mcg.

_____ 185. For which of the following will naloxone reverse the drug effects?
A. Fentanyl
B. Morphine
C. Nalbuphine
D. Diazepam
E. A, B, and C

_____ 186. The "C" in the acronym RICE used by athletic trainers stands for
A. circulation.
B. compression.
C. complexion.
D. communication.
E. composure.

Chapter 8: Thoracic Trauma

_____ 187. In vehicular crashes, chest trauma accounts for
A. the greatest cause of mortality.
B. 25 percent of the mortality.
C. the third greatest cause of mortality.
D. a minor incidence of mortality.
E. none of the above.

Paramedic Care: Principles & Practice, Vol. 5, 4th Ed.

_____188. Which of the following is located within the thorax?
- A. Vagus nerve
- B. Aortic arch
- C. Superior vena cava
- D. Bronchi
- E. All of the above

_____189. Which muscle(s) lift(s) the sternum and, with it, the thoracic cage to assist with respiration?
- A. Intercostals
- B. Diaphragm
- C. Sternocleidomastoids
- D. Scalenes
- E. Rectus abdominis

_____190. At the beginning of and during most of inhalation the pressure within the thorax is
- A. less than that of the environment.
- B. more than that of the environment.
- C. equal to that of the environment.
- D. first lower than and then higher than that of the environment.
- E. first higher than and then lower than that of the environment.

_____191. The location where the pulmonary arteries and the mainstem bronchus enter the lung is the
- A. pleura.
- B. pulmonary hilum.
- C. ligamentum arteriosum.
- D. cardiac notch.
- E. carina.

_____192. The sac surrounding the heart is called the
- A. myocardium.
- B. endocardium.
- C. pericardium.
- D. parietal cardiac sheath.
- E. epicardium arteriosum.

_____193. The structure that connects the aorta to the pulmonary artery and holds it in position within the thorax is the
- A. pleura.
- B. pulmonary hilum.
- C. ligamentum arteriosum.
- D. epicardium pocket.
- E. vena cava.

_____194. Which of the following is NOT likely to be associated with blunt trauma?
- A. Flail chest
- B. Pneumothorax (paper bag syndrome)
- C. Open pneumothorax
- D. Aortic dissection
- E. Blunt cardiac injury

_____195. Which of the following is NOT likely to be associated with penetrating trauma?
- A. Pericardial tamponade
- B. Tracheal disruption
- C. Open pneumothorax
- D. Aortic dissection
- E. Comminuted rib fracture

_____196. Which pairs of ribs most frequently transmit kinetic energy and trauma to the tissues beneath them without fracturing?
- A. 1 and 2
- B. 3 and 4
- C. 4 through 8
- D. 9 through 12
- E. both A and B

_____197. Which of the following patients is most likely to experience rib fracture with the least force of trauma?
- A. Infant patients
- B. Adult male patients
- C. Adult female patients
- D. Elderly patients
- E. Child patients

_____ **198.** A flail segment moves in opposition to the chest wall during paradoxical movement.
    A. True
    B. False

_____ **199.** As time passes, the continuing injury and muscle fatigue with a flail chest injury will permit the amount of paradoxical movement to increase.
    A. True
    B. False

_____ **200.** Which patient is most likely to display tracheal deviation early in the course of a tension pneumothorax?
    A. Pediatric patient
    B. Young adult patient
    C. Older adult patient
    D. Pregnant patient
    E. Elderly patient

_____ **201.** Each side of the thorax can hold up to half the patient's total blood supply. Hence, hemothorax is often more of a hypovolemic problem with limited respiratory signs and symptoms.
    A. True
    B. False

_____ **202.** A dull percussion noted in the lower lobe of a lung is suggestive of
    A. pneumothorax.
    B. tension pneumothorax.
    C. hemothorax.
    D. pulmonary contusion.
    E. both A and B.

_____ **203.** Pulmonary contusion may result from
    A. a bullet's passage.
    B. traumatic chest compression.
    C. the overpressure wave of a strong explosion.
    D. a high-velocity bullet striking body armor.
    E. all of the above.

_____ **204.** Which of the following is NOT associated with a pulmonary contusion?
    A. Atelectasis
    B. Increased respiratory effort
    C. Increased rate of carbon dioxide diffusion
    D. Microhemorrhage into the alveolar tissue
    E. Decreased rate of oxygen diffusion

_____ **205.** Blunt cardiac injury may result in all of the following, EXCEPT
    A. ectopic beats.
    B. heart blocks.
    C. hematoma.
    D. subcutaneous emphysema.
    E. decreased ventricular compliance.

_____ **206.** Which of the following is the most frequent mechanism of injury causing pericardial tamponade?
    A. Blunt anterior chest trauma
    B. Penetrating chest trauma
    C. The blast pressure wave
    D. Traumatic asphyxia
    E. Lateral-impact auto crash

_____ **207.** Which of the following is a sign of pericardial tamponade?
    A. Cyanosis of the upper extremities and head
    B. Decreased JVD during inspiration
    C. Electrical alternans
    D. Pulseless electrical activity
    E. All of the above

©2013 Pearson Education, Inc.
Paramedic Care: Principles & Practice, Vol. 5, 4th Ed.

_____208. Jugular vein distention, distant heart tones, and hypotension are collectively known as
  A. Beck's triad.
  B. pulsus paradoxus.
  C. Cushing's reflex.
  D. Kussmaul's sign.
  E. electrical alternans.

_____209. Which of the following is the most frequent mechanism of injury causing traumatic aortic dissection?
  A. Blunt anterior chest trauma
  B. Penetrating chest trauma
  C. The blast pressure wave
  D. Traumatic asphyxia
  E. Lateral-impact auto crash

_____210. Which of the following is a point of fixation for the aorta in the thorax?
  A. Diaphragm
  B. Aortic annulus
  C. Aortic isthmus
  D. All of the above
  E. None of the above

_____211. The left side is the site of most diaphragmatic ruptures because most assailants are right-handed.
  A. True
  B. False

_____212. Which of the following may cause the abdomen to appear hollow?
  A. Traumatic asphyxia
  B. Tension pneumothorax
  C. Aortic dissection
  D. Diaphragmatic rupture
  E. None of the above

_____213. Tracheobronchial disruption is likely to occur at what location?
  A. More than 2.5 cm below the carina
  B. More than 2.5 cm above the carina
  C. Within 2.5 cm of the carina
  D. At the bronchial bifurcation
  E. Along the right mainstem bronchus

_____214. The greatest problems associated with traumatic asphyxia are related to the
  A. bellows system.
  B. airway.
  C. heart.
  D. vasculature.
  E. lung tissue.

_____215. While assessing a supine patient, the jugular veins are found distended. This finding alone suggests
  A. a normal patient.
  B. pericardial tamponade.
  C. tension pneumothorax.
  D. traumatic asphyxia.
  E. B, C, and D.

_____216. Overdrive ventilation (bag-valve masking) of the patient with pulmonary contusions and developing edema may help push fluids back into the lung tissues.
  A. True
  B. False

_____217. You have covered the open pneumothorax in a thoracic injury patient. You then notice that dyspnea is increasing and breath sounds on the injured side are becoming diminished. Which action would you take?
  A. Insert a needle in the 2nd intercostal space.
  B. Remove the dressing.
  C. Provide overdrive ventilation.
  D. Consider nitrous oxide administration.
  E. All of the above.

_____218. Which location is recommended for prehospital pleural decompression?
  A. 2nd intercostal space, midclavicular line
  B. 5th intercostal space, midclavicular line
  C. 5th intercostal space, midaxillary line
  D. A and B
  E. A and C

_____ 219. Which of the following drugs would be considered for the patient who has experienced traumatic asphyxia for more than 20 minutes?
  A. Decadron
  B. Sodium bicarbonate
  C. Morphine sulfate
  D. Demerol
  E. Dopamine

Chapter 9: Abdominal Trauma

_____ 220. Which of the following abdominal organs is found in the left lower quadrant?
  A. Spleen
  B. Gallbladder
  C. Appendix
  D. Sigmoid colon
  E. None of the above

_____ 221. Which of the following abdominal organs is found in the right upper quadrant?
  A. Spleen
  B. Gallbladder
  C. Appendix
  D. Sigmoid colon
  E. None of the above

_____ 222. Which of the following abdominal organs is found in all the abdominal quadrants?
  A. Spleen
  B. Gallbladder
  C. Appendix
  D. Sigmoid colon
  E. Small bowel

_____ 223. The organ storing a digestive juice created by the liver is the
  A. spleen.
  B. small bowel.
  C. pancreas.
  D. gallbladder.
  E. liver.

_____ 224. The organ where bile and pancreatic juices are mixed with the digesting food is the
  A. spleen.
  B. small bowel.
  C. stomach.
  D. gallbladder.
  E. liver.

_____ 225. The urinary bladder may contain as little as 10 mL of fluid or as much as 500 mL of fluid.
  A. True
  B. False

_____ 226. The ovary releases a fertilized egg every 28 days.
  A. True
  B. False

_____ 227. The location where fertilized eggs most commonly attach and grow is the
  A. vagina.
  B. uterus.
  C. fallopian tube.
  D. ovary.
  E. cervix.

_____ 228. Pregnancy causes what change in the maternal blood volume?
  A. 10 percent decrease
  B. 25 percent decrease
  C. 25 percent increase
  D. 45 percent increase
  E. 65 percent increase

_____ 229. The connective tissue suspending the bowel from the posterior abdominal wall is the
  A. perineum.
  B. mesentery.
  C. peritoneum.
  D. retroperitoneum.
  E. ileum.

©2013 Pearson Education, Inc.
Paramedic Care: Principles & Practice, Vol. 5, 4th Ed.

_____230. Penetrating trauma may cause which of the following injuries?
   A. Spillage of the contents of hollow organs
   B. Hemorrhage from solid organs
   C. Damage to organs
   D. Eventual irritation of the abdominal lining
   E. All of the above

_____231. Blunt mechanisms cause injuries to the spleen about what percentage of the time?
   A. 40 percent
   B. 30 percent
   C. 20 percent
   D. 10 percent
   E. 5 percent

_____232. Penetrating mechanisms injure the small bowel about what percentage of the time?
   A. 40 percent
   B. 25 percent
   C. 20 percent
   D. 10 percent
   E. 5 percent

_____233. Which of the following organs is most frequently damaged during penetrating abdominal trauma?
   A. Small bowel
   B. Liver
   C. Spleen
   D. Kidneys
   E. Pancreas

_____234. Penetration of the abdominal wall where the abdominal contents protrude is called
   A. peritonitis.
   B. chyme.
   C. evisceration.
   D. peristalsis.
   E. emulsification.

_____235. Penetrating trauma just under the right thoracic border is likely to injure the
   A. liver.
   B. spleen.
   C. bowel.
   D. bladder.
   E. left kidney.

_____236. Most abdominal vascular injuries are associated with blunt trauma.
   A. True
   B. False

_____237. Which of the following is NOT true regarding abdominal vascular injury and hemorrhage?
   A. Intra-abdominal pressure associated with those injuries does not restrict hemorrhage.
   B. Blood-induced irritation of the abdominal lining occurs quickly.
   C. Hemorrhage can accumulate without any swelling becoming apparent.
   D. Blood in the abdomen may trigger a vagal response, slowing the heart.
   E. The abdomen has many large arterial and venous structures.

_____238. An injury associated with the release of either blood or bowel contents into the abdominal cavity will result in a rapidly developing presentation of severe discomfort and pain.
   A. True
   B. False

_____239. Gastric or duodenal contents released into the abdominal space will irritate the peritoneum faster than bacteria will.
   A. True
   B. False

_____240. The late-term pregnant female is at decreased risk for vomiting and aspiration.
   A. True
   B. False

241. Supine positioning of the mother may cause hypotension due to
   A. decreased intra-abdominal pressure.
   B. compression of the inferior vena cava.
   C. increased intra-abdominal pressure.
   D. increased circulation to the uterus.
   E. none of the above.

242. The signs of abdominal trauma may become less specific due to the progression of peritonitis.
   A. True
   B. False

243. The major reason auscultation of bowel and other abdominal sounds is not recommended in the field is because
   A. the sounds are not clear.
   B. the sounds do not rule out injury.
   C. the lack of sounds does not confirm injury.
   D. it takes too long to adequately assess bowel sounds.
   E. B, C, and D.

244. The abdominal evisceration covered with a moist dressing should then be covered with a(n)
   A. dry, adherent dressing wrapped firmly.
   B. dry, nonadherent dressing wrapped loosely.
   C. damp, nonadherent dressing wrapped loosely.
   D. occlusive dressing wrapped loosely.
   E. damp, nonadherent dressing wrapped firmly.

Chapter 10: Head, Face, Neck, and Spinal Trauma

245. Which of the following groups is at the lowest risk for head injuries?
   A. Females 15 to 24 years of age
   B. Males 15 to 24 years of age
   C. Young children
   D. The elderly
   E. Infants

246. Which of the following is NOT a bone of the cranium?
   A. Frontal bone
   B. Nasal bone
   C. Parietal bone
   D. Sphenoid bone
   E. Ethmoid bone

247. The upper and immovable jaw bone is the
   A. maxilla.
   B. mandible.
   C. zygoma.
   D. stapes.
   E. pinna.

248. The external portion of the ear is the
   A. maxilla.
   B. mandible.
   C. zygoma.
   D. stapes.
   E. pinna.

249. The structure responsible for the hearing sense is the
   A. ossicle.
   B. cochlea.
   C. semicircular canal.
   D. sinus.
   E. vitreous humor.

©2013 Pearson Education, Inc.
Paramedic Care: Principles & Practice, Vol. 5, 4th Ed.

_____250. The muscular tissue surrounding the opening through which light travels to contact the light-sensing tissue in the eye is the
A. retina.
B. aqueous humor.
C. vitreous humor.
D. pupil.
E. iris.

_____251. The smooth delicate tissue that moves over the sclera is the
A. meninges.
B. conjunctiva.
C. cornea.
D. aqueous humor.
E. vitreous humor.

_____252. Which of the following structures is NOT located within the neck?
A. Jugular veins
B. Aorta
C. Vagus nerve
D. Trachea
E. Esophagus

_____253. Which region of the vertebral column has seven vertebrae?
A. Cervical
B. Thoracic
C. Lumbar
D. Sacral
E. Coccygeal

_____254. The vertebra that can be felt as the first bony prominence along the spine is
A. C-1.
B. C-7.
C. T-1.
D. C-2.
E. T-7.

_____255. The portion of the vertebral column you can palpate along the thoracic and lumbar spine is the
A. spinous process.
B. transverse process.
C. vertebral body.
D. spinal foramen.
E. lamina.

_____256. Which region of the vertebral column has the largest vertebral bodies?
A. Cervical
B. Thoracic
C. Lumbar
D. Sacral
E. Coccygeal

_____257. Injury to the connective and skeletal tissue of the spinal column does not mean the spinal cord is injured.
A. True
B. False

_____258. Which mechanism of spinal injury is likely to be involved in a frontal-impact auto collision in which the driver is restrained by a shoulder strap and lap belt?
A. Hyperextension
B. Hyperflexion
C. Lateral bending
D. Axial loading
E. Both A and B

_____259. Which mechanism of spinal injury is likely to be involved with a dive into shallow water?
A. Hyperextension
B. Hyperflexion
C. Lateral bending
D. Axial loading
E. Distraction

_____260. Which of the following is NOT a mechanism of injury likely to cause spinal injury?
A. Heel-first falls
B. High-speed motor vehicle crash
C. Lifting a heavy weight
D. Penetrating objects
E. Diving in deep water

_____ **261.** Scalp wounds may present in a manner that confounds assessment.
  A. True
  B. False

_____ **262.** The skull fracture that is related to and often involves some of the numerous natural penetrations (foramina) through the skull is the
  A. depressed skull fracture.
  B. basilar skull fracture.
  C. linear skull fracture.
  D. comminuted skull fracture.
  E. none of the above.

_____ **263.** The discoloration found just behind the ear and due to basilar skull fracture is
  A. retroauricular ecchymosis.
  B. bilateral periorbital ecchymosis.
  C. Cullen's sign.
  D. the halo sign.
  E. none of the above.

_____ **264.** According to the Le Fort criteria, a fracture involving the entire facial region below the brow ridge is classified as
  A. Le Fort I.
  B. Le Fort II.
  C. Le Fort III.
  D. Le Fort IV.
  E. Le Fort V.

_____ **265.** Which of the following mechanisms is likely to injure the tympanum?
  A. Repeated small-arms fire at close range
  B. An explosion
  C. A diving injury
  D. Objects forced into the ear
  E. All of the above

_____ **266.** The discoloration of the sclera caused by a bursting blood vessel is called
  A. hyphema.
  B. retinal detachment.
  C. acute retinal artery occlusion.
  D. anterior chamber hematoma.
  E. subconjunctival hemorrhage.

_____ **267.** The patient complains of a dark curtain over a portion of one eye's field of view after head trauma. You should suspect
  A. hyphema.
  B. retinal detachment.
  C. acute retinal artery occlusion.
  D. anterior chamber hematoma.
  E. subconjunctival hemorrhage.

_____ **268.** The most frequently injured location along the spinal column is
  A. C-1/C-2.
  B. C-7.
  C. T-12/L-1.
  D. L-4.
  E. L-5/S-1.

_____ **269.** You should discontinue attempts at neutral in-line positioning if
  A. several body segments are out of alignment.
  B. the patient feels a decrease in pain.
  C. you feel significant resistance to movement.
  D. the patient is unresponsive.
  E. the patient presents with neurological deficits.

_____ **270.** If you are unclear about the reliability of the patient to report the symptoms of spinal injury, always err on the side of caution.
  A. True
  B. False

©2013 Pearson Education, Inc.
Paramedic Care: Principles & Practice, Vol. 5, 4th Ed.

_____ 271. A patient complaint of double vision is an example of
- A. diplopia.
- B. aniscoria.
- C. consensual reactivity.
- D. synergism.
- E. photophobia.

_____ 272. Vomiting is a serious consequence of head injury that may be due either to swallowing blood or head injury.
- A. True
- B. False

_____ 273. Extraglottic airways are effective airway control methods for the patient with a suspected spinal injury.
- A. True
- B. False

_____ 274. Repeated or prolonged intubation attempts should be avoided because they may induce hypoxia and hypercarbia in the head-injured patient.
- A. True
- B. False

_____ 275. Extraglottic airways may be useful in the spinal injury patient because they permit spinal movement without endangering the cord.
- A. True
- B. False

_____ 276. Which of the following airway management methods is NOT recommended for the patient with suspected basilar skull fracture?
- A. Orotracheal intubation
- B. Directed intubation
- C. Oropharyngeal airway
- D. Nasopharyngeal airway
- E. Extraglottic airway

_____ 277. Which of the following is an acceptable method for confirming endotracheal tube placement in the head injury patient?
- A. End-tidal CO_2 detector
- B. Pulse oximeter
- C. The absence of epigastric sounds
- D. Good and bilaterally equal breath sounds
- E. All of the above

_____ 278. In some cases of facial trauma, the airway may be so damaged and distorted that cricothyrotomy is the only way to open the airway.
- A. True
- B. False

_____ 279. It may be necessary to hold direct pressure on wounds of the neck during all of care and transport to control hemorrhage.
- A. True
- B. False

_____ 280. The ideal positioning for the spine includes the patient's nose in line with which of the following?
- A. Clavicle
- B. Shoulders
- C. Navel
- D. Wrists
- E. All of the above

_____ 281. Which of the following criteria indicates that a helmet should be removed from a patient?
- A. The head is not immobilized within the helmet.
- B. The helmet prevents airway maintenance.
- C. You cannot secure the helmet firmly to the long spine board.
- D. You anticipate breathing problems.
- E. Any of the above.

_____ **282.** Proper helmet removal requires a minimum of how many care providers?
  A. Two   **D.** Five
  B. Three   **E.** No fewer than six
  C. Four

_____ **283.** Before initiating a log roll, it is preferable to place a bulky blanket between the legs.
  A. True
  B. False

_____ **284.** The log roll for the patient with spinal injuries requires a minimum of how many care providers?
  A. Two   **D.** Five
  B. Three   **E.** No fewer than 6
  C. Four

_____ **285.** You immobilize the patient's head to the long spine board before you secure his body to it.
  A. True
  B. False

_____ **286.** The most ideal position for the infant's head during spinal immobilization is
  A. 2 to 3 inches above the spine board.
  B. level with the spine board.
  C. with padding under the shoulders on the spine board.
  D. with the head slightly extended and level with the spine board.
  E. none of the above.

_____ **287.** To immobilize the patient's head to the long spine board, you should use a
  A. cervical collar.
  B. vest-type immobilization device.
  C. cervical immobilization device.
  D. vacuum splint.
  E. any of the above.

_____ **288.** If a large open scalp wound is grossly contaminated, removal of gross contaminants and irrigation are indicated.
  A. True
  B. False

Chapter 11: Nervous System Trauma

_____ **289.** Which of the following places the layers of the meninges in the correct order as they occur from the skull to the cerebrum?
  A. Dura mater, pia mater, arachnoid
  B. Dura mater, arachnoid, pia mater
  C. Arachnoid, pia mater, dura mater
  D. Arachnoid, dura mater, pia mater
  E. Pia mater, arachnoid, dura mater

_____ **290.** The protective structure that is delicate and covers the convolutions of the cerebrum is the
  A. pia mater.   **D.** dura mater.
  B. falx cerebri.   **E.** tentorium.
  C. arachnoid.

_____ **291.** The structure that separates the cerebrum from the cerebellum is the
  A. pia mater.   **D.** dura mater.
  B. falx cerebri.   **E.** tentorium.
  C. arachnoid.

©2013 Pearson Education, Inc.
Paramedic Care: Principles & Practice, Vol. 5, 4th Ed.

_____292. The cerebrum fine tunes motor control and is responsible for balance and muscle tone.
 A. True
 B. False

_____293. Which of the following is a function of the hypothalamus?
 A. Control of heart rate   D. Sleep
 B. Balance   E. Speech
 C. Thirst

_____294. Which of the following is a function of the medulla oblongata?
 A. Control of respiration   D. Sleep
 B. Balance   E. None of the above
 C. Thirst

_____295. The brain needs a constant supply of blood to provide oxygen, glucose, and thiamine. Without this supply unconsciousness follows in 10 seconds and death occurs in 4 to 6 minutes.
 A. True
 B. False

_____296. Which of the following nerves is responsible for pupillary dilation?
 A. CN I   D. CN X
 B. CN III   E. CN XII
 C. CN VIII

_____297. Which of the following nerves is responsible for the sense of smell?
 A. CN I   D. CN X
 B. CN III   E. CN XII
 C. CN VIII

_____298. The nerve tissue(s) responsible for communicating motor impulses from the brain is (are) the
 A. white matter.   D. descending nerve tracts.
 B. gray matter.   E. none of the above.
 C. ascending nerve tracts.

_____299. The nerve tissue(s) consisting mostly of nerve cell bodies that make(s) up the central portion of the spinal cord is (are) the:
 A. white matter.   D. descending nerve tracts.
 B. gray matter.   E. none of the above.
 C. ascending nerve tracts.

_____300. The location to use for assessment of the C-7 nerve root is the
 A. collar region.   D. umbilicus.
 B. little finger.   E. small toe.
 C. nipple line.

_____301. The location to use for assessment of the T-4 nerve root is the
 A. collar region.   D. umbilicus.
 B. little finger.   E. small toe.
 C. nipple line.

_____302. During your assessment of a patient, you find sensation is lost as you move from the lower extremities all the way up to the level of the umbilicus. This is probably due to an injury at which spinal level?
 A. C-3   D. T-10
 B. C-7   E. S-1
 C. T-4

_____303. The injury that causes the brain to be damaged on the side of the impact is called a
   A. coup.
   B. subdural hematoma.
   C. subluxation.
   D. contrecoup.
   E. concussion.

_____304. Which of the following is considered a diffuse injury?
   A. Cerebral contusion
   B. Epidural hematoma
   C. Subdural hematoma
   D. Intracerebral hemorrhage
   E. None of the above

_____305. Bleeding between the dura mater and the interior of the cranium is a(n)
   A. cerebral contusion.
   B. epidural hematoma.
   C. subdural hematoma.
   D. intracerebral hemorrhage.
   E. none of the above.

_____306. Which of the following is considered a diffuse brain injury?
   A. Concussion
   B. Cerebral contusion
   C. Epidural hematoma
   D. Intracerebral hemorrhage
   E. Subdural hematoma

_____307. The brain is one of the most perfusion-sensitive organs of the body.
   A. True
   B. False

_____308. As intracranial hemorrhage begins, it displaces venous blood and then
   A. cerebrospinal fluid.
   B. the brainstem.
   C. arterial blood.
   D. oxygen.
   E. the meninges.

_____309. In the presence of increased intracranial pressure, the body does which of the following to ensure cerebral perfusion?
   A. Decreases cardiac output
   B. Increases heart rate
   C. Increases systemic blood pressure
   D. Dilates peripheral blood vessels
   E. All of the above

_____310. Low levels of carbon dioxide in the blood will cause which of the following?
   A. Hyperventilation
   B. Cerebral artery constriction
   C. Cerebral artery dilation
   D. Hypertension
   E. None of the above

_____311. Central syndrome will cause all of the following, EXCEPT
   A. respiratory changes.
   B. changes in blood pressure.
   C. changes in heart rate.
   D. pupillary dilation.
   E. increased pulse rate.

_____312. Increasing intracranial pressure is likely to cause pupillary dilation on the contralateral side from the source of the pressure.
   A. True
   B. False

©2013 Pearson Education, Inc.
Paramedic Care: Principles & Practice, Vol. 5, 4th Ed.

_____313. Secondary injury to the spinal cord is likely to occur
     A. immediately after the injury.
     B. within hours of the injury.
     C. within days of the injury.
     D. weeks after the injury.
     E. at the same time as the initial injury.

_____314. Blood loss into the cranium in the infant can contribute significantly to shock and hypovolemia.
     A. True
     B. False

_____315. A spinal cord concussion is not likely to produce residual deficit.
     A. True
     B. False

_____316. The signs and symptoms of spinal shock are usually permanent and no recovery is expected.
     A. True
     B. False

_____317. In which type of shock can some recovery of function be expected after the initial injury?
     A. Autonomic hyperreflexia syndrome
     B. Neurogenic shock
     C. Anterior cord syndrome
     D. Central cord syndrome
     E. Brown-Sequard syndrome

_____318. Which of the following is a sign associated with neurogenic shock?
     A. Priapism
     B. Decreased heart rate
     C. Decreased peripheral vascular resistance
     D. Cool skin above the injury
     E. All of the above

_____319. Which of the following is NOT indicative of autonomic hyperreflexia syndrome?
     A. Increased heart rate
     B. Increasing blood pressure
     C. Blurred vision
     D. Sweating
     E. Nasal congestion

_____320. The relatively low incidence of spinal column injuries in pediatric patients is primarily due to the
     A. immobility of the spine.
     B. curvature of the spine.
     C. elasticity of the spine.
     D. short length of the spine.
     E. weight of the spine.

_____321. The approximate rate of ventilation for the adult head injury patient is
     A. 5 breaths per minute.
     B. 10 breaths per minute.
     C. 20 breaths per minute.
     D. 25 breaths per minute.
     E. 30 breaths per minute.

322. Capnography-guided ventilations for the patient with suspected cerebral herniation should keep the end-tidal CO_2 readings at
   A. 25 to 30 mmHg.
   B. 30 to 35 mmHg.
   C. 40 to 50 mmHg.
   D. 10 to 20 mmHg.
   E. 90 to 100 mmHg.

323. The Glasgow Coma Scale score for a completely unresponsive patient would be which of the following?
   A. 15
   B. 12
   C. 10
   D. 3
   E. 0

324. The patient with a Glasgow Coma Scale score between 9 and 12 is likely to
   A. have a mild head injury.
   B. have a moderate head injury.
   C. be in a coma.
   D. be brain-dead.
   E. none of the above.

325. A patient is very disoriented, opens his eyes on verbal command, and can localize pain. He would be assigned what Glasgow Coma Scale score?
   A. 14
   B. 12
   C. 10
   D. 8
   E. 6

326. The patient with a large gaping wound to the neck should be placed in which of the following positions?
   A. On a spine board in the Trendelenburg position
   B. With the head of the spine board elevated 30 degrees
   C. In the left lateral recumbent position
   D. Immobilized completely and rolled to his side
   E. None of the above

327. The minimum blood pressure necessary to maintain cerebral perfusion in the child (6 to 12 years) patient with serious head injury is
   A. 90 mmHg.
   B. 80 mmHg.
   C. 75 mmHg.
   D. 65 mmHg.
   E. 50 mmHg.

328. Which of the following drugs is NOT used to sedate a patient during RSI?
   A. Vecuronium
   B. Fentanyl
   C. Diazepam
   D. Etomidate
   E. Morphine

329. Which of the following paralytics increases intracranial pressure and should be used with caution, if at all, for head injury patients?
   A. Diazepam
   B. Mannitol
   C. Vecuronium
   D. Succinylcholine
   E. Midazolam

330. Mannitol may have all of the following actions, EXCEPT
   A. draw fluid into the cardiovascular system.
   B. reduce blood pressure.
   C. reduce inflammation.
   D. reduce cerebral edema.
   E. induce hypertension.

©2013 Pearson Education, Inc.
Paramedic Care: Principles & Practice, Vol. 5, 4th Ed.

Chapter 12: Environmental Trauma

_____331. The process of heat transfer via currents in liquids or gases is
  A. conduction.
  B. convection.
  C. evaporation.
  D. radiation.
  E. respiration.

_____332. At normal room temperature, an unclothed person loses approximately 60 percent of total body heat through
  A. conduction.
  B. convection.
  C. evaporation.
  D. radiation.
  E. respiration.

_____333. Which of the following locations indicates a patient's core temperature?
  A. Axillary
  B. Forehead
  C. Popliteal
  D. Rectal
  E. Carotid

_____334. The body temperature at which temperature regulation is significantly impaired is greater than _____ and less than _____.
  A. 100°F, 96°F
  B. 102°F, 96°F
  C. 103°F, 93°F
  D. 104°F, 94°F
  E. 105°F, 90°F

_____335. For each liter of fluid lost due to sweating, a patient will lose approximately
  A. 20 to 50 mEq of potassium.
  B. 20 to 50 mEq of sodium.
  C. 5 to 20 mEq of potassium.
  D. 5 to 20 mEq of sodium.
  E. 10 to 15 mEq of potassium.

_____336. _____ is (are) a usually mild, acute reaction to heat exposure.
  A. Heat cramps
  B. Heat exhaustion
  C. Heatstroke
  D. Hyperpyrexia
  E. Hot flashes

_____337. _____ commonly presents with chronic illness and an increased core temperature due to thermoregulatory insufficiency.
  A. Classic heat exhaustion
  B. Classic heatstroke
  C. Exertional heatstroke
  D. Climactic heatstroke
  E. Excitational heat cramps

_____338. Dehydration often accompanies hyperthermic conditions because it inhibits
  A. negative chronotropic effects.
  B. positive inotropic effects.
  C. thermogenesis.
  D. vasodilation.
  E. metabolism.

_____339. All of the following are signs of dehydration, EXCEPT
  A. abdominal distress.
  B. decreased blood pressure.
  C. decreased urine output.
  D. increased skin turgor.
  E. vision disturbances.

_____340. Which of the following disease processes can predispose a patient to hypothermia?
  A. Duodenal ulcers
  B. Hyperthyroidism
  C. Hypoglycemia
  D. Cirrhosis
  E. Cushing's syndrome

_____341. At what temperature will the body shiver the most in order to compensate for heat loss?
  A. 96.8°F
  B. 95.0°F
  C. 90.0°F
  D. 89.6°F
  E. 88.8°F

____342. The ECG wave that is prominent in a patient with severe hypothermia is the
    A. J wave.
    B. P wave.
    C. Q wave.
    D. U wave.
    E. S wave.

____343. A patient with severe hypothermia will
    A. be hypertensive.
    B. display tachycardia and tachypnea.
    C. have flaccid muscles.
    D. have increased shivering.
    E. lack coordination.

____344. The MOST common presenting dysrhythmia seen in the hypothermic patient with a core temperature above 86°F is
    A. atrial fibrillation.
    B. atrial tachycardia.
    C. ventricular fibrillation.
    D. ventricular tachycardia.
    E. atrial flutter.

____345. Which type of active rewarming may be used in the prehospital setting for a patient in mild hypothermia?
    A. Massage of the affected extremity
    B. Heat lights
    C. Warm peritoneal dialysis
    D. Walking the patient around
    E. Blankets and heat packs at key circulatory points

____346. Ventricular fibrillation in the hypothermic patient may be minimized by
    A. increasing the patient's exposure to the environment.
    B. avoiding aggressive or rough handling of the patient.
    C. providing active rewarming if the patient is less than 5 minutes from the hospital.
    D. stimulating the patient with caffeinated beverages.
    E. using alcohol as a general system depressant.

____347. Which of the following ALS interventions can be performed in the field on a patient in severe hypothermia who is pulseless?
    A. Intubation
    B. Lidocaine 2 mg/kg
    C. Sodium bicarbonate 1 mEq/kg
    D. Warm peritoneal lavage
    E. Precordial thump

____348. Due to reflexive laryngospasm, _____ of water usually enters the lungs.
    A. 0 mL
    B. more than 30 mLs
    C. less than 10 mLs
    D. more than 50 mLs
    E. less than 30 mLs

____349. All of the following may occur during drowning, EXCEPT
    A. atelectasis.
    B. gastric distension.
    C. pulmonary rupture.
    D. loss of surfactant.
    E. cardiac dysrhythmias.

____350. What physiological change takes place as a result of the mammalian diving reflex?
    A. Tachycardia
    B. Vasoconstriction
    C. Diversion of blood to the periphery
    D. Decrease in cerebral blood flow
    E. Cessation of oxygen delivery

____351. _____ states that a volume of gas is inversely proportional to its pressure if its temperature remains constant.
    A. Boyle's law
    B. Dalton's law
    C. Henry's law
    D. Starling's law
    E. Joule's law

©2013 Pearson Education, Inc.
Paramedic Care: Principles & Practice, Vol. 5, 4th Ed.

____352. _____ states that the total pressure of a mixture of gases is equal to the sum of the partial pressures of the individual gases.
- **A.** Boyle's law
- **B.** Dalton's law
- **C.** Henry's law
- **D.** Starling's law
- **E.** Joule's law

____353. The pressure of air at sea level is
- **A.** 160 mmHg.
- **B.** 250 mmHg.
- **C.** 500 mmHg.
- **D.** 760 mmHg.
- **E.** 840 mmHg.

____354. _____ states that the amount of gas dissolved in a given volume of fluid is proportional to the pressure of the gas above it.
- **A.** Boyle's law
- **B.** Dalton's law
- **C.** Henry's law
- **D.** Starling's law
- **E.** Joule's law

____355. Which gas tends to dissolve in the blood and tissues in the greatest quantities when a person descends below sea level?
- **A.** Argon
- **B.** Helium
- **C.** Nitrogen
- **D.** Oxygen
- **E.** Carbon dioxide

____356. The law that BEST describes the increasing dissolution of gases in the bloodstream as a person dives deeper in water is
- **A.** Boyle's law.
- **B.** Dalton's law.
- **C.** Henry's law.
- **D.** Starling's law.
- **E.** Joule's law.

____357. Pulmonary overpressure can cause all of the following, EXCEPT
- **A.** pulmonary edema.
- **B.** arterial embolism.
- **C.** pneumothorax.
- **D.** pneumomediastinum.
- **E.** ruptured alveoli.

____358. Definitive treatment for acute mountain sickness is
- **A.** supplemental oxygen.
- **B.** acetazolamide.
- **C.** hyperbaric bag.
- **D.** odansetron.
- **E.** descent.

____359. High-concentration, supplemental oxygen can completely reverse HAPE in 12 to 24 hours.
- **A.** True
- **B.** False

____360. Which demographic group is the MOST susceptible to high-altitude pulmonary edema?
- **A.** Adult men
- **B.** Adult women
- **C.** Children
- **D.** Elderly women
- **E.** Diabetics

Chapter 13: Special Considerations in Trauma

____361. Which service has been very effective through its prevention efforts?
- **A.** Policy service
- **B.** Public safety service
- **C.** Fire service
- **D.** Health service
- **E.** Military service

____362. The annual death toll from trauma is around
    A. 37,000.
    B. 44,000.
    C. 87,000.
    D. 177,000.
    E. 277,000.

____363. An EMS home inspection might examine for
    A. knowledge of children's auto seats.
    B. helmet usage.
    C. outlet covers in children's spaces.
    D. knowledge of how to access EMS.
    E. all of the above.

____364. The anticipation of specific injuries gained from the analysis of the mechanism of injury is the
    A. factor of severity.
    B. index of suspicion.
    C. revised trauma score.
    D. trauma score.
    E. none of the above.

____365. If the hazardous materials team is not yet on scene and the patient is found to have suffered serious injuries, you would be responsible for removing him from the site and to an area free of contamination.
    A. True
    B. False

____366. The risk of contamination and resultant disease from contact with body substances is greater for your patient than for you.
    A. True
    B. False

____367. A patient with airway trauma and serious airway bleeding suggests what items of personal protection for the paramedic?
    A. Gloves
    B. Gloves and goggles
    C. Gloves and gown
    D. Gloves and mask
    E. Gloves, goggles, mask, and gown

____368. Air medical service should be summoned for any serious trauma scene more than which distance/time from the trauma center?
    A. 20 minutes
    B. 4 miles
    C. 10 miles
    D. 2 miles
    E. 45 minutes

____369. Which of the following is NOT an element of the initial assessment?
    A. Spinal precautions
    B. General patient impression
    C. SAMPLE history
    D. Airway maintenance
    E. Serious hemorrhage control

____370. The "P" of the AVPU mnemonic stands for
    A. positional sense.
    B. posturing.
    C. pain.
    D. purposeful.
    E. proprioception.

©2013 Pearson Education, Inc.
Paramedic Care: Principles & Practice, Vol. 5, 4th Ed.

_____371. Which of the following correctly represents the order in which levels of orientation are lost?
- **A.** Persons, time, place
- **B.** Time, persons, place
- **C.** Place, persons, time
- **D.** Time, place, persons
- **E.** Persons, place, time

_____372. The movement by the patient to a position of muscular extension with the elbows extending is termed
- **A.** purposeful.
- **B.** purposeless.
- **C.** decorticate posturing.
- **D.** decerebrate posturing.
- **E.** painful.

_____373. If you are required to ventilate a patient, what volume of air would you use for breaths?
- **A.** 500 mL
- **B.** 600 mL
- **C.** 500 to 800 mL
- **D.** 1,000 to 1,200 mL
- **E.** 1,200 to 1,500 mL

_____374. Capillary refill is no longer of value in the assessment of the adult patient.
- **A.** True
- **B.** False

_____375. Which of the following will affect the rate of capillary refill in the adult patient?
- **A.** Smoking
- **B.** Low ambient temperatures
- **C.** Preexisting disease
- **D.** Medications
- **E.** All of the above

_____376. A patient's perception of pain levels is subjective, and different people have different pain tolerances.
- **A.** True
- **B.** False

_____377. Percussion of the chest may yield a dull response with
- **A.** blood accumulation.
- **B.** fluid accumulation.
- **C.** air.
- **D.** air under pressure.
- **E.** both A and B.

_____378. Components of the detailed physical exam are used rarely in prehospital trauma care.
- **A.** True
- **B.** False

_____379. When one eye is exposed to a strong light, the opposite pupil should
- **A.** remain as it is.
- **B.** dilate briskly.
- **C.** dilate slowly.
- **D.** constrict briskly.
- **E.** constrict slowly.

_____380. It is important to identify use of which of the following when obtaining a history of the trauma patient?
- **A.** Aspirin
- **B.** Anticoagulants
- **C.** Beta blockers
- **D.** Antibiotics
- **E.** All of the above

_____ 381. Which of the following is NOT an indication of shock compensation?
   A. Shallow respirations
   B. Increasing pulse rate
   C. Decreasing level of consciousness
   D. Increasing pulse strength
   E. Cool and clammy skin

_____ 382. A trauma patient is breathing at 24 times per minute, has normal respiratory expansion, a blood pressure of 80 systolic, delayed capillary refill of 4 seconds, and a Glasgow Coma Scale score of 12. What should you report to medical direction as the revised trauma score?
   A. 7   D. 11
   B. 9   E. 15
   C. 10

_____ 383. Reassessment should be performed every 5 minutes on the seriously injured trauma patient.
   A. True
   B. False

_____ 384. Which of the following is a term that refers to lower-than-normal blood pressure?
   A. Hypovolemia
   B. Hypoperfusion
   C. Hypotension
   D. Anemia
   E. None of the above

_____ 385. Which of the following is a word that means "shock"?
   A. Hypovolemia
   B. Hypoperfusion
   C. Hypotension
   D. Anemia
   E. Hypertension

_____ 386. Hypothermia is a common complication of shock.
   A. True
   B. False

_____ 387. Which of the following is NOT true regarding pediatric patients when compared to adults?
   A. Their limbs are shorter and less able to protect the trunk.
   B. Their skeletons are better able to protect internal organs.
   C. Their airways are smaller.
   D. They compensate for blood loss better.
   E. Their skeletal components are more flexible.

_____ 388. Which of the following is NOT true regarding the changes in vital signs with increasing age in the pediatric patient?
   A. The blood pressure increases.
   B. The pulse rate decreases.
   C. The respirations slow.
   D. The body temperature rises.
   E. The respiratory volume increases.

_____ 389. The oral airway should be inserted by rotating it 180 degrees during insertion for the pediatric patient.
   A. True
   B. False

©2013 Pearson Education, Inc.
Paramedic Care: Principles & Practice, Vol. 5, 4th Ed.

_____390. The maximum recommended fluid administration volume for a pediatric trauma patient is
  A. 1,000 mL.
  B. 2,000 mL.
  C. 20 mL/kg.
  D. 60 mL/kg.
  E. 80 mL/kg.

_____391. Which of the following is generally NOT true regarding elderly patients?
  A. Their bones are more brittle.
  B. Their renal function is decreased.
  C. Their brain mass and volume are decreased.
  D. Their pain perception is heightened.
  E. Their cardiac strike (LM1) volume is decreased.

_____392. Key elements of the verbal patient care report include all of the following, EXCEPT
  A. mechanism of injury.
  B. interventions.
  C. results of assessment.
  D. names of EMS personnel.
  E. results of interventions.

_____393. Medical helicopters may not improve trauma outcomes in patients above the age of:
  A. 25 years.
  B. 10 years.
  C. 40 years.
  D. 75 years.
  E. 55 years.

WORKBOOK ANSWER KEY

Note: Throughout Answer Key, textbook page references are shown in italic.

Chapter 1: Trauma and Trauma Systems

CONTENT SELF-EVALUATION

MULTIPLE CHOICE

1.	C	*p. 3*	7.	B	*p. 7*	13.	A	*p. 11*
2.	A	*p. 3*	8.	D	*p. 7*	14.	A	*p. 11*
3.	A	*p. 4*	9.	E	*p. 8*	15.	C	*p. 12*
4.	A	*p. 4*	10.	D	*p. 9*	16.	E	*p. 11*
5.	C	*p. 7*	11.	C	*p. 9*	17.	C	*p. 11*
6.	D	*p. 7*	12.	B	*p.10*	18.	A	*p. 13*

Chapter 2: Blunt Trauma

CONTENT SELF-EVALUATION

MULTIPLE CHOICE

1.	A	*p. 18*	15.	C	*p. 26*	29.	A	*p. 34*
2.	B	*p. 18*	16.	B	*p. 26*	30.	A	*p. 35*
3.	B	*p. 18*	17.	C	*p. 26*	31.	E	*p. 36*
4.	D	*p. 19*	18.	A	*p. 28*	32.	D	*p. 37*
5.	C	*p. 19*	19.	E	*p. 28*	33.	B	*p. 37*
6.	E	*p. 19*	20.	A	*p. 28*	34.	C	*p. 37*
7.	B	*p. 19*	21.	E	*p. 28*	35.	A	*p. 37*
8.	E	*p. 21*	22.	E	*p. 30*	36.	C	*p. 39*
9.	E	*p. 22*	23.	B	*p. 31*	37.	A	*p. 39*
10.	D	*p. 22*	24.	D	*p. 31*	38.	D	*p. 39*
11.	A	*p. 24*	25.	A	*p. 31*	39.	B	*p. 39*
12.	B	*p. 24*	26.	B	*p. 32*	40.	E	*p. 40*
13.	C	*p. 25*	27.	C	*p. 33*			
14.	B	*p. 25*	28.	A	*p. 33*			

SPECIAL PROJECT: Mechanism of Injury Analysis

A. Mechanism of injury: sports injury, blunt trauma. Anticipated injuries: head (but well protected); neck/spine, skeletal—fractures and/or dislocations; muscular—sprains, strains.

B. Mechanism of injury: frontal-impact auto crash. Anticipated injuries: head injury; cervical spine injury; chest injury; abdominal injury; foot, leg, and thigh injuries.

C. Mechanism of injury: explosion, pressure wave, projectiles, structural collapse. Anticipated injuries: pressure wave—lung, bowel, ear injuries; penetrating trauma from projectiles; burns; inhalation injuries; blunt trauma; crush injuries.

Chapter 3: Penetrating Trauma

CONTENT SELF-EVALUATION

MULTIPLE CHOICE

1.	A	*p. 46*	10.	A	*p. 50*	19.	A	*p. 54*
2.	C	*p. 46*	11.	A	*p. 50*	20.	D	*p. 54*
3.	A	*p. 46*	12.	C	*p. 51*	21.	C	*p. 55*
4.	C	*p. 47*	13.	E	*p. 51*	22.	B	*p. 55*
5.	B	*p. 47*	14.	D	*p. 51*	23.	E	*p. 55*
6.	E	*p. 48*	15.	C	*p. 52*	24.	D	*p. 55*
7.	A	*p. 48*	16.	B	*p. 53*	25.	C	*p. 56*
8.	B	*p. 49*	17.	A	*p. 53*			
9.	E	*p. 49*	18.	A	*p. 53*			

SPECIAL PROJECT: Label the Diagram

A. Zone of injury
B. Permanent cavity
C. Pressure wave
D. Temporary cavity
E. Direct injury

Chapter 4: Hemorrhage and Shock

CONTENT SELF-EVALUATION

MULTIPLE CHOICE

1.	C	*p. 62*	20.	B	*p. 69*	39.	B	*p. 77*
2.	E	*p. 62*	21.	C	*p. 69*	40.	C	*p. 77*
3.	B	*p. 62*	22.	E	*p. 69*	41.	A	*p. 78*
4.	B	*p. 62*	23.	D	*p. 69*	42.	E	*p. 79*
5.	C	*p. 62*	24.	A	*p. 70*	43.	D	*p. 78*
6.	C	*p. 63*	25.	E	*p. 70*	44.	A	*p. 79*
7.	B	*p. 63*	26.	A	*p. 70*	45.	B	*p. 80*
8.	D	*p. 63*	27.	D	*p. 71*	46.	C	*p. 80*
9.	C	*p. 63*	28.	B	*p. 71*	47.	B	*p. 81*
10.	D	*p. 64*	29.	E	*p. 71*	48.	E	*p. 81*
11.	B	*p. 64*	30.	D	*p. 73*	49.	E	*p. 81*
12.	A	*p. 64*	31.	D	*p. 73*	50.	E	*p. 82*
13.	D	*p. 64*	32.	C	*p. 75*	51.	D	*p. 83*
14.	D	*p. 64*	33.	B	*p. 75*	52.	E	*p. 84*
15.	B	*p. 64*	34.	B	*p. 75*	53.	C	*p. 85*
16.	E	*p. 65*	35.	A	*p. 75*	54.	E	*p. 85*
17.	A	*p. 66*	36.	C	*p. 75*	55.	B	*p. 85*
18.	B	*p. 67*	37.	B	*p. 76*	56.	C	*p. 86*
19.	A	*p. 69*	38.	C	*p. 77*			

SPECIAL PROJECT: Scenario-Based Problem Solving

1. The liver, kidney, large bowel, small bowel, pancreas, diaphragm
2. The agitation could be related to the nature of his injury and the attack, or he could be experiencing minor cerebral hypoxia due to hypovolemia, which will also cause some agitation.
3. An increase in peripheral vascular resistance may be the body's compensation for a decreased cardiac output due to hypovolemia.
4. The increased diastolic pressure (in the absence of an increase in the systolic blood pressure) decreases the pulse pressure. The pulse pressure is the strength of the pulse.
5. The skin becomes cool and clammy as the arterioles serving it constrict to shunt blood to more immediately critical organs such as the heart, brain, kidneys, and (to fight or flee) the skeletal muscles.

Chapter 5: Soft-Tissue Trauma

CONTENT SELF-EVALUATION

MULTIPLE CHOICE

1.	B	p. 93	20.	C	p. 101	39.	A	p. 111
2.	A	p. 94	21.	E	p. 101	40.	E	p. 111
3.	E	p. 94	22.	A	p. 101	41.	C	p. 112
4.	D	p. 94	23.	E	p. 101	42.	B	p. 112
5.	A	p. 94	24.	C	p. 102	43.	C	p. 113
6.	B	p. 94	25.	E	p. 102	44.	D	p. 113
7.	B	p. 95	26.	A	p. 102	45.	A	p. 114
8.	B	p. 96	27.	E	p. 103	46.	C	p. 114
9.	E	p. 96	28.	E	p. 103	47.	B	p. 114
10.	B	p. 96	29.	A	p. 103	48.	E	p. 115
11.	C	p. 96	30.	A	p. 103	49.	E	p. 115
12.	D	p. 98	31.	A	p. 105	50.	C	p. 116
13.	E	p. 97	32.	C	p. 105	51.	C	p. 116
14.	B	p. 97	33.	E	p. 105	52.	B	p. 116
15.	A	p. 98	34.	D	p. 106	53.	A	p. 116
16.	D	p. 98	35.	A	p. 108	54.	E	p. 116
17.	B	p. 99	36.	A	p. 108	55.	C	p. 116
18.	C	p. 100	37.	E	p. 109			
19.	B	p. 100	38.	B	p. 111			

Chapter 6: Burn Trauma

CONTENT SELF-EVALUATION

MULTIPLE CHOICE

1.	A	p. 123	11.	A	p. 127	21.	B	p. 132
2.	D	p. 123	12.	B	p. 128	22.	C	p. 132
3.	C	p. 123	13.	C	p. 128	23.	B	p. 133
4.	D	p. 124	14.	A	p. 128	24.	C	p. 133
5.	A	p. 125	15.	E	p. 128	25.	D	p. 133
6.	D	p. 125	16.	D	p. 130	26.	E	p. 133
7.	B	p. 125	17.	B	p. 130	27.	E	p. 133
8.	A	p. 126	18.	E	p. 131	28.	E	p. 135
9.	C	p. 126	19.	C	p. 131	29.	B	p. 136
10.	E	p. 127	20.	D	p. 131	30.	A	p. 137

31.	A	p. 137	41.	B	p. 140	51.	B	p. 143
32.	B	p. 136	42.	B	p. 140	52.	D	p. 144
33.	B	p. 132	43.	B	p. 141	53.	E	p. 144
34.	E	p. 133	44.	A	p. 140	54.	C	p. 144
35.	A	p. 139	45.	B	p. 141	55.	B	p. 144
36.	D	p. 139	46.	B	p. 141	56.	D	p. 144
37.	D	p. 139	47.	B	p. 141	57.	A	p. 144
38.	D	p. 139	48.	A	p. 142	58.	A	p. 145
39.	A	p. 140	49.	E	p. 142	59.	E	p. 145
40.	A	p. 140	50.	D	p. 143	60.	B	p. 145

SPECIAL PROJECT: Drip Math Worksheet 2

1. $R = ?$

   $T = 2$ hour (120 min)

   $V = 250$ mL

   $$\text{Rate} = \frac{\text{Volume}}{\text{Time}} = \frac{250 \text{ mL}}{120 \text{ min}}$$

   $$= \frac{20.8 \text{ drops}}{\text{min}} = 2.08 \text{ mL/min}$$

   A. $D = 10$ drops/mL

   $$R = V \times D = \frac{2.08 \text{ mL} \times 10 \text{ drops}}{\text{min} \times \text{mL}}$$

   $$= \frac{20.8 \text{ drops}}{\text{min}} = 2.08 \text{ mL / min}$$

   B. $D = 15$ drops/mL

   $$R = V \times D = \frac{2.08 \text{ mL} \times 15 \text{ drops}}{\text{min} \times \text{mL}}$$

   $$= \frac{31.2 \text{ drops}}{\text{min}} = 31.2 \text{ mL/min}$$

   C. $D = 60$ drops/mL

   $$R = V \times D = \frac{2.08 \text{ mL} \times 60 \text{ drops}}{\text{min} \times \text{mL}}$$

   $$= \frac{144 \text{ drops}}{\text{min}} = 144 \text{ drops /min}$$

2. $R = 30$ drops/min

   $T = ?$

   $D = 60$ drops/mL

   $$R = R / D = \frac{30 \text{ drops} \times \text{mL}}{60 \text{ min} \times \text{min}}$$

   $$= \frac{0.5 \text{ mL}}{\text{min}} = 0.5 \text{ mL/min}$$

   A. $V = 200$

   $$T = \frac{V}{R} = \frac{200 \text{ mL} \times \text{min}}{0.5 \text{ mL}}$$

   $$= 400 \text{ min} \frac{400 \text{ min} \times \text{hr}}{60 \text{ min}}$$

   $$= 6.67 \text{ hrs (6 hrs, 40 min)}$$

   B. $V = 350$

   $$T = \frac{V}{R} = \frac{350 \text{ mL} \times \text{min}}{0.5 \text{ mL}}$$

   $$= 700 \text{ min} \frac{700 \text{ min} \times \text{hr}}{60 \text{ min}}$$

   $$= 11.67 \text{ hrs (11 hrs, 40 min)}$$

3. $R = 1$ drops/sec $= 60$ drops/min

   $T = 15$ min

   $V = ?$

$$D = 15 \text{ drops/mL}$$

$$R = \frac{60 \text{ drops} \times \text{mL}}{15 \text{ drops} \times \text{min}} = \frac{4 \text{ mL}}{\text{min}}$$

$$= 4 \text{ mL/min}$$

$$V = R \times T = \frac{4 \text{ mL} \times 15 \text{ min}}{\text{min}} = 60 \text{ mL}$$

4. Note: You must determine the volume (per minute) administered with the 60 drops/mL set running at 15 drops. Then determine the drops (/min) with the 45 drops/mL set necessary to administer the same volume.

$$R = 15 \text{ drops/mL}(60 \text{ drops/mL})$$

$$= \frac{15 \text{ drops} \times \text{mL}}{60 \text{ drops} \times \text{min}}$$

$$= \frac{0.25 \text{ mL}}{\text{min}} = 0.25 \text{ mL/min}$$

$$T = 1 \text{ min}$$

$$V = ?$$

$$D = 45 \text{ drops/mL}$$

$$V = R \times T = \frac{0.25 \text{ mL} \times 1 \text{ min}}{\text{min}} = 0.25 \text{ mL}$$

$$R = \frac{0.25 \text{ mL} \times 45 \text{ drops}}{\text{min} \times \text{mL}}$$

$$= \frac{11.25 \text{ drops}}{\text{min}}$$

$$= 11.25 \text{ drops/min}$$

Chapter 7: Orthopedic Trauma

CONTENT SELF-EVALUATION

MULTIPLE CHOICE

1.	E	p. 151	25.	B	p. 162	49.	C	p. 174
2.	B	p. 152	26.	A	p. 162	50.	D	p. 176
3.	C	p. 152	27.	E	p. 164	51.	B	p. 176
4.	B	p. 152	28.	B	p. 163	52.	B	p. 176
5.	A	p. 152	29.	A	p. 164	53.	E	p. 176
6.	C	p. 153	30.	A	p. 165	54.	E	p. 176
7.	D	p. 153	31.	E	p. 165	55.	D	p. 176
8.	A	p. 153	32.	B	p. 166	56.	E	p. 178
9.	B	p. 153	33.	A	p. 166	57.	D	p. 178
10.	D	p. 153	34.	C	p. 166	58.	E	p. 179
11.	A	p. 154	35.	A	p. 167	59.	B	p. 179
12.	C	p. 154	36.	D	p. 166	60.	A	p. 179
13.	A	p. 155	37.	E	p. 168	61.	B	p. 180
14.	C	p. 156	38.	E	p. 168	62.	C	p. 180
15.	A	p. 156	39.	E	p. 169	63.	C	p. 181
16.	E	p. 156	40.	C	p. 170	64.	A	p. 181
17.	D	p. 156	41.	C	p. 170	65.	A	p. 181
18.	C	p. 157	42.	B	p. 170	66.	B	p. 181
19.	E	p. 157	43.	A	p. 171	67.	E	p. 182
20.	D	p. 160	44.	A	p. 172	68.	E	p. 183
21.	A	p. 161	45.	A	p. 172	69.	D	p. 183
22.	A	p. 161	46.	E	p. 172	70.	B	p. 183
23.	C	p. 162	47.	A	p. 174			
24.	B	p. 162	48.	D	p. 174			

SPECIAL PROJECTS: Recognizing Bones and Bone Injuries

Part I

A. mandible
B. sternum
C. scapula
D. humerus
E. radius
F. ulna
G. sacrum
H. metacarpals
I. tibia
J. fibula

Part II

A. comminuted
B. impacted
C. greenstick
D. oblique
E. spiral
F. transverse

Chapter 8: Thoracic Trauma

CONTENT SELF-EVALUATION

MULTIPLE CHOICE

1.	B	p. 189	24.	B	p. 195	47.	B	p. 203
2.	E	p. 189	25.	D	p. 196	48.	E	p. 203
3.	B	p. 190	26.	B	p. 196	49.	C	p. 203
4.	E	p. 190	27.	B	p. 197	50.	B	p. 203
5.	C	p. 190	28.	E	p. 195	51.	A	p. 204
6.	A	p. 190	29.	D	p. 198	52.	B	p. 204
7.	D	p. 190	30.	B	p. 197	53.	E	p. 204
8.	B	p. 190	31.	D	p. 198	54.	E	p. 205
9.	E	p. 190	32.	D	p. 199	55.	A	p. 206
10.	B	p. 190	33.	D	p. 199	56.	D	p. 206
11.	A	p. 190	34.	E	p. 199	57.	E	p. 207
12.	C	p. 191	35.	C	p. 199	58.	B	p. 207
13.	C	p. 191	36.	A	p. 200	59.	B	p. 207
14.	C	p. 191	37.	A	p. 200	60.	A	p. 209
15.	B	p. 191	38.	A	p. 200	61.	C	p. 209
16.	D	p. 192	39.	D	p. 202	62.	A	p. 209
17.	A	p. 192	40.	A	p. 201	63.	B	p. 209
18.	C	p. 192	41.	E	p. 202	64.	C	p. 210
19.	D	p. 194	42.	B	p. 201	65.	A	p. 210
20.	B	p. 194	43.	D	p. 202	66.	A	p. 210
21.	A	p. 194	44.	B	p. 202	67.	E	p. 212
22.	A	p. 195	45.	A	p. 202			
23.	E	p. 195	46.	C	p. 203			

SPECIAL PROJECTS: Labeling Diagrams

Part I

A. sternum
B. lung
C. heart
D. trachea
E. pleura
F. ribs
G. diaphragm
H. pleural space

Part II

1. A   5. G   9. F
2. H   6. E   10. C
3. J   7. B   11. I
4. D   8. K

PROBLEM SOLVING—CHEST INJURY

Signs and symptoms of a tension pneumothorax include: mechanism of injury, progressive dyspnea, diminished breath sounds on injured side, JVD, tracheal deviation away from injury, subcutaneous emphysema, hyperresonant percussion on injured side, signs and symptoms of shock.

A patient report should include: chest trauma patient, unequal breath sounds, side involved, progressive and significant dyspnea, JVD.

Your decompression attempt locations: between 2nd and 3rd ribs (2nd intercostal space), midclavicular line of side with decreased breath sounds.

Chapter 9: Abdominal Trauma

CONTENT SELF-EVALUATION

MULTIPLE CHOICE

1.	A	p. 216	18.	E	p. 223	35.	D	p. 227
2.	A	p. 217	19.	B	p. 224	36.	C	p. 227
3.	C	p. 217	20.	B	p. 224	37.	A	p. 227
4.	E	p. 217	21.	E	p. 224	38.	A	p. 227
5.	E	p. 218	22.	C	p. 224	39.	E	p. 227
6.	B	p. 218	23.	B	p. 224	40.	D	p. 228
7.	A	p. 218	24.	E	p. 224	41.	D	p. 228
8.	E	p. 218	25.	C	p. 224	42.	C	p. 229
9.	A	p. 220	26.	A	p. 225	43.	D	p. 230
10.	C	p. 218	27.	C	p. 225	44.	C	p. 232
11.	B	p. 220	28.	B	p. 226	45.	C	p. 233
12.	B	p. 221	29.	B	p. 225	46.	D	p. 234
13.	D	p. 221	30.	C	p. 226	47.	B	p. 234
14.	C	p. 221	31.	A	p. 226	48.	D	p. 234
15.	D	p. 222	32.	D	p. 226	49.	A	p. 234
16.	C	p. 222	33.	E	p. 226	50.	A	p. 234
17.	C	p. 223	34.	E	p. 226			

SPECIAL PROJECT: Writing a Run Report

Please review the next page and ensure that your form includes the appropriate information.

©2013 Pearson Education, Inc.
Paramedic Care: Principles & Practice, Vol. 5, 4th Ed.

SPECIAL PROJECT: Writing a Run Report

Date Today's Date	Emergency Medical Services Run Report	Run # 914

Patient Information | Service Information | Times

Patient Information	Service Information	Times
Name: Marty	Agency:	Rcvd 03:25
Address: Harborview Apts #112	Location: Harborview Apts #112	Enrt 03:25
City: St: Zip:	Call Origin: 911 Center	Scne 03:32
Age: 43 Birth: / / Sex: [M][F]	Type: Emrg[X] Non[ ] Trnsfr[ ]	LvSn 03:38
Nature of Call: Shots fired		ArHsp 03:47
Chief Complaint: "Shot by wife"		InSv 04:00

Description of Current Problem:

Shot by a 9mm handgun @ close range.

Wound to LUQ, oozing small amount of blood.

No apparent exit wound(s). Describes pain as sharp.

Surrounding area feels "burning" in nature.

Medical Problems

Past		Present
[ ]	Cardiac	[ ]
[ ]	Stroke	[ ]
[ ]	Acute Abdomen	[ ]
[ ]	Diabetes	[ ]
[ ]	Psychiatric	[ ]
[X]	Epilepsy	[ ]
[ ]	Drug/Alcohol	[ ]
[ ]	Poisoning	[ ]
[ ]	Allergy/Asthma	[ ]
[ ]	Syncope	[ ]
[ ]	Obstetrical	[ ]
[ ]	GYN	[ ]

Other:

Trauma Scr: 12   Glasgow: 15

On-Scene Care: Covered wound w/ sterile dressing, moved to stretcher – IV 14 ga angio (L) antecubital w/250 mL LR bolus	First Aid: Towel – patient seated against wall
	By Whom? unknown

O₂ @ 12 L 03:35 Via NRM	C-Collar N/A	S-Immob. N/A	Stretcher 03:36

Allergies/Meds: Phenobarbital Dilantin no allergies, Tetanus – 3 yrs ago

Past Med Hx: Seizures – controlled

Time	Pulse	Resp.	BP S/D	LOC	ECG
03:35	R: 80 [x][i]	R: 22 [s][l]	110/86	[x][v][p][u]	NSR SaO₂ 99%
Care/Comments: A/O x 3 O₂ 12 L/NRM IV 1,000 LR					
03:42	R: 86 [x][i]	R: 24 [x][l]	112/86	[x][v][p][u]	NSR SaO₂ 99%
Care/Comments: Shoulder pain & thirst; BJ: clear in all fields; no bowel sounds					
03:47	R: 88 [r][i]	R: 22 [x][l]	112/92	[x][v][p][u]	
Care/Comments: Pt. transport uneventful					
:	R: [r][i]	R: [s][l]	/	[a][v][p][u]	
Care/Comments:					

Destination: St. Joseph's Hospital	Personnel:	Certification
Reason:[ ]pt [ ]Closest [X]M.D. [ ]Other	1. Janice	[R][E][O]
Contacted: [X]Radio [ ]Tele [ ]Direct	2. Doug	[R][E][O]
Ar Status: [ ]Better [X]UnC [ ]Worse	3.	[P][E][O]

CONTENT SELF-EVALUATION

MULTIPLE CHOICE

1.	A	p. 239	25.	E	p. 254	49.	D	p. 265			
2.	D	p. 239	26.	C	p. 254	50.	E	p. 266			
3.	E	p. 240	27.	D	p. 255	51.	A	p. 268			
4.	B	p. 240	28.	B	p. 255	52.	A	p. 268			
5.	C	p. 241	29.	B	p. 255	53.	A	p. 269			
6.	B	p. 241	30.	B	p. 255	54.	E	p. 270			
7.	C	p. 241	31.	A	p. 255	55.	B	p. 270			
8.	C	p. 242	32.	A	p. 256	56.	A	p. 270			
9.	D	p. 243	33.	A	p. 256	57.	A	p. 272			
10.	A	p. 243	34.	C	p. 257	58.	E	p. 272			
11.	A	p. 243	35.	E	p. 257	59.	B	p. 273			
12.	C	p. 243	36.	E	p. 257	60.	B	p. 273			
13.	B	p. 245	37.	A	p. 258	61.	B	p. 273			
14.	E	p. 246	38.	C	p. 258	62.	E	p. 274			
15.	B	p. 246	39.	C	p. 259	63.	A	p. 274			
16.	A	p. 246	40.	A	p. 259	64.	C	p. 275			
17.	C	p. 246	41.	B	p. 260	65.	A	p. 275			
18.	B	p. 248	42.	B	p. 260	66.	A	p. 275			
19.	C	p. 249	43.	C	p. 261	67.	B	p. 276			
20.	C	p. 250	44.	D	p. 262	68.	A	p. 277			
21.	A	p. 252	45.	A	p. 263	69.	A	p. 277			
22.	E	p. 253	46.	C	p. 264	70.	E	p. 278			
23.	A	p. 253	47.	B	p. 264	71.	D	p. 279			
24.	B	p. 253	48.	B	p. 265	72.	B	p. 279			

SPECIAL PROJECT: Recognizing Spinal Regions

A. Cervical, 7
B. Thoracic, 12
C. Lumbar, 5
D. Sacral, 5 (fused into 1)
E. Coccygeal, 5 (fused into 2 or 3)

Chapter 11: Nervous System Trauma

CONTENT SELF-EVALUATION

MULTIPLE CHOICE

1.	E	p. 285	4.	B	p. 286	7.	C	p. 286
2.	D	p. 285	5.	A	p. 286	8.	A	p. 287
3.	B	p. 286	6.	B	p. 286	9.	A	p. 287

10.	E	p. 287	32.	D	p. 296	54.	C	p. 304
11.	C	p. 287	33.	B	p. 296	55.	E	p. 305
12.	C	p. 287	34.	C	p. 296	56.	B	p. 306
13.	D	p. 288	35.	A	p. 297	57.	C	p. 306
14.	E	p. 288	36.	E	p. 298	58.	B	p. 306
15.	E	p. 288	37.	A	p. 298	59.	B	p. 306
16.	C	p. 289	38.	C	p. 298	60.	D	p. 306
17.	C	p. 289	39.	B	p. 298	61.	A	p. 308
18.	A	p. 289	40.	D	p. 299	62.	E	p. 308
19.	A	p. 290	41.	B	p. 299	63.	A	p. 309
20.	B	p. 291	42.	A	p. 299	64.	B	p. 309
21.	A	p. 292	43.	A	p. 300	65.	B	p. 309
22.	E	p. 292	44.	E	p. 301	66.	B	p. 309
23.	D	p. 292	45.	A	p. 301	67.	A	p. 309
24.	A	p. 292	46.	B	p. 301	68.	D	p. 310
25.	D	p. 294	47.	B	p. 301	69.	B	p. 310
26.	E	p. 294	48.	A	p. 303	70.	B	p. 310
27.	B	p. 294	49.	E	p. 303	71.	E	p. 310
28.	C	p. 294	50.	D	p. 303	72.	E	p. 311
29.	C	p. 295	51.	C	p. 303	73.	B	p. 310
30.	E	p. 295	52.	E	p. 304	74.	C	p. 311
31.	A	p. 295	53.	E	p. 304	75.	D	p. 311

SPECIAL PROJECT: Composing a Radio Message and Run Report

Your reports should include most of the following elements.

Radio message from the scene to medical direction: Unit 765 to medical command. We are en route to community hospital with a victim of a one-car auto crash—frontal impact. The patient was reported as initially unconscious but was conscious and alert, though somewhat disoriented upon our arrival. He is now unconscious and responsive only to painful stimuli. He did complain of chest pain that varied with breathing; breath sounds are clear; ECG with NSR at 70. He has a small contusion on his forehead. Vitals are blood pressure 136/88, pulse 52, respirations 22 and deep, and SaO_2 98 percent. We have established an IV with 1,000 mL NS running TKO and have applied O_2. A cervical collar has been applied and spinal immobilization is under way.

Follow-up radio message to medical direction: Unit 765 to Medical Center. Our patient remains unconscious and responsive only to deep painful stimuli. He is orally intubated with assisted respirations via bag-valve mask at 20. Current vitals: blood pressure 142/92, pulse 62, and SaO_2 99 percent $ETCO_2$ 38 percent. ETA 15 minutes.

Ambulance report form: Please review the next page and ensure that your form includes the appropriate information.

Ambulance report form:

Date Today's Date	Emergency Medical Services Run Report		Run # 913

Patient Information	Service Information		Times

Patient Information		**Service Information**		**Times**	
Name: John		Agency: Unit 765		Rcvd	02:15
Address:		Location: Hwy 127 & Cty Tr H		Enrt	02:15
City: St: Zip:		Call Origin: 911 Center		Scne	02:32
Age: 31 Birth: / / Sex: [X][F]		Type: Emrg[X] Non[ ] Trnsfr[ ]		LvSn	02:42
Nature of Call: One-car auto accident/frontal impact				ArHsp	03:15
Chief Complaint: Chest pain which varies with resp./unconsciousness				InSv	03:35

Description of Current Problem:

Pt. is a 31 y.o. male victim of an auto accident. He impacted the steering wheel and windshield. Though initially unconscious, the pt. was conscious, alert, though disoriented, upon our arrival, and complaining of chest pain only. During extrication his left pupil dilated, his level of consciousness began to drop, and he became unresponsive. Physical assessment did reveal a small contusion on his forehead with limited swelling and no crepitation.

Trauma Scr: 12   Glasgow: 14/5

Medical Problems

Past		Present
[ ]	Cardiac	[ ]
[ ]	Stroke	[ ]
[ ]	Acute Abdomen	[ ]
[ ]	Diabetes	[ ]
[ ]	Psychiatric	[ ]
[ ]	Epilepsy	[ ]
[ ]	Drug/Alcohol	[ ]
[ ]	Poisoning	[ ]
[ ]	Allergy/Asthma	[ ]
[ ]	Syncope	[ ]
[ ]	Obstetrical	[ ]
[ ]	GYN	[ ]

Other: none

On-Scene Care: C-collar, spinal imm.

Oxygen, IV 16 ga L forearm – NS

8.0 mm ET tube digital, assisted resp @ 20

via BVM @ 15 L O$_2$

First Aid: None

Police report the patient was unconscious when they arrived.

By Whom?

O$_2$ @ 15 L 02:36 Via NRB	C-Collar 02:34	S-Immob. 02:33	Stretcher 02:42

Allergies/Meds: None

Past Med Hx: None

Time	Pulse	Resp.	BP S/D	LOC	ECG
02:36	R: 70 [X][i]	R: 20 [s][l]	124/88	[X][v][p][u]	NSR SaO$_2$ 99%
Care/Comments: Conscious and alert, chest pain on resp, clear breath sounds 16 ga IV/NS					
02:41	R: 52 [X][i]	R: 22 [s][X]	136/88	[a][v][X][u]	NSR SaO$_2$ 98%
Care/Comments: Pt. becomes unconscious, responds to painful stimuli, left pupil is dilated					
02:51	R: 62 [X][i]	R: 20 [s][X]	142/92	[a][v][X][u]	NSR SaO$_2$ 97% GCS 5
Care/Comments: Pt. is unconscious, 8.0 ET tube – BVM hyperventilating					
03:01	R: 50 [X][i]	R: 20 [s][X]	140/90	[a][v][X][u]	NSR SaO$_2$ 97%
Care/Comments: Pt. is unresponsive to all but painful stimuli					

Destination: Medical Center	Personnel:	Certification
Reason:[ ]pt [ ]Closest [X]M.D. [ ]Other	1. Jan	[R][E][O]
Contacted: [X]Radio [ ]Tele [ ]Direct	2. Steve	[R][E][O]
Ar Status: [ ]Better [ ]UnC [X]Worse	3.	[P][R][O]

Chapter 12: Environmental Trauma

CONTENT SELF-EVALUATION

MULTIPLE CHOICE

MATCHING

LISTING

51. Work-induced thermogenesis, thermoregulatory thermogenesis, diet-induced thermogenesis *p. 317*
52. Sweating, vasodilation *p. 319*
53. Shivering, vasoconstriction *p. 320*

Chapter 13: Special Considerations in Trauma

CONTENT SELF-EVALUATION

MULTIPLE CHOICE

TRAUMA: CONTENT REVIEW

CONTENT SELF-EVALUATION

CHAPTER 1: TRAUMA AND TRAUMA SYSTEMS

CHAPTER 2: BLUNT TRAUMA

CHAPTER 3: PENETRATING TRAUMA

CHAPTER 4: HEMORRHAGE AND SHOCK

CHAPTER 5: SOFT-TISSUE TRAUMA

CHAPTER 6: BURN TRAUMA

107.	B	p. 123	119.	A	p. 132	131.	B	p. 140
108.	A	p. 123	120.	C	p. 132	132.	B	p. 140
109.	D	p. 124	121.	B	p. 133	133.	A	p. 140
110.	A	p. 126	122.	C	p. 133	134.	B	p. 140
111.	C	p. 125	123.	E	p. 133	135.	D	p. 141
112.	A	p. 126	124.	B	p. 137	136.	D	p. 141
113.	A	p. 127	125.	A	p. 136	137.	B	p. 142
114.	B	p. 128	126.	E	p. 137	138.	E	p. 143
115.	B	p. 128	127.	C	p. 139	139.	C	p. 144
116.	A	p. 130	128.	B	p. 139	140.	B	p. 144
117.	C	p. 131	129.	D	p. 139	141.	C	p. 145
118.	B	p. 131	130.	C	p. 139			

CHAPTER 7: ORTHOPEDIC TRAUMA

142.	E	p. 151	157.	E	p. 162	172.	B	p. 176
143.	A	p. 152	158.	E	p. 164	173.	E	p. 176
144.	B	p. 153	159.	A	p. 165	174.	A	p. 176
145.	E	p. 152	160.	C	p. 165	175.	B	p. 177
146.	C	p. 152	161.	B	p. 167	176.	B	p. 178
147.	E	p. 153	162.	C	p. 167	177.	E	p. 179
148.	C	p. 154	163.	B	p. 168	178.	E	p. 179
149.	B	p. 156	164.	E	p. 169	179.	B	p. 181
150.	C	p. 156	165.	C	p. 170	180.	D	p. 181
151.	B	p. 157	166.	B	p. 171	181.	B	p. 181
152.	C	p. 157	167.	A	p. 172	182.	A	p. 181
153.	E	p. 160	168.	B	p. 172	183.	E	p. 182
154.	B	p. 160	169.	B	p. 174	184.	D	p. 183
155.	C	p. 160	170.	D	p. 174	185.	E	p. 183
156.	C	p. 162	171.	B	p. 176	186.	B	p. 183

CHAPTER 8: THORACIC TRAUMA

187.	B	p. 189	198.	A	p. 196	209.	E	p. 203
188.	E	p. 189	199.	A	p. 196	210.	D	p. 203
189.	C	p. 190	200.	A	p. 198	211.	A	p. 203
190.	A	p. 190	201.	A	p. 199	212.	D	p. 204
191.	B	p. 190	202.	C	p. 199	213.	C	p. 204
192.	C	p. 191	203.	E	p. 199	214.	D	p. 204
193.	C	p. 192	204.	C	p. 200	215.	A	p. 206
194.	C	p. 192	205.	D	p. 200	216.	A	p. 209
195.	D	p. 193	206.	B	p. 201	217.	B	p. 210
196.	D	p. 194	207.	E	p. 202	218.	A	p. 210
197.	D	p. 195	208.	A	p. 202	219.	B	p. 212

CHAPTER 9: ABDOMINAL TRAUMA

220.	D	p. 217	229.	B	p. 223	238.	B	p. 226
221.	B	p. 217	230.	E	p. 224	239.	A	p. 226
222.	E	p. 217	231.	A	p. 224	240.	B	p. 227
223.	D	p. 218	232.	B	p. 224	241.	B	p. 227
224.	B	p. 218	233.	B	p. 224	242.	A	p. 229
225.	A	p. 220	234.	C	p. 224	243.	E	p. 231
226.	B	p. 221	235.	A	p. 226	244.	D	p. 233
227.	B	p. 221	236.	B	p. 226			
228.	D	p. 222	237.	B	p. 226			

CHAPTER 10: HEAD, FACE, NECK, AND SPINAL TRAUMA

245.	A	p. 239	260.	E	p. 252	275.	B	p. 269
246.	B	p. 240	261.	A	p. 254	276.	D	p. 268
247.	A	p. 241	262.	B	p. 254	277.	E	p. 270
248.	E	p. 242	263.	A	p. 255	278.	A	p. 270
249.	B	p. 242	264.	C	p. 257	279.	A	p. 271
250.	E	p. 243	265.	E	p. 257	280.	C	p. 272
251.	B	p. 243	266.	E	p. 258	281.	E	p. 274
252.	B	p. 244	267.	B	p. 258	282.	A	p. 274
253.	A	p. 246	268.	A	p. 259	283.	A	p. 275
254.	B	p. 247	269.	C	p. 261	284.	C	p. 275
255.	A	p. 248	270.	A	p. 262	285.	B	p. 277
256.	C	p. 249	271.	A	p. 266	286.	C	p. 277
257.	A	p. 251	272.	A	p. 268	287.	C	p. 277
258.	B	p. 252	273.	A	p. 269	288.	A	p. 278
259.	D	p. 252	274.	A	p. 269			

CHAPTER 11: NERVOUS SYSTEM TRAUMA

289.	B	p. 285	303.	A	p. 293	317.	E	p. 299
290.	A	p. 285	304.	E	p. 295	318.	E	p. 301
291.	E	p. 286	305.	B	p. 294	319.	A	p. 301
292.	B	p. 286	306.	A	p. 295	320.	C	p. 301
293.	C	p. 286	307.	A	p. 296	321.	B	p. 303
294.	A	p. 286	308.	A	p. 296	322.	B	p. 303
295.	A	p. 287	309.	C	p. 296	323.	D	p. 306
296.	B	p. 288	310.	B	p. 296	324.	B	p. 306
297.	A	p. 288	311.	E	p. 297	325.	B	p. 306
298.	D	p. 289	312.	B	p. 298	326.	A	p. 309
299.	B	p. 289	313.	B	p. 298	327.	B	p. 309
300.	B	p. 292	314.	A	p. 298	328.	A	p. 310
301.	C	p. 292	315.	A	p. 298	329.	D	p. 310
302.	D	p. 292	316.	B	p. 300	330.	C	p. 311

CHAPTER 12: ENVIRONMENTAL TRAUMA

331.	B	p. 318	341.	C	p. 327	351.	A	p. 335
332.	D	p. 318	342.	A	p. 328	352.	B	p. 335
333.	D	p. 319	343.	E	p. 328	353.	D	p. 335
334.	E	p. 319	344.	A	p. 328	354	C	p. 335
335.	B	p. 321	345.	E	p. 328	355.	C	p. 335
336.	B	p. 321	346.	B	p. 328	356.	C	p. 335
337.	B	p. 323	347.	A	p. 330	357.	A	p. 336
338.	D	p. 324	348.	E	p. 332	358.	E	p. 342
339.	D	p. 324	349.	C	p. 332	359.	B	p. 342
340.	C	p. 325	350.	B	p. 333	360.	C	p. 342

CHAPTER 13: SPECIAL CONSIDERATIONS IN TRAUMA

361.	C	p. 348	373.	A	p. 355	385.	B	p. 363
362.	D	p. 347	374.	B	p. 355	386.	A	p. 364
363.	E	p. 348	375.	E	p. 356	387.	B	p. 367
364.	B	p. 350	376.	A	p. 356	388.	D	p. 367
365.	B	p. 351	377.	E	p. 357	389.	B	p. 367
366.	A	p. 352	378.	B	p. 358	390.	D	p. 368
367.	E	p. 352	379.	D	p. 358	391.	D	p. 372
368.	E	p. 352	380.	E	p. 359	392.	D	p. 373
369.	C	p. 353	381.	D	p. 359	393.	E	p. 374
370.	C	p. 354	382.	C	p. 362			
371.	D	p. 354	383.	A	p. 363			
372.	D	p. 354	384.	C	p. 363			

PATIENT SCENARIO FLASH CARDS

The following pages contain prepared 3" × 5" index cards. Each card presents a patient scenario with the appropriate signs and symptoms. On the reverse side are the appropriate field diagnosis and the care steps you should consider providing for your patient.

Detach the pages, cut out the cards, and review each of them in detail. If there are any discrepancies with what you have been taught in class, please review these with your instructor and medical director and employ what is appropriate for your EMS system. Record any changes directly on the cards.

Once your cards are prepared and you have reviewed them carefully, shuffle them and then read the scenario and signs and symptoms. Try to identify the patient's problem and the treatment you would employ. Compare your diagnosis and care steps with those on the reverse side of your flash card. This exercise will help you recognize and remember the common serious trauma emergencies, their presentation, and the appropriate care.

SCENARIO 1:   Your patient is a 36-year-old driver of a small auto that collided with a tree. He was wearing his seat belt, firmly impacted the steering column, and now is complaining of increasing dyspnea.

S/S: Anxiety
Apprehension
Lowering level of consciousness
Shallow rapid breaths
Pallor
Left breath sounds diminished
Trachea shifted to the right
Hyperresonant percussion right side of chest
Some subcutaneous emphysema in lower neck
Jugular vein distension

SCENARIO 2:   A 47-year-old male driver was injured in a moderate-speed crash. Lateral impact was on the driver's side of the auto.

S/S: Anxiety
Pulse deficit, left arm
Central chest pain "tearing"
Minor pain, left thorax
Contusions, left thorax
Capillary refill—2 seconds
Clear heart sounds
Pallor
Bilaterally equal breath sounds

SCENARIO 1:

Field Diagnosis: Tension pneumothorax

Management: Scene size-up—mechanism of injury/index of suspicion
  Standard Precautions—gloves
Primary assessment.
Apply spinal clearance protocol.
Calm and reassure patient.
  Airway—Maintain a patent airway.
  Breathing—Provide oxygen, guided by pulse oximetry.
  Circulation—Initiate an IV w/ large-bore catheter. Monitor ECG.
  Maintain body temperature. Control obvious hemorrhage.
Rapid trauma assessment.
  Provide pleural decompression. Reassess breath
  sounds and breathing.
Rapidly extricate from the vehicle.
Provide reassessment(s).
Provide rapid transport. Alert trauma center.

SCENARIO 2:

Field Diagnosis: Dissecting aortic aneurysm

Management: Scene size-up—mechanism of injury/index of suspicion
  Standard Precautions—gloves
Primary assessment.
  Apply spinal clearance protocol.
  Calm and reassure patient.
  Airway—Maintain a patent airway.
  Breathing—Provide oxygen, guided by pulse oximetry. Consider IPPV.
  Circulation—Initiate an IV w/ large-bore catheter. Administer fluids
  conservatively. Monitor ECG. Maintain body temperature.
Rapid trauma assessment.
  If patient deteriorates, run fluids rapidly.
Rapidly extricate from the vehicle.
Provide reassessment(s).
Provide rapid transport. Alert trauma center.

SCENARIO 3: A young male was involved in a frontal-impact auto collision in which he struck the windshield. He is found conscious and alert and seated in the auto but cannot move his legs or arms.

S/S:
Anxiety
Apprehension
Diaphragmatic breathing
Bilateral anesthesia and paralysis
Cool limbs
Blood pressure 96/76
Priapism
Arms move to hold-up position
Capillary refill—2 seconds

SCENARIO 4: A 34-year-old pedestrian was struck by an auto and thrown to the roadside. She is found complaining of bilateral hip pain and is unable to move her legs.

S/S:
Diaphoresis
Anxiety
Apprehension
Slight dyspnea
Pallor
Pelvic pain
Rapid weak pulse
Pelvic instability
Crepitation with pressure on iliac crests
Capillary refill—4 seconds

SCENARIO 5: Your patient was involved in a serious frontal-impact auto collision with deformity of the steering wheel, though the windshield did not shatter. He is a well-developed male in his mid-30s.

S/S:
Conscious, alert, and fully oriented
Crushing substernal chest pain
Anxiety
Strong but irregular pulse
Bilaterally equal breath sounds
Clear heart sounds
ECG—sinus rhythm with frequent PACs
Jugular veins—normal
No tracheal deviation

SCENARIO 3:

Field Diagnosis: Spinal cord injury (midcervical)

Management: Scene size-up—mechanism of injury/index of suspicion
  Standard Precautions—gloves
Primary assessment.
  Apply spinal clearance protocol.
  Calm and reassure patient.
  Airway—Maintain a patent airway.
  Breathing—Provide oxygen, guided by pulse oximetry. Consider IPPV.
  Circulation—Initiate a large-bore IV catheter.
  Monitor ECG. Maintain body temperature. Control obvious hemorrhage.
Rapid trauma assessment.
  Consider a fluid challenge.
Rapidly extricate from the vehicle.
Provide reassessment(s).
Provide gentle transport. Alert trauma center.

SCENARIO 4:

Field Diagnosis: Pelvic fracture

Management: Scene size-up—mechanism of injury/index of suspicion
  Standard Precautions—gloves
Primary assessment.
  Apply spinal clearance protocol.
  Calm and reassure patient.
  Airway—Maintain a patent airway.
  Breathing—Provide oxygen, guided by pulse oximetry.
  Circulation—Initiate a large-bore IV catheter.
    Monitor ECG. Maintain body temperature. Control obvious hemorrhage.
Rapid trauma assessment.
  Consider pelvic sling to stabilize pelvis.
Provide reassessment(s).
Provide rapid transport. Alert trauma center.

SCENARIO 5:

Field Diagnosis: Blunt cardiac trauma

Management: Scene size-up—mechanism of injury/index of suspicion
  Standard Precautions—gloves
Primary assessment.
  Apply spinal clearance protocol.
  Calm and reassure patient.
  Airway—Maintain patent airway.
  Breathing—Provide oxygen, guided by pulse oximetry.
  Circulation—Initiate an IV w/ large-bore catheter. Monitor ECG. Maintain body
    temperature. Control any obvious hemorrhage.
Rapid trauma assessment.
  Treat dysrhythmias as per protocol.
Provide reassessment(s).
Provide rapid transport. Alert trauma center.

SCENARIO 6:	Your patient is a logger who had his left lower extremity crushed as a tree he was cutting fell on him. It has taken several hours for fellow workers to locate and bring him to you.
S/S:	Conscious, alert, and fully oriented Severe left leg and foot pain Reduced distal pulse strength Limb integrity appears intact (no apparent fracture) Increased capillary refill time distal to the injury Pain appears out of proportion with the injury Calf seems board-like to the touch

SCENARIO 7:	Your patient (the driver) was the victim of a lateral-impact auto collision with moderate intrusion on the driver's side.
S/S:	Severe dyspnea Reddening of left lateral chest Some crepitus in the left chest on palpation Tracheal tugging (to right with inspiration) Severe left-side chest pain Chest excursion only slightly asymmetrical Some crackles on auscultation of left chest

SCENARIO 8:	A bullet from a small-caliber handgun entered your patient's chest just left of the sternum.
S/S:	Anxiety Blood pressure 122/101 Jugular vein distention Distant heart sounds Pallor Reduced level of consciousness Capillary refill—4 seconds Limited bleeding at wound

SCENARIO 6:

Field Diagnosis: Compartment syndrome

Management: Scene size-up—mechanism of injury/index of suspicion
  Standard Precautions—gloves
Primary assessment.
  Calm and reassure patient.
  Airway—Maintain a patent airway.
  Breathing—Provide oxygen, guided by pulse oximetry.
  Circulation—Initiate an IV w/ large-bore catheter. Maintain body temperature.
  Control obvious hemorrhage.
Rapid trauma assessment.
  Splint, then elevate the limb.
  Monitor distal pulses, capillary refill, and sensation.
Provide reassessment(s).
Provide rapid transport. Alert trauma center.

SCENARIO 7:

Field Diagnosis: Flail chest

Management: Scene size-up—mechanism of injury/index of suspicion
  Standard Precautions—gloves
Primary assessment.
  Apply spinal clearance protocol.
  Calm and reassure patient.
  Airway—Maintain a patent airway.
  Breathing—Provide oxygen, guided by pulse oximetry. Consider IPPV.
  Circulation—Initiate an IV w/ large-bore catheter. Monitor ECG.
  Maintain body temperature. Control obvious hemorrhage.
Rapid trauma assessment.
  Soft bulky dressing taped to immobilize flail section.
Provide reassessment(s). Reevaluate frequently to ensure adequacy of breathing.
Provide rapid transport. Alert trauma center.

SCENARIO 8:

Field Diagnosis: Pericardial tamponade

Management: Scene size-up—Ensure scene safety. Mechanism of injury/index of suspicion
  Standard Precautions—gloves
Primary assessment.
  Calm and reassure patient.
  Airway—Maintain a patent airway.
  Breathing—Provide oxygen, guided by pulse oximetry.
  Circulation—Initiate an IV w/ large-bore catheter.
Rapid trauma assessment.
  Monitor patient carefully.
Provide reassessment(s).
Provide rapid transport. Alert trauma center.